Bile Acids in Gastroenterology

Susumu Tazuma • Hajime Takikawa
Editors

Bile Acids in Gastroenterology

Basic and Clinical

Springer

Editors
Susumu Tazuma
Department of General Medicine
Hiroshima University Hospital
Hiroshima
Japan

Hajime Takikawa
Department of Medicine
Teikyo University School of Medicine
Tokyo
Japan

ISBN 978-4-431-56060-9 ISBN 978-4-431-56062-3 (eBook)
DOI 10.1007/978-4-431-56062-3

Library of Congress Control Number: 2017935470

Printed on acid-free paper

This Springer imprint is published by Springer Nature
The registered company is Springer Japan KK
The registered company address is: Chiyoda First Bldg. East, 3-8-1 Nishi-Kanda, Chiyoda-ku, Tokyo 101-0065, Japan

Preface

It is a pleasure to introduce *Bile Acids in Gastroenterology*. Research has focused on bile acids as a key player in lipid metabolism as well as a cytotoxic or protective agent for hepatobiliary and digestive diseases. Bile acids have long been one of the most popular targets for basic and clinical research in gastroenterology, and numbers of reports are still being published in major journals as novel information. Therefore, the main objective of this book is to provide updated information on bile acids for scientists and physicians to take advantage of regarding progress in basic research and for clinical application.

In principle, bile acids are soluble amphiphilic (detergent-like) molecules produced by catabolizing cholesterol in the liver, and are essential for secretion and transport of cholesterol in bile and for fat digestion and absorption in the small intestine. In biological terms, bile acid molecules are re-absolved from the intestine, followed by recruiting to the liver. This recycling system is so-called enterohepatic circulation, and thanks to such recruitment, the liver synthesizes only enough to compensate for small losses in the feces. Accordingly, biliary bile acids are derived almost entirely from the enterohepatic circulation. Bile acids are the main constituents of bile and are stored in the gall bladder, flowing into the small intestine after meal ingestion. Intestinal bile acids facilitate digestion and absorption of lipids and fat-soluble vitamins. Thus, bile acids play a role in lipid metabolism.

Recently there has been intensive interest in the revelation that bile acids are responsible not only for the digestion and absorption of lipids but also for signal transduction in various metabolic pathways as natural ligands for nuclear receptors, to participate in pathogenesis and management of various diseases such as cancer, immune disorders, and metabolic syndrome. Therefore, in this book, Part I consists mainly of biological aspects of bile acids and includes the chapters "Metabolism of Bile Acids", "Hepatobiliary Transport of Bile Acids", "Intestinal Absorption of Bile Acids", "Nuclear Receptor Regulation of Bile Acids", and "Bile Acids as

Therapeutic Agents" (Chaps. 1, 2, 3, 4, and 5). Following the precise treatment of the biological aspects of bile acids, in Part II the relationship between bile acids and diseases is described according to recent reports in the chapter "Bile Acids and Gallstones" (Chap. 6)—a traditional theme, but recently updated evidence-based clinical practice guidelines have accelerated interest in both the basic and clinical aspects. Similarly, the chapters "Bile Acids and Cholestatic Liver Disease, Primary Biliary Cholangitis (PBC), and Primary Sclerosing Cholangitis, (PSC)", and "Bile Acids and Non-alcoholic Fatty Liver Diseases/Non-alcoholic Steatohepatitis (NAFLD/NASH)" and "Bile Acids and Viral Hepatitis and HCC" (Chaps. 7, 8, 10, and 11) are also focused on through evidence-based clinical practice guidelines. In addition, other interests including "Bile Acids and Pancreatitis", "Bile Acids and Esophageal Cancer", and "Bile Acids and Colon Cancer" (Chaps. 12, 13, and 14) are introduced to provide recent findings. Taken together, this book provides excellent coverage of the current knowledge of bile acids in gastroenterology and will be of great interest to concerned readers.

Hiroshima, Japan
Tokyo, Japan
18 November 2016

Susumu Tazuma
Hajime Takikawa

Contents

Part I
Biological Aspects of Bile Acids

Chapter 1
Metabolism of Bile Acids

Hajime Takikawa

Abstract Bile acids are biosynthesized from cholesterol in the liver. Cholic acid (CA), chenodeoxycholic acid (CDCA), and deoxycholic acid (DCA) are major bile acids in humans. Neutral (classical) pathway is the major pathway of the bile acid biosynthesis in adult humans, which starts from 7α-hydroxylation of cholesterol, catalyzed by cholesterol 7α-hydroxylase (CYP7A1), the rate-limiting step of bile acid biosynthesis. In the liver, farnesoid X receptor (FXR) induces the negative nuclear receptor, small heterodimer partner (SHP), which inhibits *CYP7A1* and *CYP8B1* gene transcription. FXR and SHP are activated by bile acids in the liver. In the intestine, FXR agonists induce fibroblast growth factor 15 (FGF15; FGF19 in humans), which activates the liver FGF receptor in the liver to inhibit CYP7A1 and CYP8B1 expression. Most bile acids in the bile and serum are conjugated with glycine or taurine. In addition, sulfate and glucuronide conjugates of bile acids also exist, which are hydrophilic and useful for urinary excretion. Bile acids with less hydroxyl groups are subjected to these conjugations, which are appropriate for the detoxication of toxic bile acids.

Keywords Cholesterol 7α-hydroxylase (CYP7A1) • Sterol 12α-hydroxylase (CYP8B1) • Sterol 27-hydroxylase (CYP27A1) • Oxysterol 7α-hydroxylase (CYP7B1) • Farnesoid X receptor (FXR)

1.1 Types of Bile Acids

Bile acids are biosynthesized from cholesterol in the liver. These bile acids, called primary bile acids, are cholic acid (CA) and chenodeoxycholic acid (CDCA) (Fig. 1.1) in humans. CA and CDCA are metabolized to deoxycholic acid (DCA) and lithocholic acid (LCA), respectively, by 7α-dehydroxylase of intestinal bacteria (Fig. 1.1). CDCA is also metabolized to ursodeoxycholic acid (UDCA) via the 7-oxo-intermediate (Fig. 1.1).

H. Takikawa (✉)
Department of Medicine, Teikyo University School of Medicine, 2-11-1 Kaga, Itabashi-ku, Tokyo 173-8605, Japan
e-mail: takikawa@med.teikyo-u.ac.jp

S. Tazuma, H. Takikawa (eds.), *Bile Acids in Gastroenterology*,
DOI 10.1007/978-4-431-56062-3_1

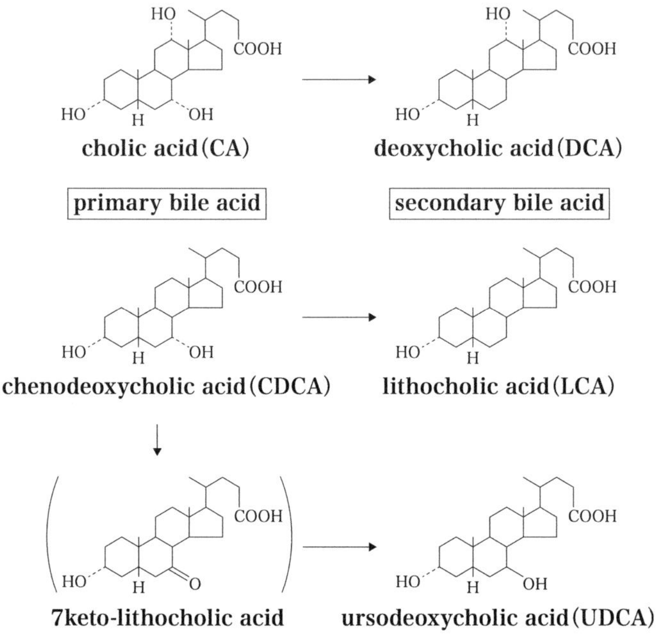

Fig. 1.1 Types of bile acids

1.2 Biosynthesis of Bile Acids

Two pathways, classical (neutral) pathway and alternative pathway, are known for the biosynthesis of bile acids [1].

Neutral pathway is the major pathway of the biosynthesis of bile acids in adult humans, which starts from 7α-hydroxylation of cholesterol, followed by the oxidative cleavage of the side chain staring from 27-hyrdoxylation (Fig. 1.2). 7α--Hydroxylation of cholesterol (1) is performed in hepatic microsomes, and 7α-hydroxycholesterol (2) is produced. This reaction is catalyzed by cholesterol 7α-hydroxylase (CYP7A1), a rate-limiting step of bile acid biosynthesis. The activity of CYP7A1 is subjected to negative feedback by bile acids returning to the liver via the portal vein. This negative feedback does not occur by external bile drainage, ileal resection, and bile acid absorbent administration, and the activity of CYP7A1 is increased and bile acid biosynthesis increases up to six- to sevenfolds. 7α-Hydroxycholesterol (2) is metabolized to 7α-hydroxycholest-4-en-3-one (3) by the oxidation of 3 ß-hydroxyl residue and the transposition of the double bond from Δ^5 to Δ^4. A part of 7α-hydroxycholest-4-en-3-one (3) is converted to 7α, 12α--dihydroxycholest-4-en-3-one (8) by microsomal sterol 12α-hydroxylase (CYP8B1). 7α-Hdroxycholest-4-en-3-one (3) and 7α, 12α-dihydroxycholest-4-en-3-one (8) are subjected to the oxidation of the Δ^4–3-keo residue and converted to the intermediates of 5ß-cholestane-3α ,7α-diol (4) and 5ß-cholestane-3α, 7α, 12α-triol (9) with the mother nucleus of CDCA and CA, respectively, and the

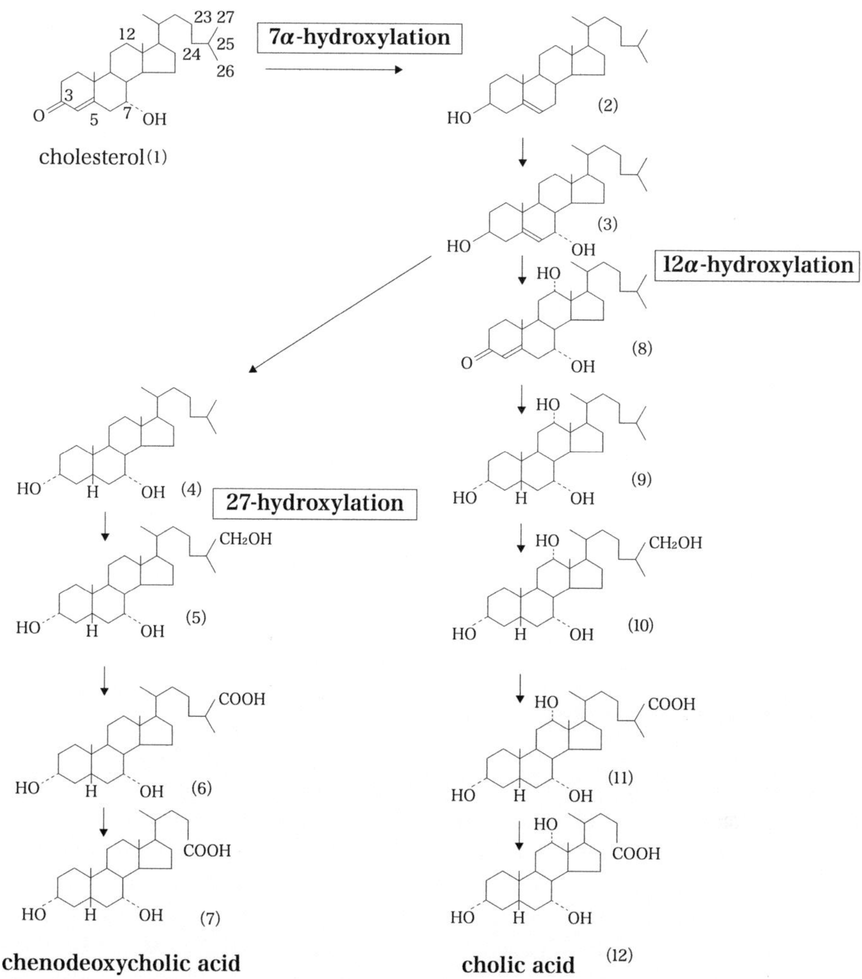

Fig. 1.2 The biosynthesis pathway of bile acids (*2*) 7α-hydroxycholesterol, (*3*) 7α--hydroxycholest-4-en-3-one, (*4*) 5ß-cholestane-3α ,7α-diol, (*5*) 5ß-cholestane-3α ,7α, 26-triol, (*6*) 3α ,7α-dihydoxy-5ß-cholestanoic acid, (*8*) 7α, 12α-dihydroxycholest-4-en-3-one, (*9*) 5-ß-cholestane-3α ,7α, 12α-triol, (*10*) 5ß-cholestane-3α ,7α, 12α, 27-tetrol, (*11*) 3α ,7α, 12 α--trihydoxy-5ß-cholestanoic acid

side chain of cholesterol, followed by the oxidized cleavage of the side chain. At first, 5ß-cholestane-3α, 7α-diol (4) and 5ß-cholestane-3α, 7α, 12α-triol (9) are converted to 5ß-cholestane-3α, 7α, 27-triol (5) and 5ß-cholestane-3α, 7α, 12α, 27-tetrol (10) by sterol 27-hydroxylase (CYP27A1) of hepatic mitochondria. Next, the hydroxyl residues of 5ß-cholestane-3α,7α, 27-triol (5) and 5-ß-cholestane-3α, 7α, 12α, 27-tetrol (10) are oxidized to the carboxyl residue via the aldehyde residue, producing 3α, 7α-dihydoxy-5ß-cholestanoic acid (6) and 3α, 7α, 12α-trihydoxy-5ß-cholestanoic acid (11). Finally, these are subjected to ß-oxidation, similar to the ß-oxidation of fatty acids, and CDCA (7) and CA (12) are produced. In fact, CDCA and CA are produced as the CoA derivatives and secreted as the glycine or taurine conjugates after the conjugation with glycine or taurine.

The acidic pathway of bile acid biosynthesis is started by CYP27A1, which produces 27-hydoxycholesterol, followed by oxysterol 7α-hydroxylase (CYP7B1), which produces 3ß,7α-dihydoxy-5-cholestenoic acid [1]. These two enzymes are expressed in most tissues and are responsible for oxidation of cholesterol. Oxysterols transported to hepatocytes are converted to bile acids. Other alternative pathways have also been reported in humans.

Farnesoid X receptor (FXR) is known to inhibit CYP7A1, CYP8B1, CYP27A1, and CYP7B1 [2]. Two mechanisms have been reported to inhibit bile acid biosynthesis by bile acids. In the liver, FXR induces the negative nuclear receptor, small heterodimer partner (SHP), which inhibits *CYP7A1* and *CYP8B1* gene transcription. FXR and SHP are activated by bile acids in the liver. In the intestine, FXR agonists induce fibroblast growth factor 15 (FGF15; FGF19 in humans), which activates the liver FGF receptor 4/β-Klotho signaling pathway in the liver to inhibit CYP7A1 and CYP8B1 expression [3]. Schaap et al. reported that hepatic FGF19 levels were increased and inversely correlated to the reduced CYP7A1 expression levels in patients with extrahepatic cholestasis [4].

1.3 Conjugation of Bile Acids

Most bile acids in the bile and serum are conjugated with glycine or taurine (Fig. 1.3). The conjugation ratio of these amino acids (G/T ratio) is about 3 in adult human bile. Although bile acid/amino acid transferase in the liver has higher affinity with taurine than glycine, glycine is used to conjugate after using up taurine, since the taurine pool in the liver is small. Thus, the G/T ratio is kept about 3.

The G/T ratio increases in patients with ileal diseases and ileal resection, since bile acid biosynthesis increases due to the inhibition of the ileal bile acid reabsorption, resulting in taurine deficiency and increased glycine conjugation of bile acids. On the other hand, the G/T ratio decreases in the conditions of decreased bile acid biosynthesis. Especially, the G/T ratio decreases markedly in patients with cerebrotendinous xanthomatosis (CTX) due to a remarkable decrease in bile acid biosynthesis.

Other than amino acid conjugates, sulfate and glucuronide conjugates of bile acids, mainly 3-hydroxy conjugates, also exist, including double conjugates with amino acid and sulfate (Fig. 1.3). These bile acid conjugates are hydrophilic and useful for urinary excretion. Bile acids with less hydroxyl groups are subjected to sulfation and glucuronidation, which are appropriate for detoxication since these bile acids are toxic. N-acetylglucosaminidation is reported to be a selective conjugation pathway for seven beta-hydroxylated bile acids [5]. Makino and coworkers reported that UDCA-N-acetylglucosaminide was detected in UDCA-treated patients, which was less than 2.5% of total serum bile acids [6].

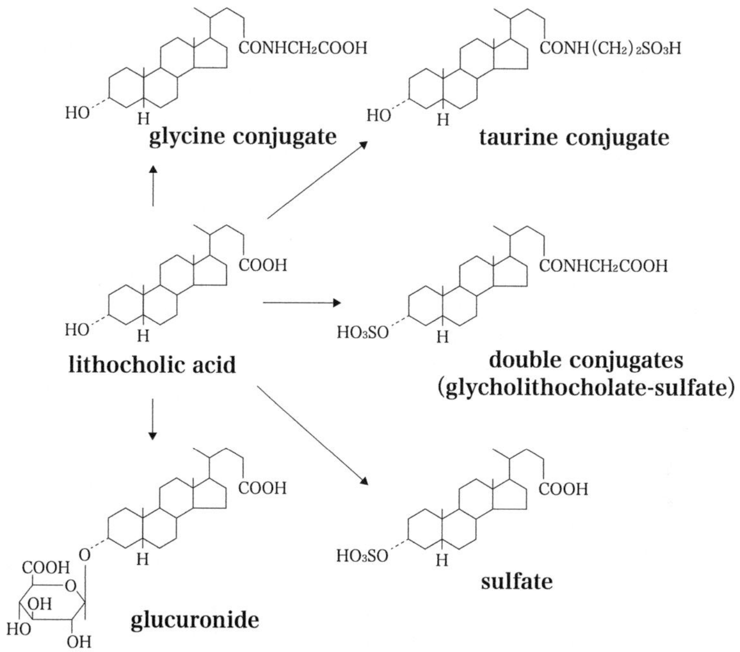

Fig. 1.3 Various conjugated forms of bile acids (shown lithocholic acid as an example)

Biliary bile acid concentrations are about 10 mg/ml and are composed mainly of CA, CDCA, and DCA, and the ratio of CA to CDCA (C/CDC ratio) is about 1.1–1.4. Because of the very efficient bile acid uptake system of the liver, serum bile acid levels in the systemic circulation are about 1–2 μg/ml. In peripheral blood, CA, CDCD, and DCA are also abundant bile acids, but the C/CDC ratio is about 0.3 due to the more efficient hepatic uptake of CA than CDCA. Serum bile acids are mainly glycine or taurine conjugates and sulfates and glucuronides comprise about 10%, respectively [7, 8].

References

1. Chiang JY. Regulation of bile acid synthesis: pathways, nuclear receptors, and mechanisms. J Hepatol. 2004;40:539–51.
2. Chiang JY. Negative feedback regulation of bile acid metabolism: impact on liver metabolism and diseases. Hepatology. 2015;62:1315–7.
3. Inagaki T, Choi M, Moschetta A, Peng L, Cummins CL, McDonald JG, et al. Fibroblast growth factor 15 functions as an enterohepatic signal to regulate bile acid homeostasis. Cell Metab. 2005;2(2):17–225.
4. Schaap FG, van der Gaag NA, Gouma DJ, Jansen PL. High expression of the bile salt-homeostatic hormone fibroblast growth factor 19 in the liver of patients with extrahepatic cholestasis. Hepatology. 2009;49:1228–35.

5. Marschall HU, Matern H, Wietholtz H, Egestad B, Matern S, Sjövall J. Bile acid N-acetylglucosaminidation. In vivo and in vitro evidence for a selective conjugation reaction of 7 beta-hydroxylated bile acids in humans. J Clin Invest. 1992;89:1981–7. See comment in PubMed Commons below
6. Kimura A, Nakamura K, Makino I. Measurement of bile acid N-acetylglucosaminides in serum and urine of patients with chronic liver diseases during ursodeoxycholic acid treatment. Nihon Shokakibyo Gakkai Zasshi. 1995;92:224–32. (in Japanese)
7. Takikawa H, Otsuka H, Beppu T, Seyama Y, Yamakawa T. Quantitative determination of bile acid glucuronides in serum by mass fragmentography. J Biochem. 1980;92:985–98.
8. Perreault M, Białek A, Trottier J, Verreault M, Caron P, Milkiewicz P, Barbier O. Role of glucuronidation for hepatic detoxification and urinary elimination of toxic bile acids during biliary obstruction. PLoS One. 2013;8:e80994.

Chapter 2
Hepatobiliary Transport of Bile Acids

Tatehiro Kagawa

Abstract Bile acids are the major driving force of bile excretion from hepatocytes; they are synthesized from cholesterol via at least 17 enzymatic reactions. They play a critical role in cholesterol disposal and the absorption of fat and fat-soluble vitamins. The concentration of intracellular bile acid is tightly regulated by modulating expression of bile acid transporters via nuclear receptors. This article provides a comprehensive overview of the characteristics and regulatory networks of hepatobiliary bile acid transporters.

Keywords Bile acid • Transporter • Cholestasis

2.1 Introduction

Bile acids are the major driving force of bile excretion from hepatocytes; they are synthesized from cholesterol via at least 17 enzymatic reactions. They play a critical role in cholesterol disposal and the absorption of fat and fat-soluble vitamins. After excretion from hepatocytes into the bile canaliculus, most bile acids (~95%) are reabsorbed in the terminal ileum and return to the liver via the portal vein (enterohepatic circulation). Influx and efflux of bile acids in organs is mediated by organ-specific transporters (Fig. 2.1). In hepatocytes, bile acids are absorbed from the sinusoid by the Na^+-taurocholate cotransporting polypeptide (NTCP, SLC10A1) and secreted into the bile canaliculus by the bile salt export pump (BSEP, ABCB11). Other bile components are secreted by their corresponding transporters: phospholipids by multidrug resistance protein 3 (MDR3, ABCB4), organic anions by multidrug resistance-associated protein 2 (MRP2, ABCC2), and cholesterol by ABCG5/G8. In the terminal ileum, bile acids are absorbed from the intestinal lumen by the apical sodium-dependent bile acid transporter (ASBT, SLC10A2) and excreted into the portal vein by the organic solute transporters (OSTα/OSTβ, SLC51A/SLC51B) that facilitate bidirectional diffusion.

T. Kagawa (✉)
Department of Internal Medicine, Division of Gastroenterology and Hepatology, Tokai University School of Medicine, Shimokasuya 143, Isehara 259-1193, Japan
e-mail: kagawa@tokai.ac.jp

S. Tazuma, H. Takikawa (eds.), *Bile Acids in Gastroenterology*,
DOI 10.1007/978-4-431-56062-3_2

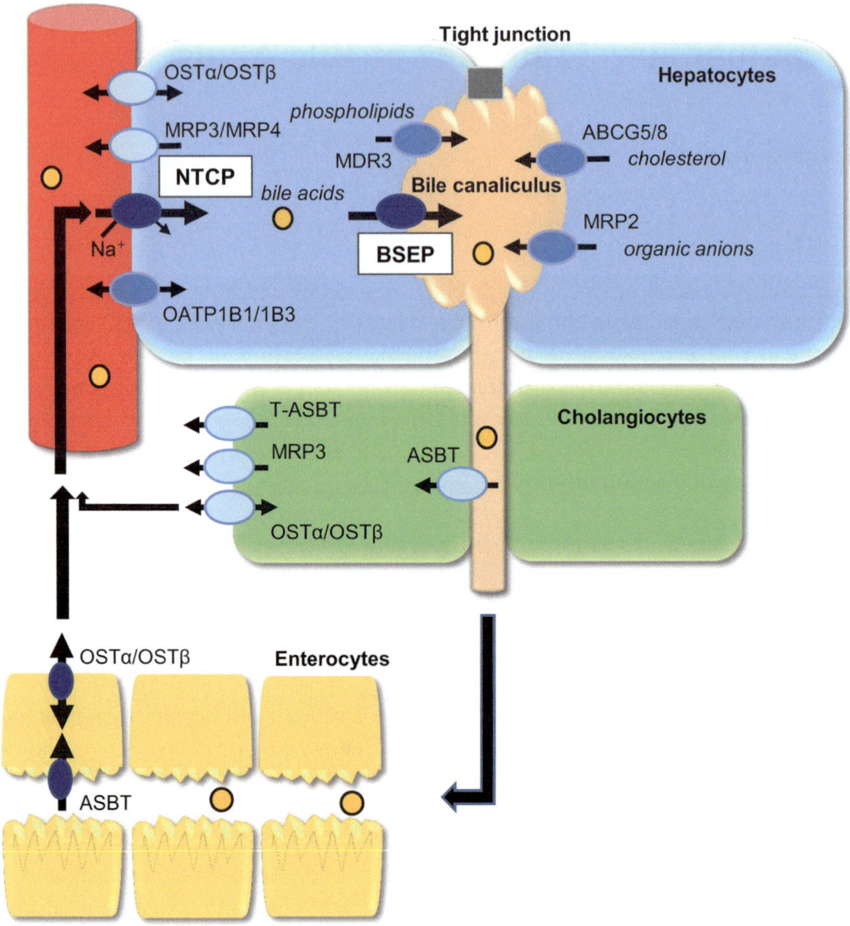

Fig. 2.1 Bile acid transporters. In hepatocytes, bile acids are absorbed from the sinusoid by NTCP, and in part by OATPs, and are secreted into the bile canaliculus by BSEP. In the terminal ileum, they are absorbed from the intestinal lumen by ASBT and excreted into the portal vein by OSTα/OSTβ to return to the liver (enterohepatic circulation). Other components of bile are secreted into the bile canaliculus by MDR3 (phospholipids), MRP2 (organic anions), and ABCG5/G8 (cholesterol). OSTα/OSTβ, MRP3, and MRP4 are involved in retrograde bile acid elimination from the basolateral membrane to the sinusoid in cholestasis. In cholangiocytes, bile acids are absorbed by ASBT and secreted into the peribiliary plexus by OSTα/OSTβ, MRP3, and a truncated ASBT (t-ASBT) (cholehepatic shunting)

Bile acids are detergents and toxic to cells at high concentrations; therefore, their cellular concentration must be tightly regulated by refined feedback systems. Bile acids, now known as a signaling molecule, activate a nuclear receptor, farnesoid X receptor (FXR, NR1H4), and the G protein-coupled bile acid receptor, TGR5, thereby triggering a number of physiological reactions (see [Chap. 4] "Nuclear Receptor

Regulation"). In hepatocytes, bile acids bind to FXR, which represses NTCP and prevents further bile acid uptake, downregulates cholesterol 7α-hydroxylase (CYP7A1) to inhibit further bile acid synthesis, and activates BSEP to induce bile acid secretion into the bile canaliculus. All of these events ultimately result in a reduction in the concentration of intracellular bile acids. This article provides a comprehensive overview of the characteristics and regulatory networks of hepatobiliary bile acid transporters.

2.2 BSEP

2.2.1 Characteristics

The human *BSEP* gene is located on chromosome 2 (2q24) and is translated into a protein comprising 1,321 amino acids, with a molecular mass of ~160 kDa [1]. BSEP belongs to the ABC subfamily B, harboring 12 potential transmembrane segments and two sets of Walker A and B motifs that bind to ATP [2–4]. BSEP is exclusively expressed in hepatocytes, where it resides along the canalicular membranes and exports bile acids into the bile canaliculus in an ATP-dependent fashion. The rat Bsep receives *N*-linked glycosylation at four asparagine residues in the first extracellular loop [5], sites that are also present in human BSEP. These glycans are required for correct trafficking to the canalicular membrane; loss of two or more glycans results in rapid degradation at the proteasome [5]. The intracellular distribution of Bsep was analyzed using pulse-chase studies in rats [6, 7]. Newly synthesized Bsep traffics directly from the Golgi to the canalicular membrane through a post-Golgi endosomal fraction. This is in contrast to other canalicular proteins, such as dipeptidyl peptidase IV and the canalicular cell adhesion molecule (cCAM105), which reach the basolateral membrane before arriving at the canalicular membrane (transcytosis) [6]. Bsep cycles between intracellular pools and the canalicular membrane, and taurocholic acid (TCA) and cAMP increase the amount of Bsep in the canalicular membrane [7]. Studies using WIFB9 cells, a stable hybrid of rat hepatoma and human fibroblasts with sealed bile canaliculi, revealed that Bsep constitutively cycles between the canalicular membrane and Rab11a-positive recycling endosomes [8]. HS-1-associated protein X-1 (HAX-1) [9] and non-muscle myosin II regulatory light chain 2a (MLC2a) [10] were identified as binding partners in a yeast two-hybrid screen. HAX-1 participates in clathrin-mediated endocytosis through interactions with cortactin [9]. MLC2a is involved in trafficking of newly synthesized Bsep to the canalicular membrane [10]. The AP2 adaptor complex is involved in clathrin-dependent endocytosis through interactions with a tyrosine motif at the carboxyl terminus of BSEP [11, 12].

p38^{MAPK} is involved in BSEP trafficking from the Golgi to the canalicular membrane, and tauroursodeoxycholic acid (TUDCA)-induced choleretic action is dependent on p38^{MAPK} activation [13]. Short-chain ubiquitination is associated with BSEP degradation and is modulated by 4-phenylbutyrate (4PBA) [14].

Human BSEP transports glycine and taurine conjugates of the two primary bile acids, cholic acid (CA) and chenodeoxycholic acid (CDCA), with high affinity and selectivity [2, 15–17].

2.2.2 Gene Regulation

BSEP expression is tightly regulated by the nuclear receptor, FXR. When bile acids bind to FXR, FXR forms a heterodimer with retinoid X receptor (RXR) [18] and induces *BSEP* upregulation via binding to the FXR-responsive element (FXRE) in the promoter region [19, 20]. Besides endogenous FXR agonists, such as CDCA, deoxycholic acid (DCA), and CA [18], more potent synthetic FXR agonists such as 6α-ethyl-CDCA (obeticholic acid, INT-747) [21], 6α-ethyl-3α,7α,23-trihydroxy-24-nor-5β-cholan-23-sulfate (INT-767) [22], and GW4064 [23] upregulate *BSEP* expression in various cell lines and animal models. As for obeticholic acid, clinical trials for primary biliary cholangitis (PBC), primary sclerosing cholangitis (PSC), and nonalcoholic steatohepatitis (NASH) are ongoing. Ursodeoxycholic acid (UDCA), which is often used to treat cholestasis, is not an FXR ligand. Notably, muricholic acid, one of the major bile acid species present in rodents but not in humans, is antagonistic to FXR [24]. In *Fxr*$^{-/-}$ mice, *Bsep* expression levels are markedly reduced at baseline and are not induced further by bile acid feeding [25], suggesting a critical role for FXR in the regulation of *BSEP* expression. Furthermore, a recent report documented four patients from two families with a homozygous loss of FXR exhibiting severe neonatal cholestasis [26].

Besides FXR, several other transcriptional factors regulate *BSEP* gene expression. Liver receptor homolog 1 (LRH-1, NR5A2), a transcriptional regulator for the biosynthesis and transport of cholesterol and bile acids, activates the BSEP promoter [27], and *Bsep* expression is reduced in LRH-1 knockout mice [28].

Nuclear factor erythroid 2-related factor 2 (Nrf2) is another transcriptional regulator for BSEP [29]. Nrf2 maintains redox homeostasis by regulating many phase I and II drug-metabolizing and detoxification enzymes. Nrf2 upregulates *BSEP* by binding to musculoaponeurotic fibrosarcoma recognition element (MARE) 1 in the BSEP promoter. Upregulation of *Bsep* expression by alpha-naphthyl isothiocyanate (ANIT) is abrogated in Nrf2-null mice [30].

Recently, Song et al. reported that 17β-estradiol (E2) repressed *BSEP* expression through direct interaction with estrogen receptor α (ERα) and FXR in the late stage of pregnancy [31], implicating a mechanistic role for the E2/ERα/FXR pathway in intrahepatic cholestasis of pregnancy (ICP).

2.2.3 BSEP-Associated Diseases

There are two types of hereditary intrahepatic cholestatic disease: progressive familial intrahepatic cholestasis (PFIC) and benign recurrent intrahepatic cholestasis (BRIC). PFIC patients progress to liver failure and require liver transplantation in childhood, whereas BRIC patients display intermittent and usually non-progressive jaundice (reviewed in [32]). PFIC1 and BRIC1 are caused by mutations in the *FIC1* (*ATB8B1*) gene, which encodes a P-type ATPase functioning as a flippase for phosphatidylserine, whereas PFIC3 is caused by mutations in the *MDR3* gene. PFIC2 and BRIC2 are caused by mutations in *BSEP*, and more than 150 genetic abnormalities, including missense, nonsense, deletions, insertions, and splice-site mutations, have been identified [3, 33–36]. Some missense mutations and single nucleotide polymorphisms (SNPs) can cause aberrant pre-mRNA splicing, resulting in impaired BSEP function [35]. PFIC2 is characterized by absent or much reduced canalicular BSEP expression [34, 37] as well as a markedly diminished concentration of biliary bile acid [37].

To elucidate the effects of these mutations and SNPs on BSEP function, a number of studies have been performed using cell lines expressing a mutated form of BSEP [38–42]. The BSEP protein harboring a disease-associated missense mutation is unstable and is degraded in the proteasome [41, 42]. TCA transport activity of BSEP was analyzed in BSEP-expressing MDCKII cells. The activity of PFIC2 mutants (D482G, E297G, K461E, G982R, R1153C, R1268Q, and 3767–3768insC) was 0–30% that of wild type, and BRIC2 mutants (A570T and R1050C) exhibited 50–60% wild-type activity [42]. The reduced activity corresponded to the stability of synthesized BSEP protein. Thus, the difference in the severity of the clinical phenotype between PFIC2 and BRIC2 may be explained by the differences in transport activity of BSEP harboring corresponding mutations [41, 42]. Several patients who had clinical and histopathological characteristics of BRIC progressed to PFIC [33, 43], suggesting a possible phenotypic progression between BRIC2 and PFIC2. Furthermore, the E297G mutation, which is responsible for PFIC2, is also found in BRIC2 patients [33]. Therefore, although the BSEP genotype appears to play an important role in determining clinical severity, other precipitating factors, including viral infection and pregnancy, may also participate [33].

Impaired BSEP function as a cause of cholestasis has been suggested for other congenital diseases. Although the exact molecular mechanism underlying cholestasis in PFIC1 is not fully understood, FIC1 deficiency may lead to a loss of asymmetric phospholipid distribution in the canalicular membrane, decreasing membrane stability, thereby disturbing the function of transporters including BSEP [44, 45]. Microvillus inclusion disease (MVID), a hereditary disorder manifesting intractable diarrhea associated with mutations in the *MYO5B* gene, occasionally accompanies PFIC-like cholestasis. Reduced BSEP expression in the canalicular membrane due to disturbed MYO5B/RAB11A apical recycling endosome pathway has been proposed as a molecular mechanism for cholestasis in this discasc [46].

An association between BSEP SNP and acquired intrahepatic cholestasis has been reported. The C-allele frequency of *BSEP* c.1331T>C (p. V444A) (rs2287622) SNP was higher among patients with ICP (67% in patients versus 54% in controls, $P < 0.001$) [47]. In a recent comprehensive study, two intronic SNPs (rs7577650 and rs3815676) were identified as significant risk alleles associated with ICP. The V444A SNP remained associated with the disease, but the association was driven by rs7577650 [48], suggesting that the V444A SNP is not causative. The effect of an amino acid substitution at position 444 on BSEP function is controversial. Western blot analysis on normal liver tissues from patients undergoing liver resection revealed that canalicular BSEP expression was slightly, but not significantly, reduced in individuals carrying the 444A polymorphism [49]. In another study that utilized a bank of human liver samples, *BSEP* mRNA, but not protein, expression was significantly attenuated in individuals with the 444A polymorphism [50]. The bile acid transport activity of 444A BSEP was not reduced when expressed in Sf9 [51] and HeLa [50] cells and was slightly reduced by up to 20% in MDCKII cells [52].

Impaired BSEP function is also involved in drug-induced liver injury; its severity is associated with dual inhibition of BSEP and mitochondrial function [53]. The association of BSEP V444A SNP in drug-induced cholestasis has been reported in European populations (76% in patients versus 57% in controls) [51]. However, this association was not reproducible among Japanese patients with drug-induced cholestasis (66% in patients versus 78% in controls) [52]. Further investigation is necessary to identify underlying causative risk alleles in the different populations.

2.2.4 Choleretic Agents

Given that bile acids are the major driving force for bile excretion, drugs that upregulate or activate BSEP are good candidates to treat intrahepatic cholestasis. UDCA is one of the drugs most commonly used for hepatobiliary diseases including PBC, PSC, cholestasis, and cholelithiasis. UDCA exerts a choleretic effect by targeting BSEP to the canalicular membrane [13, 54–56] via activation of $p38^{MAPK}$ and a Ca^{2+}-independent protein kinase C (PKC) isoform [13, 55]. In fact, UDCA administration induced remission at least transiently in children with PFIC2 by retargeting BSEP to the canalicular membrane [57].

4PBA enhanced the cell surface expression and transport capacity of wild-type BSEP and BSEP carrying a PFIC2 mutation (E297G and D482G) in MDCKII cells [58]. Administration of 4PBA also induced canalicular Bsep expression, accompanied by an increase in biliary excretion of TCA in rats [58]. These effects may be achieved by decreasing short-chain ubiquitination-mediated Bsep degradation [14] and by reducing AP2 adaptor complex-mediated clathrin-dependent endocytosis [11]. In the clinical setting, 4PBA therapy improved liver function tests, liver histology, and itching in patients with PFIC2 [59, 60] and BRIC2 [61].

2.2.5 Antibody-Induced BSEP Deficiency

Orthotopic liver transplantation usually yields a good outcome in PFIC2 patients. However, since the first case was documented by Keitel et al. [62], several cases have been reported of PFIC2 children with recurring progressive intrahepatic cholestasis in the presence of an autoantibody against BSEP after liver transplantation [63–66]. Generation of a polyclonal antibody to target the first extracellular loop of BSEP may therefore be responsible for inhibiting BSEP function [66].

2.3 NTCP

2.3.1 Characteristics

NTCP is a glycoprotein of approximately 38 kDa, consisting of 349 amino acids [67, 68]. NTCP is localized to the sinusoidal membrane of hepatocytes and functions as an electrogenic sodium-solute cotransporter [69]. Major substrates of NTCP include glycine- and taurine-conjugated bile acids, but unconjugated and sulfated bile acids can still be transported to some extent [70–72].

Other sinusoidal transporters, including organic anion transporting polypeptides (OATP) 1B1 (SLCO1B1) and OATP1B3 (SLCO1B3), are able to transport conjugated bile acids in a sodium-independent manner, as well as unconjugated species [73]. The significance of NTCP in hepatic bile acid uptake is unknown due to a lack of NTCP-null patients. Recently a case of NTCP deficiency was documented [74], a 5-year-old girl manifesting conjugated hypercholanemia without any sign of liver injury. Sequencing of the *NTCP* gene revealed a single homozygous nonsynonymous point mutation (c.755G>A, p. R252H). The R252H mutation resulted in a marked reduction in TCA uptake, along with a lack of plasma membrane expression when it was expressed in HEK293T cells. This indicates that NTCP is the major transporter for hepatocellular uptake of conjugated bile acids. However, serum bile acid concentrations were unexpectedly normal in the majority of *Slc10a1*$^{-/-}$ mice [75], suggesting differences in NTCP contribution among species.

2.3.2 Transcriptional Regulation

NCTP regulation is important for suppressing further influx of potentially toxic bile acids into hepatocytes and is repressed in patients with inflammation-induced cholestasis [76] and advanced PBC [77], as well as in several cholestatic animal models [78–80]. Although its transcriptional regulation is mediated by bile acids, hormones such as estrogen and prolactin, and pro-inflammatory cytokines may also be involved, depending on the species (reviewed in [81]). Bile acids repress *NTCP* transcription through FXR activation, which in turn induces small heterodimer partner (SHP). SHP inhibits *NTCP* upregulation by competing with coactivators for binding to hepatocyte nuclear factor 4 alpha (HNF-4α) and RXRα [80] and by suppressing retinoic acid receptor alpha (RARα) in rats [82] and glucocorticoid receptor (GR) and peroxisome proliferator-activated receptor-gamma coactivator-1 alpha (PGC-1α) in humans [83]. However, an additional SHP-independent pathway probably exists, since *Ntcp* repression was not completely abolished in $Shp^{-/-}$ mice fed with CA [84].

NTCP expression is also regulated posttranslationally. Insertion of NTCP into the plasma membrane by cAMP is mediated by the phosphoinositide-3-kinase signaling pathway [85, 86] and protein phosphatase 2B (PP2B)-induced dephosphorylation of NTCP [87]. In contrast, taurochenodeoxycholic acid (TCDCA) decreases sinusoidal NTCP expression by inducing NTCP endocytosis in a PKC- and PP2B-dependent manner [88].

2.3.3 NTCP as a Receptor for Hepatitis B and D Virus (HBV and HDV)

NTCP is attracting much attention as a functional receptor for HBV and HDV [89]. The large surface protein pre-S1 domain of HBV is a key determinant for receptor binding. In vitro studies demonstrated that myrcludex B, a myristoylated lipopeptide derived from the pre-S1 domain, blocked bile acid uptake by NTCP [90], while taurine or glycine conjugates of CA and UDCA inhibited HBV infection [13]. CYP7A1, the rate-limiting enzyme that synthesizes bile acids from cholesterol, was induced in human liver chimeric mice that were infected with HBV or were given myrcludex B and in liver biopsy samples from HBV-infected patients [91]. This may be a compensatory response against reduced bile acid uptake by HBV binding to NTCP. Interestingly, the NTCP variant p. S267F (c.800C>T, s2296651), which exhibits reduced bile acid transport capacity and has only been observed among Asians [92], is protective against HBV chronic infection [93] as well as progression to cirrhosis and hepatocellular carcinoma in patients with chronic hepatitis B [94].

2.4 Other Basolateral Bile Acid Transporters

Retrograde bile acid elimination from the basolateral membrane of hepatocytes to the sinusoid represents a rescue mechanism for avoiding intracellular bile acid overload. The relevant transporters include OSTα/OSTβ, MRP3 (ABCC3) and MRP4 (ABCC4).

OSTα comprises 340 amino acids, forms a heterodimer with OSTβ comprising 128 amino acids, and is expressed at the basolateral membrane of ileal enterocytes, hepatocytes, and cholangiocytes. Co-expression is necessary for stable expression of OSTα and OSTβ and their delivery to the plasma membrane [95, 96]. In enterocytes, OSTα/OSTβ is responsible for excreting bile acids into the portal circulation to achieve enterohepatic circulation under physiological conditions. In hepatocytes, this transporter is upregulated to transport excess bile acids back to the sinusoidal compartment in cholestasis. Hepatic OSTα/OSTβ expression was increased in patients with advanced PBC [97]. Upregulation was also observed in mice following common bile duct ligation (CBDL) [97], ANIT treatment [98], and CA feeding [99], which was dependent on FXR [100, 101].

Mrp3 and Mrp4 were upregulated in CBDL mice independently of FXR [102]. *Mrp3*$^{-/-}$ mice had normal bile acid transport function [103], whereas *Mrp4*$^{-/-}$ mice exhibited an impaired cytoprotective response to CBDL-induced cholestasis [104]. MRP4, but not MRP3, was upregulated in patients with PFIC2 and PFIC3 [105], suggesting that MRP4 plays an important role in the compensatory reaction to cholestatic liver injury. Regulatory nuclear receptors include constitutive androstane receptor (CAR), pregnane X receptor (PXR) and vitamin D receptor (VDR) for MRP3, and CAR and peroxisome proliferator-activated receptors α (PPARα) for MRP4 (reviewed in [81]).

2.5 Bile Acid Transporters in Cholangiocytes

Cholangiocytes play an important role in bile formation by secreting bicarbonate and water and possess transport systems for the influx and efflux of bile acids. Unconjugated bile acids possibly enter cholangiocytes via passive diffusion, whereas conjugated bile acids are absorbed by ASBT [106], which is also expressed in the terminal ileum to absorb bile acids from the intestinal lumen. Bile acid secretion from the basolateral membrane into the peribiliary plexus is mediated by OSTα/OSTβ, MRP3, and a truncated ASBT (t-ASBT) [106–110]. These transport systems may play a limited role under normal physiological conditions; however, "cholehepatic shunting" [111], which bypasses enterohepatic circulation along with bile duct proliferation, may help to reduce bile acid overload in cholestasis due to bile duct obstruction.

2.6 Conclusions

In this review, the characteristics and regulatory systems of hepatobiliary bile acid transporters are presented. Bile acids are among the most essential molecules to organisms. The majority of bile acids are recycled through the enterohepatic circulation, and their cellular concentration is tightly regulated by refined feedback mechanisms. Impaired function of bile acid transporters causes various types of liver injury and may be responsible for other diseases for which their causality is not yet known. Nuclear receptors regulating bile acid transporters are attractive therapeutic targets, and clinical trials for obeticholic acid are ongoing. Further understanding of bile acid transporters will likely lead to new therapeutic options for intractable liver diseases.

Acknowledgments This work was supported in part by the Japan Agency for Medical Research and Development (16mk0101045s0202). I thank Ms. Satsuki Ieda and Reiko Orii for their technical assistance.

References

1. Strautnieks SS, Kagalwalla AF, Tanner MS, Knisely AS, Bull L, Freimer N, et al. Identification of a locus for progressive familial intrahepatic cholestasis PFIC2 on chromosome 2q24. Am J Hum Genet. 1997;61(3):630–3. doi:10.1086/515501.
2. Gerloff T, Stieger B, Hagenbuch B, Madon J, Landmann L, Roth J, et al. The sister of P-glycoprotein represents the canalicular bile salt export pump of mammalian liver. J Biol Chem. 1998;273(16):10046–50.
3. Strautnieks SS, Bull LN, Knisely AS, Kocoshis SA, Dahl N, Arnell H, et al. A gene encoding a liver-specific ABC transporter is mutated in progressive familial intrahepatic cholestasis. Nat Genet. 1998;20(3):233–8. doi:10.1038/3034.
4. Green RM, Hoda F, Ward KL. Molecular cloning and characterization of the murine bile salt export pump. Gene. 2000;241(1):117–23.
5. Mochizuki K, Kagawa T, Numari A, Harris MJ, Itoh J, Watanabe N, et al. Two N-linked glycans are required to maintain the transport activity of the bile salt export pump (ABCB11) in MDCK II cells. Am J Physiol Gastrointest Liver Physiol. 2007;292(3):G818–28. doi:10.1152/ajpgi.00415.2006.
6. Kipp H, Arias IM. Newly synthesized canalicular ABC transporters are directly targeted from the Golgi to the hepatocyte apical domain in rat liver. J Biol Chem. 2000;275(21):15917–25. doi:10.1074/jbc.M909875199.
7. Kipp H, Pichetshote N, Arias IM. Transporters on demand: intrahepatic pools of canalicular ATP binding cassette transporters in rat liver. J Biol Chem. 2001;276(10):7218–24. doi:10.1074/jbc.M007794200.
8. Wakabayashi Y, Lippincott-Schwartz J, Arias IM. Intracellular trafficking of bile salt export pump (ABCB11) in polarized hepatic cells: constitutive cycling between the canalicular membrane and rab11-positive endosomes. Mol Biol Cell. 2004;15(7):3485–96. doi:10.1091/mbc.E03-10-0737.
9. Ortiz DF, Moseley J, Calderon G, Swift AL, Li S, Arias IM. Identification of HAX-1 as a protein that binds bile salt export protein and regulates its abundance in the apical membrane

of Madin-Darby canine kidney cells. J Biol Chem. 2004;279(31):32761–70. doi:10.1074/jbc.M404337200.
10. Chan W, Calderon G, Swift AL, Moseley J, Li S, Hosoya H, et al. Myosin II regulatory light chain is required for trafficking of bile salt export protein to the apical membrane in Madin-Darby canine kidney cells. J Biol Chem. 2005;280(25):23741–7. doi:10.1074/jbc.M502767200.
11. Hayashi H, Inamura K, Aida K, Naoi S, Horikawa R, Nagasaka H, et al. AP2 adaptor complex mediates bile salt export pump internalization and modulates its hepatocanalicular expression and transport function. Hepatology. 2012;55(6):1889–900. doi:10.1002/hep.25591.
12. Lam P, Xu S, Soroka CJ, Boyer JL. A C-terminal tyrosine-based motif in the bile salt export pump directs clathrin-dependent endocytosis. Hepatology. 2012;55(6):1901–11. doi:10.1002/hep.25523.
13. Kubitz R, Sutfels G, Kuhlkamp T, Kolling R, Haussinger D. Trafficking of the bile salt export pump from the Golgi to the canalicular membrane is regulated by the p38 MAP kinase. Gastroenterology. 2004;126(2):541–53.
14. Hayashi H, Sugiyama Y. Short-chain ubiquitination is associated with the degradation rate of a cell-surface-resident bile salt export pump (BSEP/ABCB11). Mol Pharmacol. 2009;75(1):143–50. doi:10.1124/mol.108.049288.
15. Byrne JA, Strautnieks SS, Mieli-Vergani G, Higgins CF, Linton KJ, Thompson RJ. The human bile salt export pump: characterization of substrate specificity and identification of inhibitors. Gastroenterology. 2002;123(5):1649–58.
16. Noe J, Stieger B, Meier PJ. Functional expression of the canalicular bile salt export pump of human liver. Gastroenterology. 2002;123(5):1659–66.
17. Hayashi H, Takada T, Suzuki H, Onuki R, Hofmann AF, Sugiyama Y. Transport by vesicles of glycine- and taurine-conjugated bile salts and taurolithocholate 3-sulfate: a comparison of human BSEP with rat Bsep. Biochim Biophys Acta. 2005;1738(1–3):54–62. doi:10.1016/j.bbalip.2005.10.006.
18. Makishima M, Okamoto AY, Repa JJ, Tu H, Learned RM, Luk A, et al. Identification of a nuclear receptor for bile acids. Science. 1999;284(5418):1362–5.
19. Ananthanarayanan M, Balasubramanian N, Makishima M, Mangelsdorf DJ, Suchy FJ. Human bile salt export pump promoter is transactivated by the farnesoid X receptor/bile acid receptor. J Biol Chem. 2001;276(31):28857–65. doi:10.1074/jbc.M011610200.
20. Plass JR, Mol O, Heegsma J, Geuken M, Faber KN, Jansen PL, et al. Farnesoid X receptor and bile salts are involved in transcriptional regulation of the gene encoding the human bile salt export pump. Hepatology. 2002;35(3):589–96. doi:10.1053/jhep.2002.31724.
21. Pellicciari R, Fiorucci S, Camaioni E, Clerici C, Costantino G, Maloney PR, et al. 6alpha-ethyl-chenodeoxycholic acid (6-ECDCA), a potent and selective FXR agonist endowed with anticholestatic activity. J Med Chem. 2002;45(17):3569–72.
22. Rizzo G, Passeri D, De Franco F, Ciaccioli G, Donadio L, Rizzo G, et al. Functional characterization of the semisynthetic bile acid derivative INT-767, a dual farnesoid X receptor and TGR5 agonist. Mol Pharmacol. 2010;78(4):617–30. doi:10.1124/mol.110.064501.
23. Yu J, Lo JL, Huang L, Zhao A, Metzger E, Adams A, et al. Lithocholic acid decreases expression of bile salt export pump through farnesoid X receptor antagonist activity. J Biol Chem. 2002;277(35):31441–7. doi:10.1074/jbc.M200474200.
24. Sayin SI, Wahlstrom A, Felin J, Jantti S, Marschall HU, Bamberg K, et al. Gut microbiota regulates bile acid metabolism by reducing the levels of tauro-beta-muricholic acid, a naturally occurring FXR antagonist. Cell Metab. 2013;17(2):225–35. doi:10.1016/j.cmet.2013.01.003.
25. Sinal CJ, Tohkin M, Miyata M, Ward JM, Lambert G, Gonzalez FJ. Targeted disruption of the nuclear receptor FXR/BAR impairs bile acid and lipid homeostasis. Cell. 2000;102(6):731–44.

26. Gomez-Ospina N, Potter CJ, Xiao R, Manickam K, Kim MS, Kim KH, et al. Mutations in the nuclear bile acid receptor FXR cause progressive familial intrahepatic cholestasis. Nat Commun. 2016;7:10713. doi:10.1038/ncomms10713.
27. Song X, Kaimal R, Yan B, Deng R. Liver receptor homolog 1 transcriptionally regulates human bile salt export pump expression. J Lipid Res. 2008;49(5):973–84. doi:10.1194/jlr.M700417-JLR200.
28. Mataki C, Magnier BC, Houten SM, Annicotte JS, Argmann C, Thomas C, et al. Compromised intestinal lipid absorption in mice with a liver-specific deficiency of liver receptor homolog 1. Mol Cell Biol. 2007;27(23):8330–9. doi:10.1128/MCB.00852-07.
29. Weerachayaphorn J, Cai SY, Soroka CJ, Boyer JL. Nuclear factor erythroid 2-related factor 2 is a positive regulator of human bile salt export pump expression. Hepatology. 2009;50 (5):1588–96. doi:10.1002/hep.23151.
30. Tanaka Y, Aleksunes LM, Cui YJ, Klaassen CD. ANIT-induced intrahepatic cholestasis alters hepatobiliary transporter expression via Nrf2-dependent and independent signaling. Toxicol Sci. 2009;108(2):247–57. doi:10.1093/toxsci/kfp020.
31. Song X, Vasilenko A, Chen Y, Valanejad L, Verma R, Yan B, et al. Transcriptional dynamics of bile salt export pump during pregnancy: mechanisms and implications in intrahepatic cholestasis of pregnancy. Hepatology. 2014;60(6):1993–2007. doi:10.1002/hep.27171.
32. Morotti RA, Suchy FJ, Magid MS. Progressive familial intrahepatic cholestasis (PFIC) type 1, 2, and 3: a review of the liver pathology findings. Semin Liver Dis. 2011;31(1):3–10. doi:10.1055/s-0031-1272831.
33. van Mil SW, van der Woerd WL, van der Brugge G, Sturm E, Jansen PL, Bull LN, et al. Benign recurrent intrahepatic cholestasis type 2 is caused by mutations in ABCB11. Gastroenterology. 2004;127(2):379–84.
34. Strautnieks SS, Byrne JA, Pawlikowska L, Cebecauerova D, Rayner A, Dutton L, et al. Severe bile salt export pump deficiency: 82 different ABCB11 mutations in 109 families. Gastroenterology. 2008;134(4):1203–14. doi:10.1053/j.gastro.2008.01.038.
35. Byrne JA, Strautnieks SS, Ihrke G, Pagani F, Knisely AS, Linton KJ, et al. Missense mutations and single nucleotide polymorphisms in ABCB11 impair bile salt export pump processing and function or disrupt pre-messenger RNA splicing. Hepatology. 2009;49 (2):553–67. doi:10.1002/hep.22683.
36. Davit-Spraul A, Fabre M, Branchereau S, Baussan C, Gonzales E, Stieger B, et al. ATP8B1 and ABCB11 analysis in 62 children with normal gamma-glutamyl transferase progressive familial intrahepatic cholestasis (PFIC): phenotypic differences between PFIC1 and PFIC2 and natural history. Hepatology. 2010;51(5):1645–55. doi:10.1002/hep.23539.
37. Jansen PL, Strautnieks SS, Jacquemin E, Hadchouel M, Sokal EM, Hooiveld GJ, et al. Hepatocanalicular bile salt export pump deficiency in patients with progressive familial intrahepatic cholestasis. Gastroenterology. 1999;117(6):1370–9.
38. Wang L, Soroka CJ, Boyer JL. The role of bile salt export pump mutations in progressive familial intrahepatic cholestasis type II. J Clin Invest. 2002;110(7):965–72. doi:10.1172/JCI15968.
39. Plass JR, Mol O, Heegsma J, Geuken M, de Bruin J, Elling G, et al. A progressive familial intrahepatic cholestasis type 2 mutation causes an unstable, temperature-sensitive bile salt export pump. J Hepatol. 2004;40(1):24–30.
40. Hayashi H, Takada T, Suzuki H, Akita H, Sugiyama Y. Two common PFIC2 mutations are associated with the impaired membrane trafficking of BSEP/ABCB11. Hepatology. 2005;41 (4):916–24. doi:10.1002/hep.20627.
41. Lam P, Pearson CL, Soroka CJ, Xu S, Mennone A, Boyer JL. Levels of plasma membrane expression in progressive and benign mutations of the bile salt export pump (Bsep/Abcb11) correlate with severity of cholestatic diseases. Am J Phys Cell Physiol. 2007;293(5): C1709–16. doi:10.1152/ajpcell.00327.2007.
42. Kagawa T, Watanabe N, Mochizuki K, Numari A, Ikeno Y, Itoh J, et al. Phenotypic differences in PFIC2 and BRIC2 correlate with protein stability of mutant Bsep and impaired

taurocholate secretion in MDCK II cells. Am J Physiol Gastrointest Liver Physiol. 2008;294(1):G58–67. doi:10.1152/ajpgi.00367.2007.
43. van Ooteghem NA, Klomp LW, van Berge-Henegouwen GP, Houwen RH. Benign recurrent intrahepatic cholestasis progressing to progressive familial intrahepatic cholestasis: low GGT cholestasis is a clinical continuum. J Hepatol. 2002;36(3):439–43.
44. Cai SY, Gautam S, Nguyen T, Soroka CJ, Rahner C, Boyer JL. ATP8B1 deficiency disrupts the bile canalicular membrane bilayer structure in hepatocytes, but FXR expression and activity are maintained. Gastroenterology. 2009;136(3):1060–9. doi:10.1053/j.gastro.2008.10.025.
45. Paulusma CC, de Waart DR, Kunne C, Mok KS, Elferink RP. Activity of the bile salt export pump (ABCB11) is critically dependent on canalicular membrane cholesterol content. J Biol Chem. 2009;284(15):9947–54. doi:10.1074/jbc.M808667200.
46. Girard M, Lacaille F, Verkarre V, Mategot R, Feldmann G, Grodet A, et al. MYO5B and bile salt export pump contribute to cholestatic liver disorder in microvillous inclusion disease. Hepatology. 2014;60(1):301–10. doi:10.1002/hep.26974.
47. Dixon PH, van Mil SW, Chambers J, Strautnieks S, Thompson RJ, Lammert F, et al. Contribution of variant alleles of ABCB11 to susceptibility to intrahepatic cholestasis of pregnancy. Gut. 2009;58(4):537–44. doi:10.1136/gut.2008.159541.
48. Dixon PH, Wadsworth CA, Chambers J, Donnelly J, Cooley S, Buckley R, et al. A comprehensive analysis of common genetic variation around six candidate loci for intrahepatic cholestasis of pregnancy. Am J Gastroenterol. 2014;109(1):76–84. doi:10.1038/ajg.2013.406.
49. Meier Y, Pauli-Magnus C, Zanger UM, Klein K, Schaeffeler E, Nussler AK, et al. Interindividual variability of canalicular ATP-binding-cassette (ABC)-transporter expression in human liver. Hepatology. 2006;44(1):62–74. doi:10.1002/hep.21214.
50. Ho RH, Leake BF, Kilkenny DM, Meyer Zu Schwabedissen HE, Glaeser H, Kroetz DL, et al. Polymorphic variants in the human bile salt export pump (BSEP; ABCB11): functional characterization and interindividual variability. Pharmacogenet Genomics. 2010;20(1):45–57. doi:10.1097/FPC.0b013e3283349eb0.
51. Lang C, Meier Y, Stieger B, Beuers U, Lang T, Kerb R, et al. Mutations and polymorphisms in the bile salt export pump and the multidrug resistance protein 3 associated with drug-induced liver injury. Pharmacogenet Genomics. 2007;17(1):47–60. doi:10.1097/01.fpc.0000230418.28091.76.
52. Kagawa T, Hirose S, Arase Y, Oka A, Anzai K, Tsuruya K, et al. No contribution of the ABCB11 p.444A polymorphism in Japanese patients with drug-induced cholestasis. Drug Metab Dispos. 2015; doi:10.1124/dmd.114.061325.
53. Aleo MD, Luo Y, Swiss R, Bonin PD, Potter DM, Will Y. Human drug-induced liver injury severity is highly associated with dual inhibition of liver mitochondrial function and bile salt export pump. Hepatology. 2014;60(3):1015–22. doi:10.1002/hep.27206.
54. Beuers U, Nathanson MH, Isales CM, Boyer JL. Tauroursodeoxycholic acid stimulates hepatocellular exocytosis and mobilizes extracellular Ca++ mechanisms defective in cholestasis. J Clin Invest. 1993;92(6):2984–93. doi:10.1172/JCI116921.
55. Kurz AK, Graf D, Schmitt M, Vom Dahl S, Haussinger D. Tauroursodesoxycholate-induced choleresis involves p38(MAPK) activation and translocation of the bile salt export pump in rats. Gastroenterology. 2001;121(2):407–19.
56. Kagawa T, Orii R, Hirose S, Arase Y, Shiraishi K, Mizutani A, et al. Ursodeoxycholic acid stabilizes the bile salt export pump in the apical membrane in MDCK II cells. J Gastroenterol. 2013; doi:10.1007/s00535-013-0833-y.
57. Varma S, Revencu N, Stephenne X, Scheers I, Smets F, Beleza-Meireles A, et al. Retargeting of bile salt export pump and favorable outcome in children with progressive familial intrahepatic cholestasis type 2. Hepatology. 2015;62(1):198–206. doi:10.1002/hep.27834.

58. Hayashi H, Sugiyama Y. 4-phenylbutyrate enhances the cell surface expression and the transport capacity of wild-type and mutated bile salt export pumps. Hepatology. 2007;45 (6):1506–16. doi:10.1002/hep.21630.
59. Naoi S, Hayashi H, Inoue T, Tanikawa K, Igarashi K, Nagasaka H, et al. Improved liver function and relieved pruritus after 4-phenylbutyrate therapy in a patient with progressive familial intrahepatic cholestasis type 2. J Pediatr. 2014;164(5):1219–27. e3 doi:10.1016/j.jpeds.2013.12.032.
60. Gonzales E, Grosse B, Schuller B, Davit-Spraul A, Conti F, Guettier C, et al. Targeted pharmacotherapy in progressive familial intrahepatic cholestasis type 2: evidence for improvement of cholestasis with 4-phenylbutyrate. Hepatology. 2015;62(2):558–66. doi:10.1002/hep.27767.
61. Hayashi H, Naoi S, Hirose Y, Matsuzaka Y, Tanikawa K, Igarashi K, et al. Successful treatment with 4-phenylbutyrate in a patient with benign recurrent intrahepatic cholestasis type 2 refractory to biliary drainage and bilirubin absorption. Hepatol Res. 2016;46 (2):192–200. doi:10.1111/hepr.12561.
62. Keitel V, Burdelski M, Vojnisek Z, Schmitt L, Haussinger D, Kubitz R. De novo bile salt transporter antibodies as a possible cause of recurrent graft failure after liver transplantation: a novel mechanism of cholestasis. Hepatology. 2009;50(2):510–7. doi:10.1002/hep.23083.
63. Jara P, Hierro L, Martinez-Fernandez P, Alvarez-Doforno R, Yanez F, Diaz MC, et al. Recurrence of bile salt export pump deficiency after liver transplantation. N Engl J Med. 2009;361(14):1359–67. doi:10.1056/NEJMoa0901075.
64. Maggiore G, Gonzales E, Sciveres M, Redon MJ, Grosse B, Stieger B, et al. Relapsing features of bile salt export pump deficiency after liver transplantation in two patients with progressive familial intrahepatic cholestasis type 2. J Hepatol. 2010;53(5):981–6. doi:10.1016/j.jhep.2010.05.025.
65. Lin HC, Alvarez L, Laroche G, Melin-Aldana H, Pfeifer K, Schwarz K, et al. Rituximab as therapy for the recurrence of bile salt export pump deficiency after liver transplantation. Liver Transpl. 2013;19(12):1403–10. doi:10.1002/lt.23754.
66. Stindt J, Kluge S, Droge C, Keitel V, Stross C, Baumann U, et al. Bile salt export pump-reactive antibodies form a polyclonal, multi-inhibitory response in antibody-induced bile salt export pump deficiency. Hepatology. 2016;63(2):524–37. doi:10.1002/hep.28311.
67. Boyer JL, Ng OC, Ananthanarayanan M, Hofmann AF, Schteingart CD, Hagenbuch B, et al. Expression and characterization of a functional rat liver Na+ bile acid cotransport system in COS-7 cells. Am J Phys. 1994;266(3 Pt 1):G382–7.
68. Hagenbuch B, Meier PJ. Molecular cloning, chromosomal localization, and functional characterization of a human liver Na+/bile acid cotransporter. J Clin Invest. 1994;93 (3):1326–31. doi:10.1172/JCI117091.
69. Hagenbuch B, Meier PJ. Sinusoidal (basolateral) bile salt uptake systems of hepatocytes. Semin Liver Dis. 1996;16(2):129–36. doi:10.1055/s-2007-1007226.
70. Hata S, Wang P, Eftychiou N, Ananthanarayanan M, Batta A, Salen G, et al. Substrate specificities of rat oatp1 and ntcp: implications for hepatic organic anion uptake. Am J Physiol Gastrointest Liver Physiol. 2003;285(5):G829–39. doi:10.1152/ajpgi.00352.2002.
71. Mita S, Suzuki H, Akita H, Stieger B, Meier PJ, Hofmann AF, et al. Vectorial transport of bile salts across MDCK cells expressing both rat Na+−taurocholate cotransporting polypeptide and rat bile salt export pump. Am J Physiol Gastrointest Liver Physiol. 2005;288(1): G159–67. doi:10.1152/ajpgi.00360.2003.
72. Mita S, Suzuki H, Akita H, Hayashi H, Onuki R, Hofmann AF, et al. Vectorial transport of unconjugated and conjugated bile salts by monolayers of LLC-PK1 cells doubly transfected with human NTCP and BSEP or with rat Ntcp and Bsep. Am J Physiol Gastrointest Liver Physiol. 2006;290(3):G550–6. doi:10.1152/ajpgi.00364.2005.
73. Hagenbuch B, Meier PJ. The superfamily of organic anion transporting polypeptides. Biochim Biophys Acta. 2003;1609(1):1–18.

74. Vaz FM, Paulusma CC, Huidekoper H, de Ru M, Lim C, Koster J, et al. Sodium taurocholate cotransporting polypeptide (SLC10A1) deficiency: conjugated hypercholanemia without a clear clinical phenotype. Hepatology. 2015;61(1):260–7. doi:10.1002/hep.27240.
75. Slijepcevic D, Kaufman C, Wichers CG, Gilglioni EH, Lempp FA, Duijst S, et al. Impaired uptake of conjugated bile acids and hepatitis b virus pres1-binding in na(+) – taurocholate cotransporting polypeptide knockout mice. Hepatology. 2015;62(1):207–19. doi:10.1002/hep.27694.
76. Zollner G, Fickert P, Zenz R, Fuchsbichler A, Stumptner C, Kenner L, et al. Hepatobiliary transporter expression in percutaneous liver biopsies of patients with cholestatic liver diseases. Hepatology. 2001;33(3):633–46. doi:10.1053/jhep.2001.22646.
77. Zollner G, Fickert P, Silbert D, Fuchsbichler A, Marschall HU, Zatloukal K, et al. Adaptive changes in hepatobiliary transporter expression in primary biliary cirrhosis. J Hepatol. 2003;38(6):717–27.
78. Gartung C, Ananthanarayanan M, Rahman MA, Schuele S, Nundy S, Soroka CJ, et al. Down-regulation of expression and function of the rat liver Na+/bile acid cotransporter in extrahepatic cholestasis. Gastroenterology. 1996;110(1):199–209.
79. Trauner M, Arrese M, Lee H, Boyer JL, Karpen SJ. Endotoxin downregulates rat hepatic ntcp gene expression via decreased activity of critical transcription factors. J Clin Invest. 1998;101(10):2092–100. doi:10.1172/JCI1680.
80. Lee YK, Dell H, Dowhan DH, Hadzopoulou-Cladaras M, Moore DD. The orphan nuclear receptor SHP inhibits hepatocyte nuclear factor 4 and retinoid X receptor transactivation: two mechanisms for repression. Mol Cell Biol. 2000;20(1):187–95.
81. Halilbasic E, Claudel T, Trauner M. Bile acid transporters and regulatory nuclear receptors in the liver and beyond. J Hepatol. 2013;58(1):155–68. doi:10.1016/j.jhep.2012.08.002.
82. Denson LA, Sturm E, Echevarria W, Zimmerman TL, Makishima M, Mangelsdorf DJ, et al. The orphan nuclear receptor, shp, mediates bile acid-induced inhibition of the rat bile acid transporter, ntcp. Gastroenterology. 2001;121(1):140–7.
83. Eloranta JJ, Jung D, Kullak-Ublick GA. The human Na+−taurocholate cotransporting polypeptide gene is activated by glucocorticoid receptor and peroxisome proliferator-activated receptor-gamma coactivator-1alpha, and suppressed by bile acids via a small heterodimer partner-dependent mechanism. Mol Endocrinol. 2006;20(1):65–79. doi:10.1210/me.2005-0159.
84. Wang L, Han Y, Kim CS, Lee YK, Moore DD. Resistance of SHP-null mice to bile acid-induced liver damage. J Biol Chem. 2003;278(45):44475–81. doi:10.1074/jbc.M305258200.
85. Webster CR, Anwer MS. Role of the PI3K/PKB signaling pathway in cAMP-mediated translocation of rat liver Ntcp. Am J Phys. 1999;277(6 Pt 1):G1165–72.
86. Webster CR, Srinivasulu U, Ananthanarayanan M, Suchy FJ, Anwer MS. Protein kinase B/Akt mediates cAMP – and cell swelling-stimulated Na+/taurocholate cotransport and Ntcp translocation. J Biol Chem. 2002;277(32):28578–83. doi:10.1074/jbc.M201937200.
87. Webster CR, Blanch C, Anwer MS. Role of PP2B in cAMP-induced dephosphorylation and translocation of NTCP. Am J Physiol Gastrointest Liver Physiol. 2002;283(1):G44–50. doi:10.1152/ajpgi.00530.2001.
88. Muhlfeld S, Domanova O, Berlage T, Stross C, Helmer A, Keitel V, et al. Short-term feedback regulation of bile salt uptake by bile salts in rodent liver. Hepatology. 2012;56(6):2387–97. doi:10.1002/hep.25955.
89. Yan H, Zhong G, Xu G, He W, Jing Z, Gao Z, et al. Sodium taurocholate cotransporting polypeptide is a functional receptor for human hepatitis B and D virus. Elife. 2012;1:e00049. doi:10.7554/eLife.00049.
90. Ni Y, Lempp FA, Mehrle S, Nkongolo S, Kaufman C, Falth M, et al. Hepatitis B and D viruses exploit sodium taurocholate co-transporting polypeptide for species-specific entry into hepatocytes. Gastroenterology. 2014;146(4):1070–83. doi:10.1053/j.gastro.2013.12.024.

91. Oehler N, Volz T, Bhadra OD, Kah J, Allweiss L, Giersch K, et al. Binding of hepatitis B virus to its cellular receptor alters the expression profile of genes of bile acid metabolism. Hepatology. 2014;60(5):1483–93. doi:10.1002/hep.27159.
92. Ho RH, Leake BF, Roberts RL, Lee W, Kim RB. Ethnicity-dependent polymorphism in Na+-taurocholate cotransporting polypeptide (SLC10A1) reveals a domain critical for bile acid substrate recognition. J Biol Chem. 2004;279(8):7213–22. doi:10.1074/jbc.M305782200.
93. Peng L, Zhao Q, Li Q, Li M, Li C, Xu T, et al. The p.Ser267Phe variant in SLC10A1 is associated with resistance to chronic hepatitis B. Hepatology. 2015;61(4):1251–60. doi:10.1002/hep.27608.
94. Hu HH, Liu J, Lin YL, Luo WS, Chu YJ, Chang CL, et al. The rs2296651 (S267F) variant on NTCP (SLC10A1) is inversely associated with chronic hepatitis B and progression to cirrhosis and hepatocellular carcinoma in patients with chronic hepatitis B. Gut. 2015; doi:10.1136/gutjnl-2015-310686.
95. Dawson PA, Hubbert M, Haywood J, Craddock AL, Zerangue N, Christian WV, et al. The heteromeric organic solute transporter alpha-beta, Ostalpha-Ostbeta, is an ileal basolateral bile acid transporter. J Biol Chem. 2005;280(8):6960–8. doi:10.1074/jbc.M412752200.
96. Li N, Cui Z, Fang F, Lee JY, Ballatori N. Heterodimerization, trafficking and membrane topology of the two proteins, Ost alpha and Ost beta, that constitute the organic solute and steroid transporter. Biochem J. 2007;407(3):363–72. doi:10.1042/BJ20070716.
97. Boyer JL, Trauner M, Mennone A, Soroka CJ, Cai SY, Moustafa T, et al. Upregulation of a basolateral FXR-dependent bile acid efflux transporter OSTalpha-OSTbeta in cholestasis in humans and rodents. Am J Physiol Gastrointest Liver Physiol. 2006;290(6):G1124–30. doi:10.1152/ajpgi.00539.2005.
98. Cui YJ, Aleksunes LM, Tanaka Y, Goedken MJ, Klaassen CD. Compensatory induction of liver efflux transporters in response to ANIT-induced liver injury is impaired in FXR-null mice. Toxicol Sci. 2009;110(1):47–60. doi:10.1093/toxsci/kfp094.
99. Zollner G, Wagner M, Moustafa T, Fickert P, Silbert D, Gumhold J, et al. Coordinated induction of bile acid detoxification and alternative elimination in mice: role of FXR-regulated organic solute transporter-alpha/beta in the adaptive response to bile acids. Am J Physiol Gastrointest Liver Physiol. 2006;290(5):G923–32. doi:10.1152/ajpgi.00490.2005.
100. Landrier JF, Eloranta JJ, Vavricka SR, Kullak-Ublick GA. The nuclear receptor for bile acids, FXR, transactivates human organic solute transporter-alpha and – beta genes. Am J Physiol Gastrointest Liver Physiol. 2006;290(3):G476–85. doi:10.1152/ajpgi.00430.2005.
101. Lee H, Zhang Y, Lee FY, Nelson SF, Gonzalez FJ, Edwards PA. FXR regulates organic solute transporters alpha and beta in the adrenal gland, kidney, and intestine. J Lipid Res. 2006;47(1):201–14. doi:10.1194/jlr.M500417-JLR200.
102. Wagner M, Fickert P, Zollner G, Fuchsbichler A, Silbert D, Tsybrovskyy O, et al. Role of farnesoid X receptor in determining hepatic ABC transporter expression and liver injury in bile duct-ligated mice. Gastroenterology. 2003;125(3):825–38.
103. Zelcer N, van de Wetering K, de Waart R, Scheffer GL, Marschall HU, Wielinga PR, et al. Mice lacking Mrp3 (Abcc3) have normal bile salt transport, but altered hepatic transport of endogenous glucuronides. J Hepatol. 2006;44(4):768–75. doi:10.1016/j.jhep.2005.07.022.
104. Mennone A, Soroka CJ, Cai SY, Harry K, Adachi M, Hagey L, et al. Mrp4−/− mice have an impaired cytoprotective response in obstructive cholestasis. Hepatology. 2006;43(5):1013–21. doi:10.1002/hep.21158.
105. Keitel V, Burdelski M, Warskulat U, Kuhlkamp T, Keppler D, Haussinger D, et al. Expression and localization of hepatobiliary transport proteins in progressive familial intrahepatic cholestasis. Hepatology. 2005;41(5):1160–72. doi:10.1002/hep.20682.
106. Lazaridis KN, Pham L, Tietz P, Marinelli RA, deGroen PC, Levine S, et al. Rat cholangiocytes absorb bile acids at their apical domain via the ileal sodium-dependent bile acid transporter. J Clin Invest. 1997;100(11):2714–21. doi:10.1172/JCI119816.

107. Kool M, van der Linden M, de Haas M, Scheffer GL, de Vree JM, Smith AJ, et al. MRP3, an organic anion transporter able to transport anti-cancer drugs. Proc Natl Acad Sci U S A. 1999;96(12):6914–9.
108. Lazaridis KN, Tietz P, Wu T, Kip S, Dawson PA, LaRusso NF. Alternative splicing of the rat sodium/bile acid transporter changes its cellular localization and transport properties. Proc Natl Acad Sci U S A. 2000;97(20):11092–7. doi:10.1073/pnas.200325297.
109. Soroka CJ, Lee JM, Azzaroli F, Boyer JL. Cellular localization and up-regulation of multidrug resistance-associated protein 3 in hepatocytes and cholangiocytes during obstructive cholestasis in rat liver. Hepatology. 2001;33(4):783–91. doi:10.1053/jhep.2001.23501.
110. Ballatori N, Christian WV, Lee JY, Dawson PA, Soroka CJ, Boyer JL, et al. OSTalpha-OSTbeta: a major basolateral bile acid and steroid transporter in human intestinal, renal, and biliary epithelia. Hepatology. 2005;42(6):1270–9. doi:10.1002/hep.20961.
111. Hofmann AF. Bile acids: trying to understand their chemistry and biology with the hope of helping patients. Hepatology. 2009;49(5):1403–18. doi:10.1002/hep.22789.

Chapter 3
Intestinal Digestion and Absorption

Akira Honda, Tadashi Ikegami, and Yasushi Matsuzaki

Abstract Bile acids are planar amphipathic molecules that have a polar and a nonpolar face. They are the end products of cholesterol metabolism and are called biological detergents. In the duodenum and upper jejunum, they participate in the digestion and absorption of lipids, including triacylglycerols, phospholipids, cholesterol, and fat-soluble vitamins. The formation of mixed micelles is the best-known property of bile acids, and the activation of pancreatic lipases is another important role. Triacylglycerols account for 90–95% of dietary lipids and are hydrolyzed to 2-monoacylglycerol and free fatty acids. Conjugated bile acids and phospholipids form mixed micelles with these hydrolysates of triacylglycerols, cholesterol, and fat-soluble vitamins. The mixed micelles effectively pass through the unstirred water layer overlying the microvillus border of the enterocytes, and all of the nutrients except for the conjugated bile acids are finally taken up by the cells. Conjugation of bile acids with glycine or taurine maintains water solubility at an acidic pH and prevents nonionic passive absorption from the proximal small intestine, which allows bile acids to be absorbed efficiently by an active transport system at the terminal ileum after the completion of their roles.

Keywords Bile acids • Digestion • Absorption • Triacylglycerols • Phospholipids • Cholesterol • Fat-soluble vitamins

3.1 Introduction

Bile acids are the end products of cholesterol metabolism and possess a number of chemical, physiological, and pathophysiological functions. The recent discovery of nuclear and transmembrane G protein-coupled bile acid receptors has interested many scientists in the regulation of lipid and carbohydrate metabolism, inflammation, fibrosis, and carcinogenesis through transcriptional networks and/or signaling cascades [1]. In contrast to the recent rapid development within these topics, the

A. Honda • T. Ikegami • Y. Matsuzaki (✉)
Department of Gastroenterology and Hepatology, Tokyo Medical University Ibaraki Medical Center, 3-20-1 Chuoh, Ami, Ibaraki 300-0395, Japan
e-mail: ymatsuzaki-gi@umin.ac.jp

S. Tazuma, H. Takikawa (eds.), *Bile Acids in Gastroenterology*,
DOI 10.1007/978-4-431-56062-3_3

roles of bile acids in digestion and absorption may be the most basic and historic subject that has been studied for more than half a century [2–5]. In this review, we will summarize the progress in our understanding of the mechanisms of digestion and absorption in the gastrointestinal tract with a particular emphasis on bile acids.

3.2 Bile Acids as Biological Detergents

Bile acids are planar amphipathic molecules having a polar and a nonpolar face [6]. The polar face contains hydroxyl and carboxyl groups and is water soluble, while the other face contains two methyl groups and is fat soluble. Thus, bile acids are called biological detergents. In water or a low salt concentration, bile acids form smaller micelles relative to classical detergent micelles because of the planar polarity. However, bile acids also form mixed micelles with a variety of other soluble and insoluble lipidic substances [7].

In human bile, bile acids are almost completely conjugated with either glycine or taurine [8] at the carboxyl group of the side chain through an amide bond. The pKa values of free (unconjugated) bile acids are between 5 and 6.5, while those of glycine- and taurine-conjugated bile acids are approximately 4 and 2, respectively [7]. It indicates that amino acid conjugation promotes ionization and increases the aqueous solubility of bile acids at an acidic pH [9]. Because the postprandial pH of the duodenum is between 3 and 5 [10], the conjugation allows bile acids to maintain water solubility to facilitate digestion in the duodenum and upper jejunum. In addition, the conjugation prevents nonionic passive absorption of bile acids [11]. Patients with genetic defects in bile acid conjugation experience fat-soluble vitamin deficiency because of an inability to form mixed micelles due to rapid nonionic passive absorption of unconjugated bile acids from the proximal small intestine [12]. Thus, conjugation with glycine or taurine allows bile acids to be actively absorbed in the terminal ileum after the completion of their roles.

3.3 Digestion and Absorption of Lipids

Typical adult Japanese and American diets contain approximately 54 and 85 g of fat per day, providing approximately 26% and 35% of the calorie intake of each individual, respectively [13, 14]. Approximately 90–95% of the dietary lipids are triacylglycerols (triglycerides) that consist of three fatty acids esterified to a glycerol. Dietary lipids also include phospholipids (predominantly phosphatidylcholine), sterols (cholesterol and plant sterols), and other lipids (e.g., fat-soluble vitamins). Phospholipids (essentially phosphatidylcholine) and cholesterol are also provided endogenously via the bile. Daily 7–22 g of phospholipids and approximately 1 g of cholesterol are loaded on the duodenum by biliary secretion, while 4–8 g of phospholipids and 200–400 mg of cholesterol per day are of dietary origin [5, 13, 15].

Digestion and absorption of lipids are complex processes with sequential and interdependent steps [3]. Emulsification, hydrolysis (lipolysis), and solubilization (micellization) are intraluminal key steps before the translocation of lipids across the apical membranes of enterocytes (absorption) [16, 17].

Emulsification mainly takes place in the stomach. A coarse emulsion (chyme) is produced by antral peristalsis against a closed pylorus, and the squirting of the antral contents through a partially opened pyloric canal into the duodenum produces a fine emulsion [5]. In the duodenum, the fine emulsion particles are generally less than 500 nm in diameter and are extremely stable.

Hydrolysis is carried out enzymatically by preduodenal and pancreatic lipases (Fig. 3.1). Preduodenal lipases are secreted from the tongue, pharynx, and stomach depending on the species; humans possess predominantly gastric lipase [18]. Human gastric lipase hydrolyzes triacylglycerols, but does not hydrolyze phospholipids or cholesterol ester. It has a pH optimum of 3–6, and conjugated bile acids inhibit the reaction [19, 20]. Pancreatic triacylglycerol lipase (EC 3.1.1.3) is secreted into the duodenum with colipase (as a procolipase) and conjugated bile acids. Most of the dietary triacylglycerols are hydrolyzed by pancreatic triacylglycerol lipase rather than gastric lipase [18]. This enzyme works at the interface between oil and water and an optimum pH optimum of 8–9. The presence

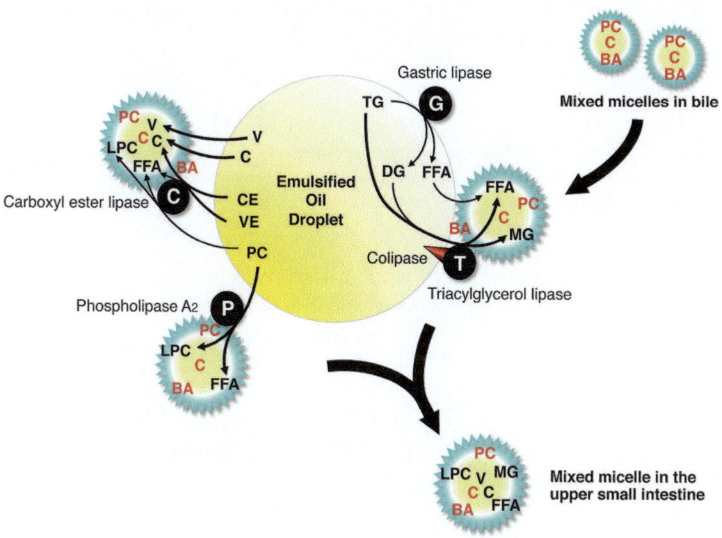

Fig. 3.1 Enzymatic hydrolysis and micellar solubilization of dietary lipids. *BA* conjugated bile acid, *C* cholesterol, *CE* cholesterol ester, *DG* diacylglycerol, *FFA* free fatty acid, *LPC* lysophosphatidylcholine, *MG* monoacylglycerol, *PC* phosphatidylcholine, *TG* triacylglycerol, *V* fat-soluble vitamin, *VE* fat-soluble vitamin ester

of conjugated bile acids inhibits the lipase activity, but colipase overcomes the inhibition with a shift in the pH optimum to 6–7 [21] (see Sect. 3.3.1.1). In general, pancreatic lipases include phospholipase A_2 (EC 3.1.1.4) and carboxyl ester lipase (EC 3.1.1.13) [16]. The latter is also called pancreatic nonspecific lipase or cholesterol esterase [5]. Phospholipase A_2 preferentially hydrolyzes phospholipids, whereas carboxyl ester lipase has a wide substrate specificity hydrolyzing cholesterol esters; tri-, di-, and monoacylglycerols; phospholipids; lysophospholipids; ceramide; and fat-soluble vitamins [22].

Solubilization of lipids and lipolytic products due to the formation of mixed micelles is a critical step for the absorption. Conjugated bile acids play a key role in this process, but polar lipids, including fatty acids and monoglycerides, are also important to increase the solubility of nonpolar lipids such as cholesterol. In contrast to emulsion, mixed micelle solution is optically clear. The diameter of the mixed micelles is 4–5 nm, which means that they have an approximately 100-fold reduced size and 10,000-fold increased surface area relative to the fine emulsion particle. It is also estimated that one fine emulsion particle can form approximately 1×10^6 micelles [23]. The unstirred water layer overlying the microvillus border of the epithelial cells is an intestinal diffusion barrier (Fig. 3.2). The mixed micelles effectively pass into the intermicrovillous spaces and are able to reach to the epithelial cells [24]. However, it seems to be an

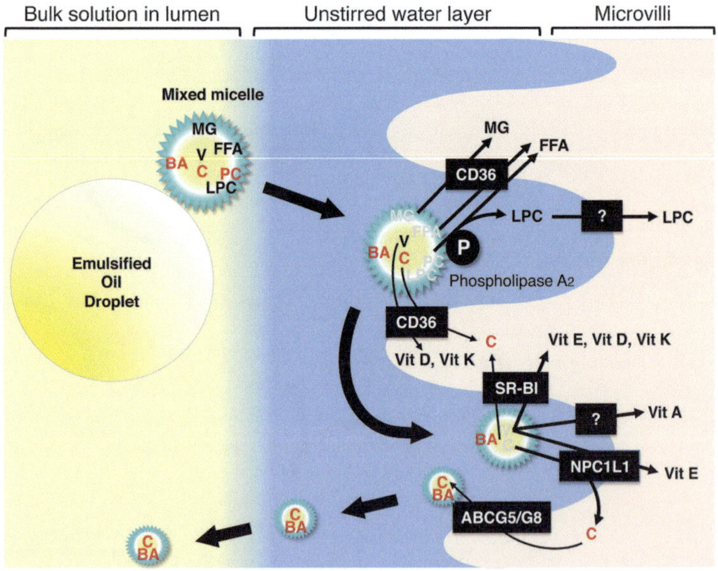

Fig. 3.2 Micellar solubilization and absorption of lipids in the upper small intestine. *ABCG5/ABCG8* ATP-binding cassette G5 and G8, *BA* conjugated bile acid, *C* cholesterol, *CD36* cluster determinant 36, *FFA* free fatty acid, *LPC* lysophosphatidylcholine, *MG* monoacylglycerol, *NPC1L1* Niemann-Pick C1-like 1, *PC* phosphatidylcholine, *SR-BI* scavenger receptor class B type I, *V* fat-soluble vitamin

oversimplification to divide the intestinal phase of lipids into an emulsion and mixed micelles. Under an adequate concentration of bile acids, the lipids are incorporated into mixed micelles. When the bile acid concentration is relatively low but still exceeds the critical micellar concentration, large mixed disclike micelles are formed at approximately 40 nm in diameter. Furthermore, when the relative bile acid concentration is much lower, this results in the formation of vesicles (liposomes) with a diameter of approximately 80–120 nm [5]. Because patients with low upper intestinal bile acid concentration show reasonably good absorption of lipids [25, 26], vesicles may play an important role in the uptake of free fatty acids and monoglycerides by enterocytes [5]. However, the relative roles of the mixed micelles and the vesicles have not been clarified [16].

3.3.1 Triacylglycerols

Most of the triacylglycerols found in food have long-chain fatty acids with 16–18 carbon atoms. However, a small but variable proportion of triacylglycerols contain fatty acids with only 6–10 carbon atoms and are called medium-chain triacylglycerols [27]. Because medium-chain triacylglycerols are less hydrophobic than long-chain triacylglycerols, the processes of digestion and absorption of these two types of triacylglycerols are somewhat different.

3.3.1.1 Long-Chain Triacylglycerols

The digestion of dietary triacylglycerols begins in the stomach. In addition to emulsification, gastric lipase hydrolyzes a significant portion of dietary triacylglycerols. This enzyme hydrolyzes medium-chain triacylglycerols better than long-chain triacylglycerols [28] and preferentially acts on the *sn*-3 position of the triacylglycerols [29] to release diacylglycerols and free fatty acids [19, 20, 30]. The relative contributions of gastric lipase and pancreatic triacylglycerol lipase to the hydrolysis of dietary triacylglycerols were reported to be approximately 1:3, and approximately 40% of the hydrolysis by gastric lipase occurred in the duodenum [31].

In the duodenum and proximal jejunum, the rest of triacylglycerols and diacylglycerols are hydrolyzed by pancreatic triacylglycerol lipase. This enzyme works at the oil-water interface of the emulsion. Conjugated bile acids adsorb onto fat droplets and remove proteins, emulsifiers, and lipolysis products from the lipid surface [32]. However, only triacylglycerol lipase is not removed from the oil-water interface and instigates lipolysis because colipase binds a bile-acid-covered oil-water interface and provides a high-affinity anchor site for triacylglycerol lipase [5, 21, 32]. Pancreatic triacylglycerol lipase preferentially cleaves the ester bond in the *sn*-1 and *sn*-3 positions of the triacylglycerols at equal rates [29, 33] so that 2-monoacylglycerol and free fatty acids are formed. A part of 2-monoacylglycerol is further hydrolyzed into glycerol and a free fatty acid by pancreatic triacylglycerol lipase either directly or after isomerization to 1-monoacylglycerol [33, 34]. Carboxyl ester lipase also hydrolyzes the acyl group at the *sn*-2 position to release glycerol and free fatty acid [35]. However, 80–90% of dietary glycerides retain their fatty acid in the *sn*-2 position during the entire digestion and absorption process [33].

Long-chain triacylglycerols and diacylglycerols are insoluble in aqueous solution regardless of whether bile acids are present [3]. Therefore, most of these acylglycerols reside in emulsified oil phase. In contrast, monoacylglycerols and free fatty acids possess polar groups that make them highly soluble in the presence of conjugated bile acids to form mixed micelles. The mixed micelles effectively pass through the unstirred water layer overlying the microvillus border of the enterocytes, and monoacylglycerols and free fatty acids are finally taken up by the cells [24].

The mechanisms by which free fatty acids and monoacylglycerols are translocated into the enterocytes have not been elucidated completely. Cluster determinant 36 (CD36) or fatty acid translocase (FAT) is known to be a membrane protein that facilitates cellular uptake of long-chain fatty acids. This protein is also highly expressed on the luminal surface of enterocytes in the proximal small intestine [36, 37]. However, CD36-null mice exhibited normal overall absorption of long-chain fatty acids and impaired chylomicron secretion. These findings suggest that CD36 plays critical roles for the absorption of long-chain fatty acids and the formation of chylomicron in the proximal small intestine, but CD36-independent absorption mechanisms predominate in the distal segments [37]. In comparison to free fatty acids, studies on intestinal uptake of monoacylglycerols are limited. An in vitro study using human intestinal Caco-2 cells showed that long-chain fatty acid and 2-monoacylglycerol were taken up in a saturable and competitive manner. The results suggest that long-chain fatty acids and 2-monoacylglycerol are transported into the enterocyte, at least in part, via a protein-mediated pathway that is shared by both lipids [38].

3.3.1.2 Medium-Chain Triacylglycerols

Higher concentrations of medium-chain length fatty acids are found in coconut oil (14%) and palm kernel oil (7%), butter (3%), and fresh cream (2%); cow and breast milk fat (1–3%) also contain significant amounts of the fatty acids [39]. However, the ingestion of medium-chain fatty acids is reported to be less than 2% of the total fatty acid intake in the United States [40].

Gastric lipase and pancreatic triacylglycerol lipase work more efficiently with medium-chain triacylglycerols than long-chain triacylglycerols. As a consequence, medium-chain triacylglycerols are absorbed mainly as free fatty acids and glycerol and only rarely as mono- or diacylglycerols [41]. Because of their smaller molecular size, medium-chain fatty acids and glycerol have greater solubility in water, and micellization with bile acids is unnecessary. In contrast to long-chain fatty acids that are resynthesized to triacylglycerol in the enterocytes and follow the lymphatic system as chylomicrons, medium-chain fatty acids are bound with albumin and follow the portal venous system [41].

3.3.2 *Phospholipids*

Dietary phospholipids are not hydrolyzed by gastric lipase but aid the emulsification of dietary fat. Therefore, they are forwarded to the duodenum as a component of emulsified oil droplets. In contrast, biliary phospholipids (essentially phosphatidylcholine) are supplied in mixed micelles along with cholesterol and conjugated bile acids. In the upper small intestine, dietary phospholipids are redistributed much in favor of the micellar phase [42].

The digestion of phospholipids is carried out mainly by pancreatic phospholipase A_2, but carboxyl ester lipase may contribute to the hydrolysis of phosphatidylcholine and lysophosphatidylcholine to some extent [22]. In fact, mice deficient in phospholipase A_2 show no abnormality in dietary phospholipid absorption [43]. Phospholipase A_2 undergoes a substantial increase in the catalytic activity on binding to the surface of phospholipid membranes or micelles [44] and the presence of bile acids [45]. However, the enzyme shows a low activity on biliary phosphatidylcholine because the high bile acid/phosphatidylcholine molar ratio in native bile presents unfavorable conditions for hydrolysis [46]. Phospholipase A_2 preferentially cleaves the ester bond in the *sn*-2 position of the phospholipids to yield lysophosphatidylcholine and free fatty acid [47].

Deacylation of lysophosphatidylcholine in the gut lumen is believed to be quite limited, and lysophosphatidylcholine and free fatty acids are taken up by enterocytes and resynthesized to phospholipids or triacylglycerols, which follow the lymphatic system as chylomicrons. The remaining absorbed lysophosphatidylcholine is hydrolyzed to form glycero-3-phosphorylcholine by phospholipase A_2/lysophospholipase (phospholipase B) [48–50], which is readily transported via the portal blood for use in the liver [51]. Although specific intestinal transporters for phosphatidylcholine and lysophosphatidylcholine have not been identified, lysophosphatidylcholine uptake by enterocytes is much greater than phosphatidylcholine absorption [52, 53].

3.3.3 *Cholesterol and Plant Sterols*

Most dietary cholesterol is present in the free form, but 10–15% exists as cholesterol ester [16]. Gastric lipase does not hydrolyze cholesterol ester; rather, the hydrolysis is performed by pancreatic carboxyl ester lipase (cholesterol esterase). In this process, bile acids strongly stimulate the lipase activity [54, 55]. Chemical modification studies suggest that positive-charged arginine residues in carboxyl ester lipase are important for its interaction with bile acids [56–59, 22]. In contrast, biliary cholesterol is exclusively free form and is secreted as mixed micelles with phosphatidylcholine and conjugated bile acids. In the proximal small intestine, dietary cholesterol is initially emulsified with triglycerides in oil droplets, but free cholesterol originated from the diet is finally incorporated into mixed micelles or vesicles with biliary cholesterol [60].

In humans, cholesterol absorption is not complete, and the percent of absorption varies from 15% to 75% [61]. Relative to monoacylglycerols, free fatty acids, and lysophosphatidylcholine, the aqueous solubility of cholesterol is extremely low. Therefore, the formation of mixed micelles and vesicles is critically important for the transport of cholesterol through the unstirred water layer overlying the microvillus border of enterocytes. Therefore, intestinal cholesterol absorption is markedly affected by coexisting bile acids, phospholipids, free fatty acids, and plant sterols.

It has been reported that trihydroxy bile acids more effectively promote cholesterol absorption than dihydroxy bile acids [62–64], and the size of the cholic acid pool significantly correlates with cholesterol absorption in patients with liver cirrhosis [65]. On the other hand, the intestinal uptake of cholesterol was linearly dependent on micellar cholesterol concentration and was not dependent on the bile acid concentration [64]. However, taurochenodeoxycholic acid is a better micellar solubilizer of cholesterol than taurocholic acid, although the latter is a better promoter of cholesterol absorption [66–68]. In addition, when cholesterol was completely solubilized in micelles with a nontoxic nonionic detergent, Pluronic F68, cholesterol was not taken up by enterocytes [64]. These results suggest that not only the solubilization capacity but also the interaction between micelle and acceptor (transporter) serves as determinants of the absorption efficiency of cholesterol.

There are at least four transporters that are key players in the control of cholesterol absorption from the intestine. Niemann-Pick C1-like 1 (NPC1L1) is a major cholesterol uptake transporter [69], while scavenger receptor class B type I (SR-BI) also plays a role in cholesterol uptake to a lesser extent [70, 71]. On the other hand, ATP-binding cassette (ABC) proteins ABCG5 and ABCG8 are cholesterol efflux transporters [72]. Although little is known about the direct effects of bile acids on intestinal NPC1L1 and SR-BI activities, ABCG5-/ABCG8-specific cholesterol efflux is stimulated by bile acids in cell models [73, 74]. ABCG5/ABCG8 transfers cholesterol in an ATP-dependent manner, and the hydrolysis of ATP is stimulated by bile acids [75]. It has been suggested that bile acids may promote an active conformation of ABCG5/ABCG8 either by global stabilization of the transporter or by binding to a specific site on ABCG5/ABCG8. Furthermore, CD36 may also play a role in cholesterol uptake. Overexpression of CD36 enhanced cholesterol uptake from micellar substrates in COS-7 cells [76]. Conversely, CD36-null mice showed significant reduced cholesterol transport from the intestinal lumen to the lymphatic system [77]. However, its absence was not sufficient to cause an overall reduction in intestinal cholesterol uptake.

Although phospholipids are essential molecules for the effective solubilization of cholesterol in the bile and intestine, excess phospholipids cause the suppression of cholesterol absorption. There are at least three possible mechanisms [15]. First, excess phospholipids may interfere with efficient hydrolysis of micellar phospholipids, which is a prerequisite for efficient mucosal uptake of cholesterol. Second, surplus phospholipids may alter the physicochemical properties of mixed micelles resulting in reduced absorption of cholesterol. Third, phospholipids may act on the membrane characteristics of enterocytes or have a direct effect on cellular cholesterol transporters. Free fatty acids may also affect intestinal cholesterol absorption. Mixed micelles containing medium-chain fatty acids have a reduced solubilizing capacity for cholesterol relative to those containing long-chain fatty acids [78].

Food of a plant origin includes plant sterols that are structurally related to cholesterol but differ from cholesterol only in their unsaturation level and/or side-chain configuration [76]. Typical Western diets contain approximately 300 mg of plant sterols per day [79, 80], but the absorption percentage of plant sterols is less than 2% in humans [81], which is considerably lower than that of cholesterol (15–75%). Plant sterols transported into enterocytes with cholesterol via NPC1L1 are pumped back to the lumen via ABCG5/ABCG8, whereas a significant proportion of the internalized cholesterol is esterified and incorporated into chylomicrons [82, 83]. Plant sterols are known to inhibit cholesterol absorption, but the mechanisms are not fully understood. Because the digestion process of plant sterols and cholesterol is virtually the same, it has been suggested that plant sterols compete with intestinal cholesterol for incorporation into mixed micelles [84, 85], but other possible mechanisms have also been proposed [86].

3.3.4 Fat-Soluble Vitamins

Because vitamins A, D, E, and K are fat soluble, micelle formation is required for intestinal absorption. Vitamins A, D, and E have hydroxyl groups that can be esterified with fatty acid, and pancreatic carboxyl ester lipase catalyzes the hydrolysis under the presence of bile acids [35]. While most dietary vitamin E (tocopherol and tocotrienol) is in the free form, vitamin A (retinol) is often esterified and must be hydrolyzed to retinol and fatty acid before absorption [22, 87]. Except for carboxyl ester lipase, pancreatic triacylglycerol lipase and intestinal phospholipase B also contribute to the hydrolysis of retinyl esters [22]. Free retinol is then incorporated with other lipids into the mixed micelles, passes through the unstirred water layer, and is taken up by enterocytes [87]. Although the intestinal retinol-specific transporter has not been clarified, stimulated by retinoic acid 6 (STRA6) [88] and retinol-binding protein 4-receptor 2 (RBPR2) [89] are candidate proteins.

Micelle formation is also required for the absorption of vitamins E, D, and K [12, 90]. It has been reported that intestinal cholesterol transporters, NPC1L1 and SR-BI, play a role in the uptake of micellar vitamin E [91, 92]. However, recent report suggests that additional intestinal transporters are also involved in the uptake of vitamin E [93]. In addition, there are reports that both SR-BI and CD36 contribute to the intestinal absorption of vitamins D [94] and K [95].

3.4 Protein Digestion

In addition to promoting lipid digestion and absorption, conjugated bile acids also bind to dietary proteins in the small intestine. The binding of bile acids denatures the protein and dramatically enhances the proteolysis by pancreatic proteases [96]. The effect was most pronounced in the presence of dihydroxy bile acids and was observed at concentrations below the critical micellar concentration.

3.5 Absorption of Polyvalent Metals

Polyvalent metals such as calcium (Ca^{2+}) and iron (Fe^{2+}) are poorly soluble at the intestinal pH. However, premicellar concentrations of taurocholic acid solubilize calcium [97] and iron [98, 99] in the proximal small intestine and promote their absorption. The mechanism of solubilization is explained by high-affinity binding of these polyvalent cations to the interposition between terminal carboxyl and 7- or 12-hydroxyl groups of the steroid ring of taurocholic acid. Taurodehydrocholic acid, lacking ring hydroxyl groups, did not bind either cation with a high affinity and did not promote their absorption [100].

3.6 Conclusions

In the duodenum and upper jejunum, the conjugated bile acids facilitate lipolysis by pancreatic lipases and formation of mixed micelles with phospholipids, lipolytic products of triacylglycerols (2-monoacylglycerols and free fatty acids), cholesterol, and fat-soluble vitamins. The mixed micelles can effectively approach the enterocytes, and each nutrient is finally taken up by the cells primarily by protein-mediated processes. Conjugated bile acids also promote digestion of proteins and absorption of polyvalent metals, such as calcium and iron. In addition to these direct effects on digestion and absorption, duodenal conjugated bile acids are known to inhibit the release of cholecystokinin [101] and motilin [102], which modulate contractions of the gallbladder and indirectly control digestion and absorption. Conjugated bile acids maintain water solubility at an acidic pH in the upper small intestine and are not absorbed together with the solubilized lipids, which allows for efficient active absorption of bile acids from the terminal ileum after the completion of their roles.

References

1. Schaap FG, Trauner M, Jansen PL. Bile acid receptors as targets for drug development. Nat Rev Gastroenterol Hepatol. 2014;11:55–67. doi:10.1038/nrgastro.2013.151.
2. Hofmann AF. The function of bile salts in fat absorption. The solvent properties of dilute micellar solutions of conjugated bile salts. Biochem J. 1963;89:57–68.
3. Hofmann AF. A physicochemical approach to the intraluminal phase of fat absorption. Gastroenterology. 1966;50:56–64.
4. Friedman HI, Nylund B. Intestinal fat digestion, absorption, and transport. A review. Am J Clin Nutr. 1980;33:1108–39.
5. Carey MC, Small DM, Bliss CM. Lipid digestion and absorption. Annu Rev Physiol. 1983;45:651–77. doi:10.1146/annurev.ph.45.030183.003251.
6. Hofmann AF, Hagey LR. Bile acids: chemistry, pathochemistry, biology, pathobiology, and therapeutics. Cell Mol Life Sci. 2008;65:2461–83. doi:10.1007/s00018-008-7568-6.
7. Carey MC, Small DM. Micelle formation by bile salts. Physical-chemical and thermodynamic considerations. Arch Intern Med. 1972;130:506–27.
8. Matoba N, Une M, Hoshita T. Identification of unconjugated bile acids in human bile. J Lipid Res. 1986;27:1154–62.
9. Hofmann AF, Mysels KJ. Bile acid solubility and precipitation in vitro and in vivo: the role of conjugation, pH, and Ca2+ ions. J Lipid Res. 1992;33:617–26.
10. Ovesen L, Bendtsen F, Tage-Jensen U, Pedersen NT, Gram BR, Rune SJ. Intraluminal pH in the stomach, duodenum, and proximal jejunum in normal subjects and patients with exocrine pancreatic insufficiency. Gastroenterology. 1986;90:958–62.
11. Hofmann AF, Roda A. Physicochemical properties of bile acids and their relationship to biological properties: an overview of the problem. J Lipid Res. 1984;25:1477–89.
12. Setchell KD, Heubi JE, Shah S, Lavine JE, Suskind D, Al-Edreesi M, et al. Genetic defects in bile acid conjugation cause fat-soluble vitamin deficiency. Gastroenterology. 2013;144:945–55 e6. quiz e14-5 doi:10.1053/j.gastro.2013.02.004.
13. National Health and Nutrition Survey Japan 2013 Ministry of Health, Labour and Welfare, Japan. http://www.mhlw.go.jp/stf/houdou/0000067890.html/. Accessed 15 Dec 2015.
14. Freedman MR, King J, Kennedy E. Popular diets: a scientific review. Obes Res. 2001;9(Suppl 1):1S–40S. doi:10.1038/oby.2001.113.
15. Cohn JS, Kamili A, Wat E, Chung RW, Tandy S. Dietary phospholipids and intestinal cholesterol absorption. Nutrients. 2010;2:116–27. doi:10.3390/nu2020116.
16. Phan CT, Tso P. Intestinal lipid absorption and transport. Front Biosci. 2001;6:D299–319.
17. Iqbal J, Hussain MM. Intestinal lipid absorption. Am J Physiol Endocrinol Metab. 2009;296: E1183–94. doi:10.1152/ajpendo.90899.2008.
18. Verger R, Aoubala M, Carriere F, Ransac S, Dupuis L, De Caro J, et al. Regulation of lumen fat digestion: enzymic aspects. Proc Nutr Soc. 1996;55:5–18.
19. Hamosh M, Scanlon JW, Ganot D, Likel M, Scanlon KB, Hamosh P. Fat digestion in the newborn. Characterization of lipase in gastric aspirates of premature and term infants. J Clin Invest. 1981;67:838–46.
20. Abrams CK, Hamosh M, Lee TC, Ansher AF, Collen MJ, Lewis JH, et al. Gastric lipase: localization in the human stomach. Gastroenterology. 1988;95:1460–4.
21. Borgström B, Erlanson C. Pancreatic lipase and co-lipase. Interactions and effects of bile salts and other detergents. Eur J Biochem. 1973;37:60–8.
22. Hui DY, Howles PN. Carboxyl ester lipase: structure-function relationship and physiological role in lipoprotein metabolism and atherosclerosis. J Lipid Res. 2002;43:2017–30.
23. Ganguly J. Biochemistry of vitamin A. Boca Raton: CRC Press, Inc.; 1989.
24. Thomson AB, Schoeller C, Keelan M, Smith L, Clandinin MT. Lipid absorption: passing through the unstirred layers, brush-border membrane, and beyond. Can J Physiol Pharmacol. 1993;71:531–55.

25. Porter HP, Saunders DR, Tytgat G, Brunser O, Rubin CE. Fat absorption in bile fistula man. A morphological and biochemical study. Gastroenterology. 1971;60:1008–19.
26. Mansbach 2nd CM, Newton D, Stevens RD. Fat digestion in patients with bile acid malabsorption but minimal steatorrhea. Dig Dis Sci. 1980;25:353–62.
27. Scheig R. What is dietary fat? Am J Clin Nutr. 1969;22:651–3.
28. Liao TH, Hamosh P, Hamosh M. Fat digestion by lingual lipase: mechanism of lipolysis in the stomach and upper small intestine. Pediatr Res. 1984;18:402–9.
29. Paltauf F, Esfandi F, Holasek A. Stereospecificity of lipases. Enzymic hydrolysis of enantiomeric alkyl diacylglycerols by lipoprotein lipase, lingual lipase and pancreatic lipase. FEBS Lett. 1974;40:119–23.
30. Cohen M, Morgan RG, Hofmann AF. Lipolytic activity of human gastric and duodenal juice against medium and long chain triglycerides. Gastroenterology. 1971;60:1–15.
31. Carriere F, Barrowman JA, Verger R, Laugier R. Secretion and contribution to lipolysis of gastric and pancreatic lipases during a test meal in humans. Gastroenterology. 1993;105:876–88.
32. Gargouri Y, Julien R, Bois AG, Verger R, Sarda L. Studies on the detergent inhibition of pancreatic lipase activity. J Lipid Res. 1983;24:1336–42.
33. Borgström B. Influence of bile salt, pH, and time on the action of pancreatic lipase; physiological implications. J Lipid Res. 1964;5:522–31.
34. Hofmann AF, Borgstrom B. Hydrolysis of long-chain monoglycerides in micellar solution by pancreatic lipase. Biochim Biophys Acta. 1963;70:317–31.
35. Lombardo D, Guy O. Studies on the substrate specificity of a carboxyl ester hydrolase from human pancreatic juice. II. Action on cholesterol esters and lipid-soluble vitamin esters. Biochim Biophys Acta. 1980;611:147–55.
36. Chen M, Yang Y, Braunstein E, Georgeson KE, Harmon CM. Gut expression and regulation of FAT/CD36: possible role in fatty acid transport in rat enterocytes. Am J Physiol Endocrinol Metab. 2001;281:E916–23.
37. Nassir F, Wilson B, Han X, Gross RW, Abumrad NA. CD36 is important for fatty acid and cholesterol uptake by the proximal but not distal intestine. J Biol Chem. 2007;282:19493–501. doi:10.1074/jbc.M703330200.
38. Murota K, Storch J. Uptake of micellar long-chain fatty acid and sn-2-monoacylglycerol into human intestinal Caco-2 cells exhibits characteristics of protein-mediated transport. J Nutr. 2005;135:1626–30.
39. Takeuchi H, Sekine S, Kojima K, Aoyama T. The application of medium-chain fatty acids: edible oil with a suppressing effect on body fat accumulation. Asia Pac J Clin Nutr. 2008;17 (Suppl 1):320–3.
40. U.S. Department of Agriculture ARS. Nutrient intakes from foods: mean amounts consumed per individual, one day, 2011–2012 http://www.ars.usda.gov/Services/docs.htm?docid=18349 Accessed 15 Dec 2015.
41. Bach AC, Babayan VK. Medium-chain triglycerides: an update. Am J Clin Nutr. 1982;36:950–62.
42. Arnesjo B, Nilsson A, Barrowman J, Borgstrom B. Intestinal digestion and absorption of cholesterol and lecithin in the human. Intubation studies with a fat-soluble reference substance. Scand J Gastroenterol. 1969;4:653–65.
43. Richmond BL, Boileau AC, Zheng S, Huggins KW, Granholm NA, Tso P, et al. Compensatory phospholipid digestion is required for cholesterol absorption in pancreatic phospholipase A2-deficient mice. Gastroenterology. 2001;120:1193–202. doi:10.1053/gast.2001.23254.
44. Tatulian SA. Toward understanding interfacial activation of secretory phospholipase A2 (PLA2): membrane surface properties and membrane-induced structural changes in the enzyme contribute synergistically to PLA2 activation. Biophys J. 2001;80:789–800. doi:10.1016/S0006-3495(01)76058-4.

45. Arnesjo B, Grubb A. The activation, purification and properties of rat pancreatic juice phospholipase A 2. Acta Chem Scand. 1971;25:577–89.
46. Nalbone G, Lairon D, Charbonnier-Augeire M, Vigne JL, Leonardi J, Chabert C, et al. Pancreatic phospholipase A2 hydrolysis of phosphatidylcholines in various physicochemical states. Biochim Biophys Acta. 1980;620:612–25.
47. van den Bosch H, Postema NM, de Haas GH, van Deenen LL. On the positional specificity of phospholipase A from pancreas. Biochim Biophys Acta. 1965;98:657–9.
48. Ottolenghi A. Estimation and subcellular distribution of lecithinase activity in rat intestinal mucosa. J Lipid Res. 1964;5:532–7.
49. Subbaiah PV, Ganguly J. Studies on the phospholipases of rat intestinal mucosa. Biochem J. 1970;118:233–9.
50. Gassama-Diagne A, Fauvel J, Chap H. Purification of a new, calcium-independent, high molecular weight phospholipase A2/lysophospholipase (phospholipase B) from guinea pig intestinal brush-border membrane. J Biol Chem. 1989;264:9470–5.
51. Le Kim D, Betzing H. Intestinal absorption of polyunsaturated phosphatidylcholine in the rat. Hoppe Seylers Z Physiol Chem. 1976;357:1321–31.
52. Reynier MO, Lafont H, Crotte C, Sauve P, Gerolami A. Intestinal cholesterol uptake: comparison between mixed micelles containing lecithin or lysolecithin. Lipids. 1985;20:145–50.
53. Homan R, Hamelehle KL. Phospholipase A2 relieves phosphatidylcholine inhibition of micellar cholesterol absorption and transport by human intestinal cell line Caco-2. J Lipid Res. 1998;39:1197–209.
54. Erlanson C. Purification, properties, and substrate specificity of a carboxylesterase in pancreatic juice. Scand J Gastroenterol. 1975;10:401–8.
55. Blackberg L, Lombardo D, Hernell O, Guy O, Olivecrona T. Bile salt-stimulated lipase in human milk and carboxyl ester hydrolase in pancreatic juice: are they identical enzymes? FEBS Lett. 1981;136:284–8.
56. Lombardo D, Campese D, Multigner L, Lafont H, De Caro A. On the probable involvement of arginine residues in the bile-salt-binding site of human pancreatic carboxylic ester hydrolase. Eur J Biochem. 1983;133:327–33.
57. Blackberg L, Hernell O. Bile salt-stimulated lipase in human milk. Evidence that bile salt induces lipid binding and activation via binding to different sites. FEBS Lett. 1993;323:207–10.
58. Gjellesvik DR, Lorens JB, Male R. Pancreatic carboxylester lipase from Atlantic salmon (*Salmo salar*). cDNA sequence and computer-assisted modelling of tertiary structure. Eur J Biochem. 1994;226:603–12.
59. Liang Y, Medhekar R, Brockman HL, Quinn DM, Hui DY. Importance of arginines 63 and 423 in modulating the bile salt-dependent and bile salt-independent hydrolytic activities of rat carboxyl ester lipase. J Biol Chem. 2000;275:24040–6. doi:10.1074/jbc.M003187200.
60. Yao L, Heubi JE, Buckley DD, Fierra H, Setchell KD, Granholm NA, et al. Separation of micelles and vesicles within lumenal aspirates from healthy humans: solubilization of cholesterol after a meal. J Lipid Res. 2002;43:654–60.
61. Grundy SM. Absorption and metabolism of dietary cholesterol. Annu Rev Nutr. 1983;3:71–96. doi:10.1146/annurev.nu.03.070183.000443.
62. Swell L, Flick DF, Field Jr H, Treadwell CR. Influence of dietary bile salts on blood cholesterol levels. Proc Soc Exp Biol Med. 1953;84:428–31.
63. Gallo-Torres HE, Miller ON, Hamilton JG. Further studies on the role of bile salts in cholesterol esterification and absorption from the gut. Arch Biochem Biophys. 1971;143:22–36.
64. Watt SM, Simmonds WJ. The specificity of bile salts in the intestinal absorption of micellar cholesterol in the rat. Clin Exp Pharmacol Physiol. 1976;3:305–22.
65. Ponz de Leon M, Loria P, Iori R, Carulli N. Cholesterol absorption in cirrhosis: the role of total and individual bile acid pool size. Gastroenterology. 1981;80:1428–37.

66. Cohen BI, Raicht RF, Mosbach EH. Sterol metabolism studies in the rat. Effects of primary bile acids (sodium taurochenodeoxycholate and sodium taurocholate) on sterol metabolism. J Lipid Res. 1977;18:223–31.
67. Reynier MO, Montet JC, Gerolami A, Marteau C, Crotte C, Montet AM, et al. Comparative effects of cholic, chenodeoxycholic, and ursodeoxycholic acids on micellar solubilization and intestinal absorption of cholesterol. J Lipid Res. 1981;22:467–73.
68. Watt SM, Simmonds WJ. Effects of four taurine-conjugated bile acids on mucosal uptake and lymphatic absorption of cholesterol in the rat. J Lipid Res. 1984;25:448–55.
69. Altmann SW, Davis Jr HR, Zhu LJ, Yao X, Hoos LM, Tetzloff G, et al. Niemann-Pick C1 like 1 protein is critical for intestinal cholesterol absorption. Science. 2004;303:1201–4. doi:10.1126/science.1093131.
70. Altmann SW, Davis Jr HR, Yao X, Laverty M, Compton DS, Zhu LJ, et al. The identification of intestinal scavenger receptor class B, type I (SR-BI) by expression cloning and its role in cholesterol absorption. Biochim Biophys Acta. 2002;1580:77–93.
71. Bietrix F, Yan D, Nauze M, Rolland C, Bertrand-Michel J, Comera C, et al. Accelerated lipid absorption in mice overexpressing intestinal SR-BI. J Biol Chem. 2006;281:7214–9. doi:10.1074/jbc.M508868200.
72. Lee MH, Lu K, Hazard S, Yu H, Shulenin S, Hidaka H, et al. Identification of a gene, ABCG5, important in the regulation of dietary cholesterol absorption. Nat Genet. 2001;27:79–83. doi:10.1038/83799.
73. Vrins C, Vink E, Vandenberghe KE, Frijters R, Seppen J, Groen AK. The sterol transporting heterodimer ABCG5/ABCG8 requires bile salts to mediate cholesterol efflux. FEBS Lett. 2007;581:4616–20. doi:10.1016/j.febslet.2007.08.052.
74. Tachibana S, Hirano M, Hirata T, Matsuo M, Ikeda I, Ueda K, et al. Cholesterol and plant sterol efflux from cultured intestinal epithelial cells is mediated by ATP-binding cassette transporters. Biosci Biotechnol Biochem. 2007;71:1886–95.
75. Johnson BJ, Lee JY, Pickert A, Urbatsch IL. Bile acids stimulate ATP hydrolysis in the purified cholesterol transporter ABCG5/G8. Biochemistry. 2010;49:3403–11. doi:10.1021/bi902064g.
76. van Bennekum A, Werder M, Thuahnai ST, Han CH, Duong P, Williams DL, et al. Class B scavenger receptor-mediated intestinal absorption of dietary beta-carotene and cholesterol. Biochemistry. 2005;44:4517–25. doi:10.1021/bi0484320.
77. Nauli AM, Nassir F, Zheng S, Yang Q, Lo CM, Vonlehmden SB, et al. CD36 is important for chylomicron formation and secretion and may mediate cholesterol uptake in the proximal intestine. Gastroenterology. 2006;131:1197–207. doi:10.1053/j.gastro.2006.08.012.
78. von Bonsdorff-Nikander A, Christiansen L, Huikko L, Lampi AM, Piironen V, Yliruusi J, et al. A comparison of the effect of medium- vs. long-chain triglycerides on the in vitro solubilization of cholesterol and/or phytosterol into mixed micelles. Lipids. 2005;40:181–90.
79. Klingberg S, Andersson H, Mulligan A, Bhaniani A, Welch A, Bingham S, et al. Food sources of plant sterols in the EPIC Norfolk population. Eur J Clin Nutr. 2008;62:695–703. doi:10.1038/sj.ejcn.1602765.
80. Valsta LM, Lemstrom A, Ovaskainen ML, Lampi AM, Toivo J, Korhonen T, et al. Estimation of plant sterol and cholesterol intake in Finland: quality of new values and their effect on intake. Br J Nutr. 2004;92:671–8.
81. Ostlund Jr RE, McGill JB, Zeng CM, Covey DF, Stearns J, Stenson WF, et al. Gastrointestinal absorption and plasma kinetics of soy Delta(5)-phytosterols and phytostanols in humans. Am J Physiol Endocrinol Metab. 2002;282:E911–6. doi:10.1152/ajpendo.00328.2001.
82. Calandra S, Tarugi P, Speedy HE, Dean AF, Bertolini S, Shoulders CC. Mechanisms and genetic determinants regulating sterol absorption, circulating LDL levels, and sterol elimination: implications for classification and disease risk. J Lipid Res. 2011;52:1885–926. doi:10.1194/jlr.R017855.
83. Gylling H, Plat J, Turley S, Ginsberg HN, Ellegard L, Jessup W, et al. Plant sterols and plant stanols in the management of dyslipidaemia and prevention of cardiovascular disease. Atherosclerosis. 2014;232:346–60. doi:10.1016/j.atherosclerosis.2013.11.043.

84. Nissinen M, Gylling H, Vuoristo M, Miettinen TA. Micellar distribution of cholesterol and phytosterols after duodenal plant stanol ester infusion. Am J Physiol Gastrointest Liver Physiol. 2002;282:G1009–15. doi:10.1152/ajpgi.00446.2001.
85. Ikeda I. Factors affecting intestinal absorption of cholesterol and plant sterols and stanols. J Oleo Sci. 2015;64:9–18. doi:10.5650/jos.ess14221.
86. De Smet E, Mensink RP, Plat J. Effects of plant sterols and stanols on intestinal cholesterol metabolism: suggested mechanisms from past to present. Mol Nutr Food Res. 2012;56:1058–72. doi:10.1002/mnfr.201100722.
87. Reboul E. Absorption of vitamin A and carotenoids by the enterocyte: focus on transport proteins. Nutrients. 2013;5:3563–81. doi:10.3390/nu5093563.
88. Isken A, Golczak M, Oberhauser V, Hunzelmann S, Driever W, Imanishi Y, et al. RBP4 disrupts vitamin A uptake homeostasis in a STRA6-deficient animal model for Matthew-Wood syndrome. Cell Metab. 2008;7:258–68. doi:10.1016/j.cmet.2008.01.009.
89. Alapatt P, Guo F, Komanetsky SM, Wang S, Cai J, Sargsyan A, et al. Liver retinol transporter and receptor for serum retinol-binding protein (RBP4). J Biol Chem. 2013;288:1250–65. doi:10.1074/jbc.M112.369132.
90. Goncalves A, Gontero B, Nowicki M, Margier M, Masset G, Amiot MJ, et al. Micellar lipid composition affects micelle interaction with class B scavenger receptor extracellular loops. J Lipid Res. 2015;56:1123–33. doi:10.1194/jlr.M057612.
91. Reboul E, Klein A, Bietrix F, Gleize B, Malezet-Desmoulins C, Schneider M, et al. Scavenger receptor class B type I (SR-BI) is involved in vitamin E transport across the enterocyte. J Biol Chem. 2006;281:4739–45. doi:10.1074/jbc.M509042200.
92. Narushima K, Takada T, Yamanashi Y, Suzuki H. Niemann-pick C1-like 1 mediates alpha-tocopherol transport. Mol Pharmacol. 2008;74:42–9. doi:10.1124/mol.107.043034.
93. Reboul E, Soayfane Z, Goncalves A, Cantiello M, Bott R, Nauze M, et al. Respective contributions of intestinal Niemann-Pick C1-like 1 and scavenger receptor class B type I to cholesterol and tocopherol uptake: in vivo v. in vitro studies. Br J Nutr. 2012;107:1296–304. doi:10.1017/S0007114511004405.
94. Reboul E, Borel P. Proteins involved in uptake, intracellular transport and basolateral secretion of fat-soluble vitamins and carotenoids by mammalian enterocytes. Prog Lipid Res. 2011;50:388–402. doi:10.1016/j.plipres.2011.07.001.
95. Goncalves A, Margier M, Roi S, Collet X, Niot I, Goupy P, et al. Intestinal scavenger receptors are involved in vitamin K1 absorption. J Biol Chem. 2014;289:30743–52. doi:10.1074/jbc.M114.587659.
96. Gass J, Vora H, Hofmann AF, Gray GM, Khosla C. Enhancement of dietary protein digestion by conjugated bile acids. Gastroenterology. 2007;133:16–23. doi:10.1053/j.gastro.2007.04.008.
97. Sanyal AJ, Hirsch JI, Moore EW. Premicellar taurocholate enhances calcium uptake from all regions of rat small intestine. Gastroenterology. 1994;106:866–74.
98. Sanyal AJ, Hirsch JI, Moore EW. Premicellar taurocholate avidly binds ferrous (Fe++) iron: a potential physiologic role for bile salts in iron absorption. J Lab Clin Med. 1990;116:76–86.
99. Sanyal AJ, Shiffmann ML, Hirsch JI, Moore EW. Premicellar taurocholate enhances ferrous iron uptake from all regions of rat small intestine. Gastroenterology. 1991;101:382–9.
100. Sanyal AJ, Hirsch JI, Moore EW. High-affinity binding is essential for enhancement of intestinal Fe2+ and Ca2+ uptake by bile salts. Gastroenterology. 1992;102:1997–2005.
101. Koop I, Schindler M, Bosshammer A, Scheibner J, Stange E, Koop H. Physiological control of cholecystokinin release and pancreatic enzyme secretion by intraduodenal bile acids. Gut. 1996;39:661–7.
102. Portincasa P, Peeters TL, van Berge-Henegouwen GP, van Solinge WW, Palasciano G, van Erpecum KJ. Acute intraduodenal bile salt depletion leads to strong gallbladder contraction, altered antroduodenal motility and high plasma motilin levels in humans. Neurogastroenterol Motil. 2000;12:421–30.

Chapter 4
Nuclear Receptor Regulation

Makoto Makishima

Abstract Bile acids are essential for the intestinal digestion and absorption of lipid-soluble nutrients. Bile acids, which are synthesized from cholesterol in the liver, have been identified as signaling molecules that act as ligands for nuclear receptors, farnesoid X receptor (FXR), pregnane X receptor (PXR), and vitamin D receptor (VDR). FXR is activated by chenodeoxycholic acid, deoxycholic acid, lithocholic acid, cholic acid, and their taurine and glycine conjugates and regulates bile acid synthesis and enterohepatic circulation. PXR and VDR respond to the secondary bile acids, such as lithocholic acid or deoxycholic acid, and stimulate xenobiotic metabolism of bile acids. The oxysterol receptor liver X receptor-α and the orphan nuclear receptors short heterodimeric partner, liver receptor homolog-1, and hepatocyte nuclear factor 4α are also involved in regulation of bile acid metabolism. These nuclear receptors regulate various physiological processes other than bile acid metabolism, such as glucose and lipid metabolism, cellular growth and differentiation, and immunity. Bile acid metabolism by intestinal microflora modulates nuclear receptor function in host cells. Bile acid-activated G protein-coupled receptors have also been identified. Bile acids may play a role in various physiological mechanisms by binding to cellular receptors as "prototypes" of steroid hormones.

Keywords Farnesoid X receptor • Pregnane X receptor • Vitamin D receptor • Transcription • Regulation

4.1 Nuclear Receptors

Transcription factors of the nuclear receptor superfamily regulate numerous biological processes including cell growth and differentiation, embryonic development, endocrine regulation, and metabolic homeostasis [1, 2]. Forty-eight nuclear receptors have been identified in human, while there are 49 receptors in the mouse

M. Makishima (✉)
Division of Biochemistry, Department of Biomedical Sciences, Nihon University School of Medicine, 30-1 Oyaguchi-kamicho, Itabashi-ku, Tokyo 173-8610, Japan
e-mail: makishima.makoto@nihon-u.ac.jp

S. Tazuma, H. Takikawa (eds.), *Bile Acids in Gastroenterology*,
DOI 10.1007/978-4-431-56062-3_4

genome. Nuclear receptors are classified into three groups based on their ligand-responding characteristics. The first group consists of nuclear receptors for steroid hormones, such as estrogen, progesterone, androgen, glucocorticoid, and mineralocorticoid, which act as homodimers and mediate endocrine signals. The second group includes metabolic sensors, which were initially identified as orphan receptors [1, 3]. This class of receptors form heterodimers with retinoid X receptor (RXR; NR2B) and are activated by retinoic acid, vitamin D, thyroid hormone, bile acids, oxysterols, fatty acids, and xenobiotics. Among this group of receptors, liver X receptor-α (LXRα; NR1H3), farnesoid X receptor (FXR; NR1H4), pregnane X receptor (PXR; NR1I2), constitutive androstane receptor (CAR; NR1I3), and vitamin D receptor (VDR; NR1I1) regulate bile acid metabolism by sensing the metabolic environment [4, 5] (Fig. 4.1). The third group includes orphan receptors that have no known physiological ligands or may be regulated by ligand-independent mechanisms. In this group, short heterodimeric partner (SHP; NR0B2), liver receptor homolog-1 (LRH-1; NR5A2), and hepatocyte nuclear factor 4α (HNF4α; NR2A1) are involved in regulation of bile acid metabolism [4] (Fig. 4.1). SHP is an unusual nuclear receptor that lacks a DNA-binding domain [5]. Although phospholipids and fatty acids have been reported to bind to LRH-1 and HNF4α, respectively, the physiological relevance of these interactions remains unclear [6].

Nuclear receptors, including LXR, FXR, PXR, CAR, and VDR, have a structure comprised of an activation function 1 (AF1) region, a DNA-binding region with a C4-type zinc finger structure, a hinge region, and a ligand-binding domain containing an AF2 region [3]. Ligand binding alters the AF2 surface, leading to dissociation of a corepressor complex and recruitment of a coactivator complex [7]. These structural rearrangements allow the receptors to induce transcription of specific target genes. Nuclear receptors also exhibit transrepression effects and non-genomic actions through poorly characterized mechanisms. Both steroid hormones and bile acids are steroid compounds synthesized from cholesterol and act as ligands of nuclear receptors. Bile acids are essential factors for the ingestion and intestinal absorption of hydrophobic nutrients, such as cholesterol, fatty acids, and lipid-soluble vitamins, including vitamin D [8], and act as "prototypes" of steroid hormones by binding to nuclear receptors.

4.2 Bile Acid Metabolism

Primary bile acids, such as cholic acid (CA) and chenodeoxycholic acid (CDCA), are generated from cholesterol in the liver and are secreted in bile as glycine and taurine conjugates (in humans; glyco-CA, tauro-CA (TCA), glyco-CDCA, and tauro-CDCA (TCDCA)) [9, 10]. The synthesis of bile acids is mediated by at least 16 enzymes. The first step for cholesterol catabolism is initiated by one of two mechanisms, the classic pathway and the alternate pathway [9] (Fig. 4.2). In the classic pathway, cholesterol is converted to 7α-hydroxycholesterol by cholesterol

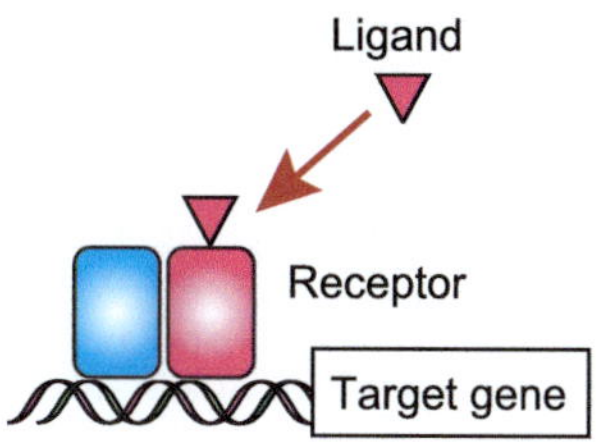

Nuclear receptor	Ligand	Target gene involved in bile acid metabolism
LXRα	Oxysterols	CYP7A1 (rodent)
LRH-1	(Phospholipids?)	CYP7A1, CYP8B1
HNF4α	(Fatty acids?)	CYP7A1, CYP8B1
SHP	-	[CYP7A1, CYP8B1]
FXR	CDCA > DCA = LCA > CA (Antagonists: TαMCA, TβMCA, LCA, UDCA)	SHP, FGF15/19 BSEP, OSTα, OSTβ I-BABP (CYP7A1, CYP8B1, NTCP)
PXR	Xenobiotics 3-Keto-LCA > LCA > DCA = CA	FGF15/19 OATP1A4, MRP3 CYP3A4, SULT2A1, PAPSS2 (CYP7A1, CYP8B1)
CAR	Xenobiotics	CYP3A4, MRP3
VDR	1,25(OH)2D3 3-Keto-LCA > LCA	CYP3A4, SULT2A1 MRP2, MRP3, MRP4 FGF15/19 (CYP7A1)

Fig. 4.1 Nuclear receptors regulate bile acid metabolism. Nuclear receptors that regulate expression of genes involved in bile acid metabolism are shown. FXR, PXR, and VDR respond to bile acids. SHP does not have a DNA-binding domain and represses expression of CYP7A1 and CYP8B1 as a corepressor. FXR, PXR, and VDR repress expression of CYP7A1, CYP8B1, or NTCP through indirect mechanisms

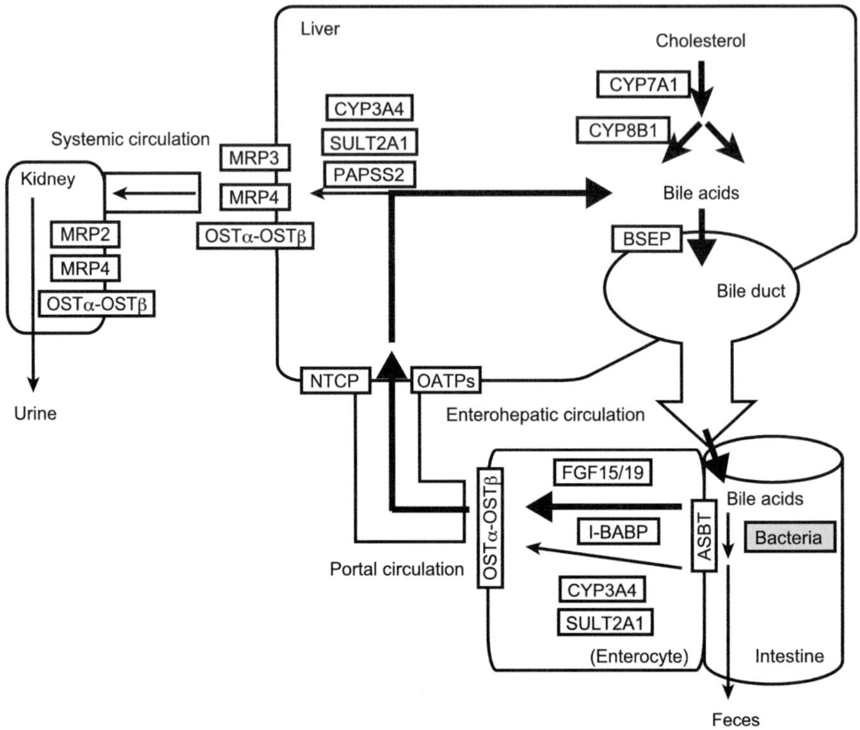

Fig. 4.2 Bile acid synthesis, enterohepatic circulation, and catabolism through the xenobiotic metabolic pathway. Nuclear receptor target gene products involved in bile acid metabolism are shown. Primary bile acids are synthesized by several enzymes, including CYP7A1 and CYP8B1, in the liver. Conjugated bile acids are secreted into bile via the canalicular transporter BSEP. Most bile acids are reabsorbed in the intestine, which expresses transporters, ASBT and OSTα–OSTβ, and an intracellular binding protein, I-BABP, and enter the enterohepatic circulation via portal circulation and hepatic uptake via NTCP and OATPs. Bile acids that escape reabsorption are converted to the secondary bile acids by intestinal bacteria. These bile acids are detoxified by CYP3A4 and SULT2A1. PAPSS2 provides the sulfate donor PAPS to SULT2A1. Hepatocytes can dispose bile acids through xenobiotic metabolism enzymes, such as CYP3A4 and SULT2A1, and basolateral transporters, MRP3, MRP4, and OSTα–OSTβ, leading to excretion into urine via renal transporters, MRP2, MRP4, and OSTα–OSTβ. FGF15/FGF19 is a hormone that regulates bile acid synthesis

7α-hydroxylase (CYP7A1), a microsomal P450 enzyme. In humans, the classical pathway accounts for more than 50% of total bile acid production. In the alternate pathway, cholesterol is converted to 25-hydroxycholesterol and 27-hydroxycholesterol prior to being 7α-hydroxylated by oxysterol 7α-hydroxylase (CYP7B1). CYP27A1 hydroxylates cholesterol to 27-hydroxycholesterol and, to a lesser extent, 25-hydroxycholesterol, while a non-P450 enzyme, cholesterol 25-hydroxylase, produces 25-hydroxycholesterol. The alternate pathway is thought to produce less than 10% of the total bile acids under physiological conditions.

The initial step of 7α-hydroxylation of sterol precursors is followed by modification of ring structures, side chain oxidation, and conjugation with taurine or glycine. The ring structure modification catalyzed by sterol 12α-hydroxylase (CYP8B1) finally produces CA, while the CYP8B1-independent pathway results in CDCA. CYP27A1, an enzyme that is involved in the alternate pathway, is also involved in the side chain oxidation of all intermediates regardless of their source. Oxidation by CYP27A1 is followed by side chain shortening and finally conjugation with taurine or glycine. In mice, CDCA is converted to α-muricholic acid (αMCA) and βMCA by unknown mechanisms.

Conjugated primary bile acids are secreted into the bile via the bile salt export pump (BSEP; ABCB11), an ATP-binding cassette (ABC) transporter that is localized in the canalicular membrane of hepatocytes [11] (Fig. 4.2). As the major components in bile, bile acids solubilize dietary lipids and promote their digestion and absorption in the small intestine. About 90–95% of conjugated bile acids are reabsorbed in the intestine and recirculate to the liver through the portal vein in a mechanism called the enterohepatic circulation. Less than 5% of bile acids escape reabsorption and are subjected to deconjugation, 7α-dehydroxylation, and other modifications by intestinal microflora, yielding the secondary bile acids, such as deoxycholic acid (DCA) and lithocholic acid (LCA) [12]. A portion of the secondary bile acids can enter the enterohepatic circulation from the ileum and colon and enter the bile acid pool. Because taurine conjugation is predominant in rodents, the major bile acids in mouse bile are TCA, tauro-αMCA (TαMCA), TβMCA, TDCA, and TωMCA [13, 14]. Ursodeoxycholic acid (UDCA) is generated from CDCA by intestinal bacteria [12, 15]. Interestingly, UDCA and tauro-UDCA (TUDCA) concentrations are higher in germ-free mice than in conventional mice, suggesting the presence of UDCA-generating enzyme(s) in mouse hepatocytes [14, 16].

Intestinal bile acid reabsorption is mainly mediated by the apical sodium-dependent bile salt transporter (ASBT; SLC10A2) expressed in the terminal ileum [11] (Fig. 4.2). Intracellular bile acids are bound to the intestinal bile acid-binding protein (I-BABP), then shuttled to the basolateral membrane, and effluxed into the portal circulation via the heterodimer organic solute transporter-α (OSTα) and OSTβ [4, 17]. The majority of circulating bile acids are taken up by hepatocytes via the Na^+/taurocholate-cotransporting polypeptide (NTCP; SLC10A1) and organic anion-transporting polypeptides (OATPs). In addition to canalicular excretion by BSEP, the basolateral (sinusoidal) transporters multidrug resistance-associated protein 3 (MRP3), MRP4, and OSTα–OSTβ play a role in the alternative excretion of bile acids from hepatocytes into the systemic circulation. Renal MRP2, MRP4, and OSTα–OSTβ are thought to be involved in urinary bile acid excretion [18, 19].

4.3 LXR and FXR

Bile acids have been identified as regulatory signaling molecules for the transcription of genes involved in their synthesis (e.g., CYP7A1, CYP8B1) and transport (e.g., BSEP, NTCP). LXRα, originally identified as an orphan receptor, is activated by oxysterol intermediates in the bile acid synthetic pathway, such as 7-α-hydroxycholesterol, 25-hydroxychoelsterol, and 27-hydroxycholesterol, while the more potent oxysterol for LXRα, 24(*S*),25-epoxycholsterol, is derived in a shunt pathway of cholesterol biosynthesis [20, 21]. Oxysterol-activated LXRα induces the transcription of mouse *Cyp7a1*, the rate-limiting enzyme in the classic pathway of bile acid synthesis by binding to a specific promoter element that consists of a two-hexanucleotide (AGGTCA or a related sequence) direct repeat motif separated by four nucleotides (direct repeat 4; DR4) [22] (Fig. 4.1). The ABC transporters ABCG5 and ABCG8, which mediate biliary excretion of cholesterol, are also induced by LXRα activation. A high cholesterol diet increases bile acid pool size in wild-type mice but not in LXRα-null mice [21]. Thus, LXRα plays a role in the feed-forward induction of bile acid synthesis in rodents. The expression of the human *CYP7A1* gene is not regulated by LXRα due to an alternate sequence in the DR4 element [23].

LXRα acts as an RXR heterodimer, which can be activated by ligands for either LXRα or RXR [3]. According to this characteristic of the LXRα–RXR heterodimer, it had been predicted that treatment of mice with an RXR agonist could increase hepatic *Cyp7a1* expression. Surprisingly, contrary to this prediction, RXR agonist treatment decreases *Cyp7a1* expression in both wild-type and LXR-α-null mice [24]. This finding led to the hypothesis that a distinct RXR heterodimeric partner might respond to bile acids, since bile acids have been known to induce feedback regulation in their synthesis by repressing *Cyp7a1* expression [9]. Indeed, FXR was found to function as a bile acid receptor [25]. FXR was originally characterized as an orphan receptor that is weakly activated by farnesol, an intermediate in cholesterol synthesis, and juvenile hormone III, an insect hormone [26]. FXR belongs to the NR1H nuclear receptor subfamily along with LXRα; is expressed in the liver, intestine, kidney, and adrenal gland; and recognizes a two-hexanucleotide (AGGTCA or a related sequence) inverted repeat motif with one spacer nucleotide (inverted repeat 1; IR1) as an RXR heterodimer [5]. FXR is activated by both primary and secondary bile acids in their free and conjugated forms with relative potency CDCA > DCA = LCA > CA, but not by αMCA, βMCA, or UDCA [25, 27, 28] (Fig. 4.1). LCA, UDCA, TαMCA, and TβMCA have been reported to act as FXR antagonists [16, 29–31].

FXR regulates the synthesis and enterohepatic circulation of bile acids by both direct and indirect mechanisms [4, 32]. The orphan nuclear receptors HNF4α and LRH-1 are involved in transcription of the bile acid synthetic enzymes CYP7A1 and CYP8B1 [4, 33, 34] (Fig. 4.1). FXR represses the expression of CYP7A1 and CYP8B1 by inducing the transcriptional repressor SHP [35–38]. FXR appears to also repress expression of CYP7A1 and CYP8B1 via a SHP-independent mechanism, because significant *Cyp7a1* and *Cyp8b1* repression is retained in SHP-null mice fed cholic acid [38]. FXR induces the expression of fibroblast growth factor 19 (FGF19; or FGF15, the mouse ortholog of human FGF19) in enterocytes. FGF15/19 represses the expression of CYP7A1 by binding to a heterodimeric receptor composed of FGF receptor 4 and β-Klotho in hepatocytes through both SHP-dependent and -independent mechanisms [34, 39–41]. There are IR1 elements identified in human *SHP* and *FGF19* genes [35, 42]. Thus, FXR activation suppresses bile acid synthesis through multiple mechanisms.

The hepatic bile acid transport system is also regulated by FXR. The basolateral transporter NTCP is negatively regulated by FXR through a SHP-mediated mechanism [37, 43], while its expression is induced by retinoic acid receptor and HNF4α [44, 45] (Fig. 4.1). The canalicular transporter BSEP is induced by FXR activation [37]. Human *BSEP* contains an IR1 element in the promoter [46]. FXR activation by a synthetic ligand protects hepatocytes from cholestatic liver damage by repressing bile acid synthesis and hepatocellular uptake and stimulating bile acid export from cells [47]. Despite this finding, FXR-null mice exhibit resistance to obstructive cholestasis [48]. FXR deletion protects hepatocytes by facilitating bile acid export into blood and renal excretion via a compensatory mechanism such as PXR activation. These findings suggest that protection of hepatocytes from cholestatic damage by FXR activation requires sufficient bile flow. FXR also induces the sinusoidal bile acid transporters OSTα and OSTβ [49], while PXR is involved in expression of MRP3 in mice [50]. FXR-null mice exhibit reduced fecal bile acid excretion as well as dysregulated bile acid synthesis [37]. Although FXR–RXR has been reported to bind to an everted repeat motif with 8-nucleotide spacer called ER-8 in the rat *Mrp2* promoter [51], FXR deletion does not change *Mrp2* expression in mice [52]. Multidrug resistance protein 3 MDR3 (ABCB4; corresponding to the murine MDR2), which is involved in phosphatidylcholine transport through the canalicular membrane, is induced by FXR through its binding to an IR1 element in the promoter [53, 54]. The cholesterol transporters ABCG5 and ABCG8 are also induced by cholic acid treatment of mice in an FXR-dependent manner [55].

FXR activation induces the bile acid transporter OSTα–OSTβ in the intestine and kidney [49] (Fig. 4.1). The intestinal intracellular bile acid-binding protein I-BABP is also a FXR target gene [25, 56]. IR1 elements have been identified in the promoters of these human genes [49, 56]. In contrast to the hepatic phenotype, FXR-null mice have efficient intestinal absorption of bile acids [52]. The physiological role of FXR in intestinal bile acid absorption remains to be elucidated.

Studies using pharmacological FXR activation and FXR-null mice have shown that FXR regulates triglyceride, cholesterol, and carbohydrate metabolism [4, 5, 32]. FXR deletion in mice has been reported to induce both increased and decreased glucose tolerance [57, 58]. FXR activation increases expression of genes involved in gluconeogenesis in hepatocytes [59], supporting the role of FXR in decreasing glucose tolerance. Recently, intestinal microflora have been found to play a role in energy metabolism through bile acid metabolism [16, 31]. Compared to conventionally raised mice, germ-free mice have decreased expression of the FXR targets *Shp* and *Fgf15* in the distal ileum [16]. Germ-free mice have decreased secondary bile acids and increased TαMCA and TβMCA, which act as FXR antagonists, and show increased glucose tolerance, a similar phenotype to intestine-specific FXR-knockout mice [31]. Intestinal FXR-null mice are also resistant to diet-induced obesity. It is unknown how intestinal FXR antagonism or deletion induces metabolic effects. Bile acids have bacteriostatic effects and also protect the intestine from bacterial invasion through an FXR-dependent mechanism [60]. Thus, there are reciprocal interactions between host and bacteria through FXR regulation.

FXR exhibits immune modulatory action through a transrepression mechanism [61]. FXR agonist treatment attenuates inflammation in mouse models of hepatitis and colitis [61, 62]. The physiological relevance of bile acid in these FXR functions remains unclear. Elevated bile acid levels after partial hepatectomy accelerate liver regeneration in an FXR-dependent manner [63]. FXR activates the forkhead box M1 transcription factor, a cell cycle regulator controlling the G1/S and G2/M transitions, through binding to an IR0 element located in an intron of its gene [64]. The FGF15 signaling pathway induced by intestinal FXR activation is also involved in liver regeneration [65].

4.4 PXR, CAR, and VDR

PXR, CAR, and VDR belong to the NR1I nuclear receptor subfamily [1, 2]. PXR can respond to numerous structurally diverse compounds, including drugs, environmental contaminants, and bile acids, induces expression of transporters and enzymes involved in xenobiotic metabolism, and plays an important role in the detoxification and clearance of xenobiotics [4, 5, 66] (Fig. 4.1). PXR is activated by bile acids in potency order: 3-keto-LCA $>$ LCA $>$ DCA $=$ CA [67, 68]. PXR activation represses expression of the bile acid synthetic genes, *CYP7A1* and *CYP8B1*, without inducing *SHP* expression [69, 70]. PXR agonist treatment increases *Cyp7a1* expression in wild-type mice but not in PXR-null mice [68]. PXR induces expression of human *FGF19* and mouse *Fgf15* genes [71], suggesting that FGF15/19 signaling plays a role in hepatic CYP7A1 suppression by PXR. PXR agonist treatment enhances bile acid detoxification by inducing the import transporter *Oatp1a4* (*Slco1a4*; also called *Oatp2*), the detoxifying enzyme *Cyp3a11*, and the basolateral export transporter *Mrp3* in the liver, leading to decreased serum bile acids and increased urinary bile acid excretion [50, 68, 72] (Fig. 4.2). CYP3A4, a human ortholog of mouse CYP3A11, is involved in the metabolism of 50–60% of pharmaceuticals as well as natural compounds such as steroids and herbal supplements [73]. CYP3A4 metabolizes LCA to 3-keto-LCA by 3-oxidation and hyodeoxycholic acid by 6α-hydroxylation [67, 74]. 3-Keto-LCA is a more potent PXR ligand than LCA, an interaction that enhances xenobiotic metabolism. PXR-binding elements have been identified in the *CYP3A4* and *OATP1B1* (*SLCO1B1*) promoters [75, 76]. Sulfation of LCA is mediated primarily by dehydroepiandrosterone sulfotransferase 2 (SULT2), which requires 3-′-phosphoadenosine-5′-phosphosulfate (PAPS) as a donor molecule. The expression of *Sult2* and PAPS synthase 2 (*Papss2*) is induced by PXR [77]. PXR is a candidate drug target for the treatment of cholestasis.

CAR is a nuclear receptor that regulates the transcription of genes involved in xenobiotic metabolism, cooperatively with PXR, and is abundantly expressed in the liver and intestine [78]. Although there is no evidence to date that endogenous bile acids are ligands for CAR, CAR has been shown to regulate bile acid metabolism (Fig. 4.1). CAR activation induces *Cyp3a11* expression in PXR/FXR double knockout mice fed cholic acid [79]. Comparison of PXR-null mice, CAR-null mice, and PXR/CAR double knockout mice shows that CAR predominantly mediates induction of *Cyp3a11* and *Mrp3*, while PXR is the major regulator of *Oatp1a4* [80]. CAR is also involved in the induction of *Sult2a*, *Papss2*, and *Mrp4* [81, 82]. In a bile duct ligation model of cholestasis, hepatic damage is increased in both PXR-null mice and CAR-null mice. PXR and CAR are required for elimination of toxic bile acids. Although these receptors have been reported to be involved in regulation of glucose and lipid metabolism [33], the role of bile acid signaling remains unknown.

VDR has been identified as a receptor for 1α,25-dihydroxyvitamin D_3 (1,25 $(OH)_2D_3$), the active form of vitamin D [33]. The secosteroid vitamin D_3 is synthesized from 7-dehydrocholesterol through a photochemical reaction induced by sunlight exposure. Vitamin D_3 is hydroxylated at the 25-position by CYP2R1 and CYP27A1 to yield 25-hydroxyvitamin D_3 in the liver. CYP27A1 is a key enzyme in the alternate bile acid synthetic pathway and in side chain oxidation [9]. 25-Hydroxyvitamin D_3 is further hydroxylated at the 1α-position by CYP27B1 to yield the active metabolite $1,25(OH)_2D_3$ in the kidney [33]. The 1-α-hydroxylation reaction is tightly regulated positively by parathyroid hormone and negatively by FGF23 and $1,25(OH)_2D_3$. VDR activation induces feedback regulation by repressing *CYP27B1* transcription through a poorly characterized mechanism. $1,25(OH)_2D_3$ is also synthesized in extrarenal cells and tissues, such as macrophages. Dietary vitamin D_2 and vitamin D_3 are activated by the same processes, including hepatic 25-hydroxylation and renal 1α-hydroxylation. 1,25 $(OH)_2D_2$ activates VDR as well as $1,25(OH)_2D_3$ and has a different catabolic pathway than $1,25(OH)_2D_3$. The VDR–RXR heterodimer binds preferentially to a two-hexanucleotide (AGGTCA or a related sequence) direct repeat motif separated by three nucleotides (DR3). Everted repeat elements separated by six, seven, eight, or nine nucleotides (ER6, ER7, ER8, or ER9) have also been identified as vitamin D response elements in genes including *CYP3A4* [83, 84]. Pharmacological experiments using $1,25(OH)_2D_3$ and its derivatives and animal studies using VDR-null mice have demonstrated that VDR regulates many physiological processes, including cellular growth and differentiation, hair cycle, immunity, cardiovascular function, lipid and xenobiotic metabolism, and neuronal function as well as bone and calcium metabolism [85, 86]. An understanding of VDR regulation of bile acid metabolism has been emerging since the discovery that VDR is activated by the secondary bile acid LCA and more effectively by 3-keto-LCA [87] (Fig. 4.1). Because CYP3A4 metabolizes LCA to 3-keto-LCA by 3-oxidation and hyodeoxycholic acid by 6α-hydroxylation [67, 74], LCA-activated VDR induces both enhanced VDR activation by 3-keto-LCA and detoxification to hyodeoxycholic acid, a mechanism similar to PXR (Fig. 4.2). Vitamin D signaling can induce this LCA detoxification mechanism [87]. Intestine-specific VDR knockout mice show increased contents of TCA and TDCA in the liver homogenate, a phenotype reversed by CYP3A4 transgene expression [88]. VDR also induces expression of other xenobiotic metabolism enzymes, such as MRP2, MRP3, MRP4, and SULT2A1 [89–91]. 1,25(OH)$_2$D$_3$ treatment does not induce hepatocyte target gene expression due to low VDR expression [92], suggesting a limited role of VDR in bile acid metabolism in the liver. Pharmacological activation of VDR enhances urinary excretion of bile acid by increasing the expression of bile acid transporters, such as MRP4, in the kidney [93] (Fig. 4.2) and does not alter bile acid accumulation in bile duct-ligated mice, but represses proinflammatory cytokine expression [94]. Interestingly, VDR ligand treatment represses hepatic *Cyp7a1* expression in an FGF15-dependent mechanism, because *Fgf15* is a VDR target gene [95]. In contrast, repeated administration of 1α-hydroxyvitamin D$_3$, which is rapidly converted to 1,25(OH)$_2$D$_3$ in mice, increases *Cyp7a1* expression [93]. This may be due to decreased bile acid pool sizes and subsequent relief from bile acid-induced suppression. Thus, VDR is involved in regulation of bile acid metabolism mainly in the intestine and kidney.

Apart from the direct effect on vitamin D absorption, a physiologic link connecting bile acids and calcium metabolism has not been demonstrated. LCA-derived ligands may exhibit selective non-calcemic VDR activity. Crystal structures of rat VDR with LCA and its derivatives show that they bind to the VDR–LBP with an orientation opposite to that of 1,25(OH)$_2$D$_3$ in both horizontal and vertical planes [33, 96]. The side chain carboxyl group is directed toward the β-turn side, the A ring faces helix 12, and the β-face of the steroid is directed toward helix 7 in the bottom of the ligand-binding pocket. The crystal structure of zebrafish VDR with LCA reveals the binding of two LCA molecules [97]. While one LCA binds to the canonical LBP, the second one is anchored to a site located on the VDR surface and is suggested to promote stabilization of the active conformation. LCA acetate and LCA propionate are more potent VDR agonists than LCA and can induce differentiation of myeloid leukemia cells, a useful cellular assay for pharmacological effects of 1,25(OH)$_2$D$_3$ and its derivatives [98, 99]. Administration of LCA acetate or LCA propionate to mice effectively induces tissue VDR activation without causing hypercalcemia [99]. Intestine-specific VDR deletion induces a change in the intestinal microbial flora and increases susceptibility to colitis in a mouse model of inflammatory bowel disease [100]. LCA can substitute for vitamin D in elevating serum calcium levels, mobilizing calcium from bone, and inducing expression in the kidney of the VDR target gene CYP24A1 only in vitamin D-deficient rats [101]. The VDRs of non-mammalian species, such as lamprey, zebrafish, and *Xenopus laevis*, are insensitive to bile acids and bile alcohols [13]. The ability of VDR to respond to LCA may be a more recent evolutionary development, occurring after appearance of the synthetic pathway of CDCA in hepatocytes and its conversion to LCA in bacteria. LCA may be involved in selective VDR functions, such as regulation of intestinal microbial colonization.

4.5 Other Receptors

UDCA is used in the treatment of cholestatic disease, such as primary biliary cirrhosis [102]. Glucocorticoid receptor (GR; NR3C1) responds to UDCA in a ligand-independent way [103]. Although it remains unclear whether GR mediates the pharmacological action of UDCA, the combination of UDCA and a FXR or PXR activator may be useful in the treatment of cholestasis. Bile acid-activated G protein-coupled receptors, such as TGR5 and sphingosine-1-phosphate receptor 2, have also been identified [4]. Elucidation of the bile acid signaling network should provide insight into pathophysiology of metabolic diseases and development of novel therapeutics.

4.6 Conclusion

Bile acids are important not only as bile components for lipid digestion and absorption but also as signaling molecules for nuclear receptors, such as FXR, PXR, and VDR. Bile acids regulate bile acid and lipid metabolism through activation of these receptors and also exhibit other physiological actions. Intestinal bacteria metabolize bile acids and can influence host metabolism by changing nuclear receptor activities. Bile acids might represent "prototypes" of steroid hormones and also serve as signaling molecules for communication between host and bacteria. The bile acid receptors FXR, PXR, and VDR are promising drug targets for metabolic diseases.

Acknowledgments The author thanks Dr. Andrew I. Shulman for editorial assistance.

References

1. Evans RM, Mangelsdorf DJ. Nuclear receptors, RXR, and the big bang. Cell. 2014;157(1):255–66. doi:10.1016/j.cell.2014.03.012.
2. Makishima M. Nuclear receptors as targets for drug development: regulation of cholesterol and bile acid metabolism by nuclear receptors. J Pharmacol Sci. 2005;97(2):177–83. doi:10.1254/jphs.FMJ04008X4.
3. Shulman AI, Mangelsdorf DJ. Retinoid x receptor heterodimers in the metabolic syndrome. N Engl J Med. 2005;353(6):604–15. doi:10.1056/NEJMra043590.
4. Li T, Chiang JY. Bile acid signaling in metabolic disease and drug therapy. Pharmacol Rev. 2014;66(4):948–83. doi:10.1124/pr.113.008201.
5. Makishima M. Nuclear receptors sense bile acid metabolism: a hormal action of bile acids. In: Morikawa K, Take S, editors. Functional and structural biology on the lipo-network. Kerala: Transworld Research Network; 2006. p. 17–35.
6. Huang P, Chandra V, Rastinejad F. Structural overview of the nuclear receptor superfamily: insights into physiology and therapeutics. Annu Rev Physiol. 2010;72:247–72. doi:10.1146/annurev-physiol-021909-135917.

7. Rosenfeld MG, Lunyak VV, Glass CK. Sensors and signals: a coactivator/corepressor/epigenetic code for integrating signal-dependent programs of transcriptional response. Genes Dev. 2006;20(11):1405–28. doi:10.1101/gad.1424806.
8. Hofmann AF. The continuing importance of bile acids in liver and intestinal disease. Arch Intern Med. 1999;159(22):2647–58. doi:10.1001/archinte.159.22.2647.
9. Russell DW. The enzymes, regulation, and genetics of bile acid synthesis. Annu Rev Biochem. 2003;72(1):137–74. doi:10.1146/annurev.biochem.72.121801.161712.
10. Russell DW. Fifty years of advances in bile acid synthesis and metabolism. J Lipid Res. 2009 (50 Suppl):S120–5. doi:10.1194/jlr.R800026-JLR200.
11. Trauner M, Boyer JL. Bile salt transporters: molecular characterization, function, and regulation. Physiol Rev. 2003;83(2):633–71. doi:10.1152/physrev.00027.2002.
12. Ridlon JM, Kang DJ, Hylemon PB. Bile salt biotransformations by human intestinal bacteria. J Lipid Res. 2006;47(2):241–59. doi:10.1194/jlr.R500013-JLR200.
13. Hofmann AF, Hagey LR, Krasowski MD. Bile salts of vertebrates: structural variation and possible evolutionary significance. J Lipid Res. 2010;51(2):226–46. doi:10.1194/jlr.R000042.
14. Selwyn FP, Csanaky IL, Zhang Y, Klaassen CD. Importance of large intestine in regulating bile acids and glucagon-like peptide-1 in germ-free mice. Drug Metab Dispos. 2015;43(10):1544–56. doi:10.1124/dmd.115.065276.
15. Fromm H, Sarva RP, Bazzoli F. Formation of ursodeoxycholic acid from chenodeoxycholic acid in the human colon: studies of the role of 7-ketolithocholic acid as an intermediate. J Lipid Res. 1983;24(7):841–53.
16. Sayin SI, Wahlstrom A, Felin J, Jantti S, Marschall HU, Bamberg K, et al. Gut microbiota regulates bile acid metabolism by reducing the levels of tauro-beta-muricholic acid, a naturally occurring FXR antagonist. Cell Metab. 2013;17(2):225–35. doi:10.1016/j.cmet.2013.01.003.
17. Dawson PA, Lan T, Rao A. Bile acid transporters. J Lipid Res. 2009;50(12):2340–57. doi:10.1194/jlr.R900012-JLR200.
18. Zollner G, Marschall HU, Wagner M, Trauner M. Role of nuclear receptors in the adaptive response to bile acids and cholestasis: pathogenetic and therapeutic considerations. Mol Pharm. 2006;3(3):231–51. doi:10.1021/mp060010s.
19. Alrefai WA, Gill RK. Bile acid transporters: structure, function, regulation and pathophysiological implications. Pharm Res. 2007;24(10):1803–23. doi:10.1007/s11095-007-9289-1.
20. Janowski BA, Willy PJ, Devi TR, Falck JR, Mangelsdorf DJ. An oxysterol signalling pathway mediated by the nuclear receptor LXR alpha. Nature. 1996;383(6602):728–31. doi:10.1038/383728a0.
21. Peet DJ, Turley SD, Ma W, Janowski BA, Lobaccaro JM, Hammer RE, et al. Cholesterol and bile acid metabolism are impaired in mice lacking the nuclear oxysterol receptor LXR alpha. Cell. 1998;93(5):693–704. doi:10.1016/S0092-8674(00)81432-4.
22. Calkin AC, Tontonoz P. Transcriptional integration of metabolism by the nuclear sterol-activated receptors LXR and FXR. Nat Rev Mol Cell Biol. 2012;13(4):213–24. doi:10.1038/nrm3312.
23. Agellon LB, Drover VA, Cheema SK, Gbaguidi GF, Walsh A. Dietary cholesterol fails to stimulate the human cholesterol 7alpha-hydroxylase gene (CYP7A1) in transgenic mice. J Biol Chem. 2002;277(23):20131–4. doi:10.1074/jbc.C200105200.
24. Repa JJ, Turley SD, Lobaccaro JA, Medina J, Li L, Lustig K, et al. Regulation of absorption and ABC1-mediated efflux of cholesterol by RXR heterodimers. Science. 2000;289(5484):1524–9. doi:10.1126/science.289.5484.1524.
25. Makishima M, Okamoto AY, Repa JJ, Tu H, Learned RM, Luk A, et al. Identification of a nuclear receptor for bile acids. Science. 1999;284(5418):1362–5. doi:10.1126/science.284.5418.1362.

26. Forman BM, Goode E, Chen J, Oro AE, Bradley DJ, Perlmann T, et al. Identification of a nuclear receptor that is activated by farnesol metabolites. Cell. 1995;81(5):687–93. doi:10.1016/0092-8674(95)90530-8.
27. Parks DJ, Blanchard SG, Bledsoe RK, Chandra G, Consler TG, Kliewer SA, et al. Bile acids: natural ligands for an orphan nuclear receptor. Science. 1999;284(5418):1365–8. doi:10.1126/science.284.5418.1365.
28. Wang H, Chen J, Hollister K, Sowers LC, Forman BM. Endogenous bile acids are ligands for the nuclear receptor FXR/BAR. Mol Cell. 1999;3(5):543–53. doi:10.1016/S1097-2765(00)80348-2.
29. Yu J, Lo JL, Huang L, Zhao A, Metzger E, Adams A, et al. Lithocholic acid decreases expression of bile salt export pump through farnesoid X receptor antagonist activity. J Biol Chem. 2002;277(35):31441–7. doi:10.1074/jbc.M200474200.
30. Campana G, Pasini P, Roda A, Spampinato S. Regulation of ileal bile acid-binding protein expression in Caco-2 cells by ursodeoxycholic acid: role of the farnesoid X receptor. Biochem Pharmacol. 2005;69(12):1755–63. doi:10.1016/j.bcp.2005.03.019.
31. Li F, Jiang C, Krausz KW, Li Y, Albert I, Hao H, et al. Microbiome remodelling leads to inhibition of intestinal farnesoid X receptor signalling and decreased obesity. Nat Commun. 2013;4:2384. doi:10.1038/ncomms3384.
32. Mazuy C, Helleboid A, Staels B, Lefebvre P. Nuclear bile acid signaling through the farnesoid X receptor. Cell Mol Life Sci. 2015;72(9):1631–50. doi:10.1007/s00018-014-1805-y.
33. Makishima M, Yamada S. The bile acid derivatives lithocholic acid acetate and lithocholic acid propionate are functionally selective vitamin D receptor ligands. In: Feldman D, Pike JW, Adams JS, editors. Vitamin D. 3rd ed. Waltham: Academic; 2011. p. 1509–24.
34. Kir S, Zhang Y, Gerard RD, Kliewer SA, Mangelsdorf DJ. Nuclear receptors HNF4alpha and LRH-1 cooperate in regulating Cyp7a1 in vivo. J Biol Chem. 2012;287(49):41334–41. doi:10.1074/jbc.M112.421834.
35. Lu TT, Makishima M, Repa JJ, Schoonjans K, Kerr TA, Auwerx J, et al. Molecular basis for feedback regulation of bile acid synthesis by nuclear receptors. Mol Cell. 2000;6(3):507–15. doi:10.1016/S1097-2765(00)00050-2.
36. Goodwin B, Jones SA, Price RR, Watson MA, McKee DD, Moore LB, et al. A regulatory cascade of the nuclear receptors FXR, SHP-1, and LRH-1 represses bile acid biosynthesis. Mol Cell. 2000;6(3):517–26. doi:10.1016/S1097-2765(00)00051-4.
37. Sinal CJ, Tohkin M, Miyata M, Ward JM, Lambert G, Gonzalez FJ. Targeted disruption of the nuclear receptor FXR/BAR impairs bile acid and lipid homeostasis. Cell. 2000;102(6):731–44. doi:10.1016/S0092-8674(00)00062-3.
38. Wang L, Lee YK, Bundman D, Han Y, Thevananther S, Kim CS, et al. Redundant pathways for negative feedback regulation of bile acid production. Dev Cell. 2002;2(6):721–31. doi:10.1016/S1534-5807(02)00187-9.
39. Inagaki T, Choi M, Moschetta A, Peng L, Cummins CL, McDonald JG, et al. Fibroblast growth factor 15 functions as an enterohepatic signal to regulate bile acid homeostasis. Cell Metab. 2005;2(4):217–25. doi:10.1016/j.cmet.2005.09.001.
40. Potthoff MJ, Kliewer SA, Mangelsdorf DJ. Endocrine fibroblast growth factors 15/19 and 21: from feast to famine. Genes Dev. 2012;26(4):312–24. doi:10.1101/gad.184788.111.
41. Kong B, Wang L, Chiang JY, Zhang Y, Klaassen CD, Guo GL. Mechanism of tissue-specific farnesoid X receptor in suppressing the expression of genes in bile-acid synthesis in mice. Hepatology. 2012;56(3):1034–43. doi:10.1002/hep.25740.
42. Holt JA, Luo G, Billin AN, Bisi J, McNeill YY, Kozarsky KF, et al. Definition of a novel growth factor-dependent signal cascade for the suppression of bile acid biosynthesis. Genes Dev. 2003;17(13):1581–91. doi:10.1101/gad.1083503.
43. Kerr TA, Saeki S, Schneider M, Schaefer K, Berdy S, Redder T, et al. Loss of nuclear receptor SHP impairs but does not eliminate negative feedback regulation of bile acid synthesis. Dev Cell. 2002;2(6):713–20. doi: 10.1016/S1534-5807(02)00154-5.

44. Denson LA, Sturm E, Echevarria W, Zimmerman TL, Makishima M, Mangelsdorf DJ, et al. The orphan nuclear receptor, shp, mediates bile acid-induced inhibition of the rat bile acid transporter, ntcp. Gastroenterology. 2001;121(1):140–7. doi:10.1053/gast.2001.25503.
45. Hayhurst GP, Lee YH, Lambert G, Ward JM, Gonzalez FJ. Hepatocyte nuclear factor 4alpha (nuclear receptor 2A1) is essential for maintenance of hepatic gene expression and lipid homeostasis. Mol Cell Biol. 2001;21(4):1393–403. doi:10.1128/MCB.21.4.1393-1403.2001.
46. Ananthanarayanan M, Balasubramanian N, Makishima M, Mangelsdorf DJ, Suchy FJ. Human bile salt export pump promoter is transactivated by the farnesoid X receptor/bile acid receptor. J Biol Chem. 2001;276(31):28857–65. doi:10.1074/jbc.M011610200.
47. Liu Y, Binz J, Numerick MJ, Dennis S, Luo G, Desai B, et al. Hepatoprotection by the farnesoid X receptor agonist GW4064 in rat models of intra- and extrahepatic cholestasis. J Clin Invest. 2003;112(11):1678–87. doi:10.1172/JCI18945.
48. Stedman C, Liddle C, Coulter S, Sonoda J, Alvarez JG, Evans RM, et al. Benefit of farnesoid X receptor inhibition in obstructive cholestasis. Proc Natl Acad Sci U S A. 2006;103 (30):11323–8. doi:10.1073/pnas.0604772103.
49. Lee H, Zhang Y, Lee FY, Nelson SF, Gonzalez FJ, Edwards PA. FXR regulates organic solute transporters alpha and beta in the adrenal gland, kidney, and intestine. J Lipid Res. 2006;47(1): 201–14. doi:10.1194/jlr.M500417-JLR200.
50. Staudinger JL, Madan A, Carol KM, Parkinson A. Regulation of drug transporter gene expression by nuclear receptors. Drug Metab Dispos. 2003;31(5):523–7. doi:10.1124/dmd.31.5.523.
51. Kast HR, Goodwin B, Tarr PT, Jones SA, Anisfeld AM, Stoltz CM, et al. Regulation of multidrug resistance-associated protein 2 (ABCC2) by the nuclear receptors pregnane X receptor, farnesoid X-activated receptor, and constitutive androstane receptor. J Biol Chem. 2002; 277(4):2908–15. doi:10.1074/jbc.M109326200.
52. Kok T, Hulzebos CV, Wolters H, Havinga R, Agellon LB, Stellaard F, et al. Enterohepatic circulation of bile salts in farnesoid X receptor-deficient mice: efficient intestinal bile salt absorption in the absence of ileal bile acid-binding protein. J Biol Chem. 2003;278(43): 41930–7. doi:10.1074/jbc.M306309200.
53. Huang L, Zhao A, Lew JL, Zhang T, Hrywna Y, Thompson JR, et al. Farnesoid X receptor activates transcription of the phospholipid pump MDR3. J Biol Chem. 2003;278(51): 51085–90. doi:10.1074/jbc.M308321200.
54. Moschetta A, Bookout AL, Mangelsdorf DJ. Prevention of cholesterol gallstone disease by FXR agonists in a mouse model. Nat Med. 2004;10(12):1352–8. doi:10.1038/nm1138.
55. Yu L, Gupta S, Xu F, Liverman AD, Moschetta A, Mangelsdorf DJ, et al. Expression of ABCG5 and ABCG8 is required for regulation of biliary cholesterol secretion. J Biol Chem. 2005;280(10):8742–7. doi:10.1074/jbc.M411080200.
56. Grober J, Zaghini I, Fujii H, Jones SA, Kliewer SA, Willson TM, et al. Identification of a bile acid-responsive element in the human ileal bile acid-binding protein gene. Involvement of the farnesoid X receptor/9-cis-retinoic acid receptor heterodimer. J Biol Chem. 1999; 274(42):29749–54. doi:10.1074/jbc.274.42.29749.
57. Ma K, Saha PK, Chan L, Moore DD. Farnesoid X receptor is essential for normal glucose homeostasis. J Clin Invest. 2006;116(4):1102–9. doi:10.1172/JCI25604.
58. Duran-Sandoval D, Cariou B, Percevault F, Hennuyer N, Grefhorst A, van Dijk TH, et al. The farnesoid X receptor modulates hepatic carbohydrate metabolism during the fasting-refeeding transition. J Biol Chem. 2005;280(33):29971–9. doi:10.1074/jbc.M501931200.
59. Stayrook KR, Bramlett KS, Savkur RS, Ficorilli J, Cook T, Christe ME, et al. Regulation of carbohydrate metabolism by the farnesoid X receptor. Endocrinology. 2005;146(3):984–91. doi:10.1210/en.2004-0965.
60. Inagaki T, Moschetta A, Lee YK, Peng L, Zhao G, Downes M, et al. Regulation of antibacterial defense in the small intestine by the nuclear bile acid receptor. Proc Natl Acad Sci U S A. 2006;103(10):3920–5. doi:10.1073/pnas.0509592103.

61. Vavassori P, Mencarelli A, Renga B, Distrutti E, Fiorucci S. The bile acid receptor FXR is a modulator of intestinal innate immunity. J Immunol. 2009;183(10):6251–61. doi:10.4049/jimmunol.0803978.
62. Mencarelli A, Renga B, Migliorati M, Cipriani S, Distrutti E, Santucci L, et al. The bile acid sensor farnesoid X receptor is a modulator of liver immunity in a rodent model of acute hepatitis. J Immunol. 2009;183(10):6657–66. doi:10.4049/jimmunol.0901347.
63. Huang W, Ma K, Zhang J, Qatanani M, Cuvillier J, Liu J, et al. Nuclear receptor-dependent bile acid signaling is required for normal liver regeneration. Science. 2006;312(5771):233–6. doi:10.1126/science.1121435.
64. Chen WD, Wang YD, Zhang L, Shiah S, Wang M, Yang F, et al. Farnesoid X receptor alleviates age-related proliferation defects in regenerating mouse livers by activating forkhead box m1b transcription. Hepatology. 2010;51(3):953–62. doi:10.1002/hep.23390.
65. Zhang L, Wang YD, Chen WD, Wang X, Lou G, Liu N, et al. Promotion of liver regeneration/repair by farnesoid X receptor in both liver and intestine in mice. Hepatology. 2012; 56(6):2336–43. doi:10.1002/hep.25905.
66. Gao J, Xie W. Pregnane X receptor and constitutive androstane receptor at the crossroads of drug metabolism and energy metabolism. Drug Metab Dispos. 2010;38(12):2091–5. doi:10.1124/dmd.110.035568.
67. Xie W, Radominska-Pandya A, Shi Y, Simon CM, Nelson MC, Ong ES, et al. An essential role for nuclear receptors SXR/PXR in detoxification of cholestatic bile acids. Proc Natl Acad Sci U S A. 2001;98(6):3375–80. doi:10.1073/pnas.051014398.
68. Staudinger JL, Goodwin B, Jones SA, Hawkins-Brown D, MacKenzie KI, LaTour A, et al. The nuclear receptor PXR is a lithocholic acid sensor that protects against liver toxicity. Proc Natl Acad Sci U S A. 2001;98(6):3369–74. doi:10.1073/pnas.051551698.
69. Bhalla S, Ozalp C, Fang S, Xiang L, Kemper JK. Ligand-activated pregnane X receptor interferes with HNF-4 signaling by targeting a common coactivator PGC-1alpha. Functional implications in hepatic cholesterol and glucose metabolism. J Biol Chem. 2004;279(43): 45139–47. doi:10.1074/jbc.M405423200.
70. Li T, Chiang JY. Mechanism of rifampicin and pregnane X receptor inhibition of human cholesterol 7 alpha-hydroxylase gene transcription. Am J Physiol Gastrointest Liver Physiol. 2005;288(1):G74–84. doi:10.1152/ajpgi.00258.2004.
71. Wang H, Venkatesh M, Li H, Goetz R, Mukherjee S, Biswas A, et al. Pregnane X receptor activation induces FGF19-dependent tumor aggressiveness in humans and mice. J Clin Invest. 2011;121(8):3220–32. doi:10.1172/JCI41514.
72. Wagner M, Halilbasic E, Marschall HU, Zollner G, Fickert P, Langner C, et al. CAR and PXR agonists stimulate hepatic bile acid and bilirubin detoxification and elimination pathways in mice. Hepatology. 2005;42(2):420–30. doi:10.1002/hep.20784.
73. Xie W, Evans RM. Orphan nuclear receptors: the exotics of xenobiotics. J Biol Chem. 2001; 276(41):37739–42. doi:10.1074/jbc.R100033200.
74. Bodin K, Lindbom U, Diczfalusy U. Novel pathways of bile acid metabolism involving CYP3A4. Biochim Biophys Acta. 2005;1687(1–3):84–93. doi:10.1016/j.bbalip.2004.11.003.
75. Goodwin B, Hodgson E, Liddle C. The orphan human pregnane X receptor mediates the transcriptional activation of CYP3A4 by rifampicin through a distal enhancer module. Mol Pharmacol. 1999;56(6):1329–39. doi: 10.1124/mol.56.6.1329.
76. Frank C, Makkonen H, Dunlop TW, Matilainen M, Vaisanen S, Carlberg C. Identification of pregnane X receptor binding sites in the regulatory regions of genes involved in bile acid homeostasis. J Mol Biol. 2005;346(2):505–19. doi:10.1016/j.jmb.2004.12.003.
77. Sonoda J, Xie W, Rosenfeld JM, Barwick JL, Guzelian PS, Evans RM. Regulation of a xenobiotic sulfonation cascade by nuclear pregnane X receptor (PXR). Proc Natl Acad Sci U S A. 2002;99(21):13801–6. doi:10.1073/pnas.212494599.
78. Timsit YE, Negishi M. CAR and PXR: the xenobiotic-sensing receptors. Steroids. 2007; 72(3):231–46. doi:10.1016/j.steroids.2006.12.006.

79. Guo GL, Lambert G, Negishi M, Ward JM, Brewer Jr HB, Kliewer SA, et al. Complementary roles of farnesoid X receptor, pregnane X receptor, and constitutive androstane receptor in protection against bile acid toxicity. J Biol Chem. 2003;278(46):45062–71. doi:10.1074/jbc.M307145200.
80. Zhang J, Huang W, Qatanani M, Evans RM, Moore DD. The constitutive androstane receptor and pregnane X receptor function coordinately to prevent bile acid-induced hepatotoxicity. J Biol Chem. 2004;279(47):49517–22. doi:10.1074/jbc.M409041200.
81. Saini SP, Sonoda J, Xu L, Toma D, Uppal H, Mu Y, et al. A novel constitutive androstane receptor-mediated and CYP3A-independent pathway of bile acid detoxification. Mol Pharmacol. 2004;65(2):292–300. doi:10.1124/mol.65.2.292.
82. Assem M, Schuetz EG, Leggas M, Sun D, Yasuda K, Reid G, et al. Interactions between hepatic Mrp4 and Sult2a as revealed by the constitutive androstane receptor and Mrp4 knockout mice. J Biol Chem. 2004;279(21):22250–7. doi:10.1074/jbc.M314111200.
83. Thummel KE, Brimer C, Yasuda K, Thottassery J, Senn T, Lin Y, et al. Transcriptional control of intestinal cytochrome P-4503A by 1alpha,25-dihydroxy vitamin D3. Mol Pharmacol. 2001;60(6):1399–406. doi:10.1124/mol.60.6.1399.
84. Makishima M. Cooperative regulation of expression of cytochrome P450 enzymes by aryl hydrocarbon recetpor and vitamin D receptor. In: Yamazaki H, editor. Fifty years of cytochrome P450 research. Tokyo: Springer Japan; 2014. p. 277–90.
85. Takada I, Makishima M. Therapeutic application of vitamin D receptor ligands: an updated patent review. Expert Opin Ther Pat. 2015; doi:10.1517/13543776.2015.1093113.
86. Nagpal S, Na S, Rathnachalam R. Noncalcemic actions of vitamin D receptor ligands. Endocr Rev. 2005;26(5):662–87. doi:10.1210/er.2004-0002.
87. Makishima M, Lu TT, Xie W, Whitfield GK, Domoto H, Evans RM, et al. Vitamin D receptor as an intestinal bile acid sensor. Science. 2002;296(5571):1313–6. doi:10.1126/science.1070477.
88. Cheng J, Fang Z-Z, Kim J-H, Krausz KW, Tanaka N, Chiang JYL, et al. Intestinal CYP3A4 protects against lithocholic acid-induced hepatotoxicity in intestine-specific VDR-deficient mice. J Lipid Res. 2014;55(3):455–65. doi:10.1194/jlr.M044420.
89. McCarthy TC, Li X, Sinal CJ. Vitamin D receptor-dependent regulation of colon multidrug resistance-associated protein 3 gene expression by bile acids. J Biol Chem. 2005;280(24):23232–42. doi:10.1074/jbc.M411520200.
90. Fan J, Liu S, Du Y, Morrison J, Shipman R, Pang KS. Up-regulation of transporters and enzymes by the vitamin D receptor ligands, 1alpha,25-dihydroxyvitamin D3 and vitamin D analogs, in the Caco-2 cell monolayer. J Pharmacol Exp Ther. 2009;330(2):389–402. doi:10.1124/jpet.108.149815.
91. Echchgadda I, Song CS, Roy AK, Chatterjee B. Dehydroepiandrosterone sulfotransferase is a target for transcriptional induction by the vitamin D receptor. Mol Pharmacol. 2004;65(3):720–9. doi:10.1124/Mol.65.3.720.
92. Gascon-Barre M, Demers C, Mirshahi A, Neron S, Zalzal S, Nanci A. The normal liver harbors the vitamin D nuclear receptor in nonparenchymal and biliary epithelial cells. Hepatology. 2003;37(5):1034–42. doi:10.1053/jhep.2003.50176.
93. Nishida S, Ozeki J, Makishima M. Modulation of bile acid metabolism by 1alpha-hydroxyvitamin D3 administration in mice. Drug Metab Dispos. 2009;37(10):2037–44. doi:10.1124/dmd.109.027334.
94. Ogura M, Nishida S, Ishizawa M, Sakurai K, Shimizu M, Matsuo S, et al. Vitamin D3 modulates the expression of bile acid regulatory genes and represses inflammation in bile duct-ligated mice. J Pharmacol Exp Ther. 2009;328(2):564–70. doi:10.1124/jpet.108.145987.
95. Schmidt DR, Holmstrom SR, Fon Tacer K, Bookout AL, Kliewer SA, Mangelsdorf DJ. Regulation of bile acid synthesis by fat-soluble vitamins A and D. J Biol Chem. 2010;285(19):14486–94. doi:10.1074/jbc.M110.116004.

96. Masuno H, Ikura T, Morizono D, Orita I, Yamada S, Shimizu M, et al. Crystal structures of complexes of vitamin D receptor ligand-binding domain with lithocholic acid derivatives. J Lipid Res. 2013;54(8):2206–13. doi:10.1194/jlr.M038307.
97. Belorusova AY, Eberhardt J, Potier N, Stote RH, Dejaegere A, Rochel N. Structural insights into the molecular mechanism of vitamin D receptor activation by lithocholic acid involving a new mode of ligand recognition. J Med Chem. 2014;57(11):4710–9. doi:10.1021/jm5002524.
98. Adachi R, Honma Y, Masuno H, Kawana K, Shimomura I, Yamada S, et al. Selective activation of vitamin D receptor by lithocholic acid acetate, a bile acid derivative. J Lipid Res. 2005;46(1):46–57. doi:10.1194/jlr.M400294-JLR200.
99. Ishizawa M, Matsunawa M, Adachi R, Uno S, Ikeda K, Masuno H, et al. Lithocholic acid derivatives act as selective vitamin D receptor modulators without inducing hypercalcemia. J Lipid Res. 2008;49(4):763–72. doi:10.1194/jlr.M700293-JLR200.
100. Wu S, Zhang Y-g, Lu R, Xia Y, Zhou D, Petrof EO, et al. Intestinal epithelial vitamin D receptor deletion leads to defective autophagy in colitis. Gut. 2015;64(7):1082–94. doi:10.1136/gutjnl-2014-307436.
101. Nehring JA, Zierold C, DeLuca HF. Lithocholic acid can carry out in vivo functions of vitamin D. Proc Natl Acad Sci U S A. 2007;104(24):10006–9. doi:10.1073/pnas.0703512104.
102. Beuers U, Trauner M, Jansen P, Poupon R. New paradigms in the treatment of hepatic cholestasis: from UDCA to FXR. PXR Beyond J Hepatol. 2015;62(1 Suppl):S25–37. doi:10.1016/j.jhep.2015.02.023.
103. Tanaka H, Makino Y, Miura T, Hirano F, Okamoto K, Komura K, et al. Ligand-independent activation of the glucocorticoid receptor by ursodeoxycholic acid. Repression of IFN-gamma-induced MHC class II gene expression via a glucocorticoid receptor-dependent pathway. J Immunol. 1996;156(4):1601–8.

Chapter 5
Bile Acid as Therapeutic Agents

Yoshihide Yamanashi, Tappei Takada, and Hiroshi Suzuki

Abstract Bile acids are the amphipathic compounds produced as the end products of cholesterol metabolism in the liver. Due to their detergent properties, bile acids play important roles in micelle formation and in intestinal lipid absorption. Besides such classical functions, bile acids modulate a number of intracellular signaling cascades involved in apoptosis, immune response, and carcinogenesis. In addition, recent findings showed that bile acids are endogenous ligands of the farnesoid X receptor (FXR; nuclear receptor (NR) subfamily 1 group H member 4 (NR1H4)) and the membrane-bound G-protein-coupled bile acid receptor 1 (GP-BAR1, commonly known as TGR5), indicating that bile acids themselves are signaling molecules. Taken together with the fact that both FXR and TGR5 regulate various physiological processes, including lipid metabolism, glucose metabolism, and energy expenditure, these findings suggest that modulation of bile acid metabolism and/or signaling would be a potential therapeutic strategy for the treatment of several diseases. In this context, bile acid-related drugs (agents) such as ursodeoxycholic acid, bile acid mimetics, and bile acid sequestrants have garnered the attention as therapeutic agents with pleiotropic properties. This chapter aims to provide an overview of the clinical efficacy and limitations of pharmacotherapies with bile acid-related drugs and to discuss molecular mechanisms underlying their pharmacological activities.

Keywords Bile acid sequestrant • Dyslipidemia • Liver disease • Ursodeoxycholic acid • Type 2 diabetes mellitus

5.1 Physiological Properties and Functions of Bile Acids

Bile acids are amphipathic compounds synthesized in the body. Based on their synthetic host, bile acids are divided into two groups, primary bile acids and secondary bile acids. Primary bile acids are synthesized from cholesterol in the

---

Y. Yamanashi • T. Takada • H. Suzuki (✉)
Department of Pharmacy, The University of Tokyo Hospital, Faculty of Medicine, The University of Tokyo, 7-3-1 Hongo, Bukyoku, Tokyo 113-8655, Japan
e-mail: suzukihi-tky@umin.ac.jp

S. Tazuma, H. Takikawa (eds.), *Bile Acids in Gastroenterology*,
DOI 10.1007/978-4-431-56062-3_5

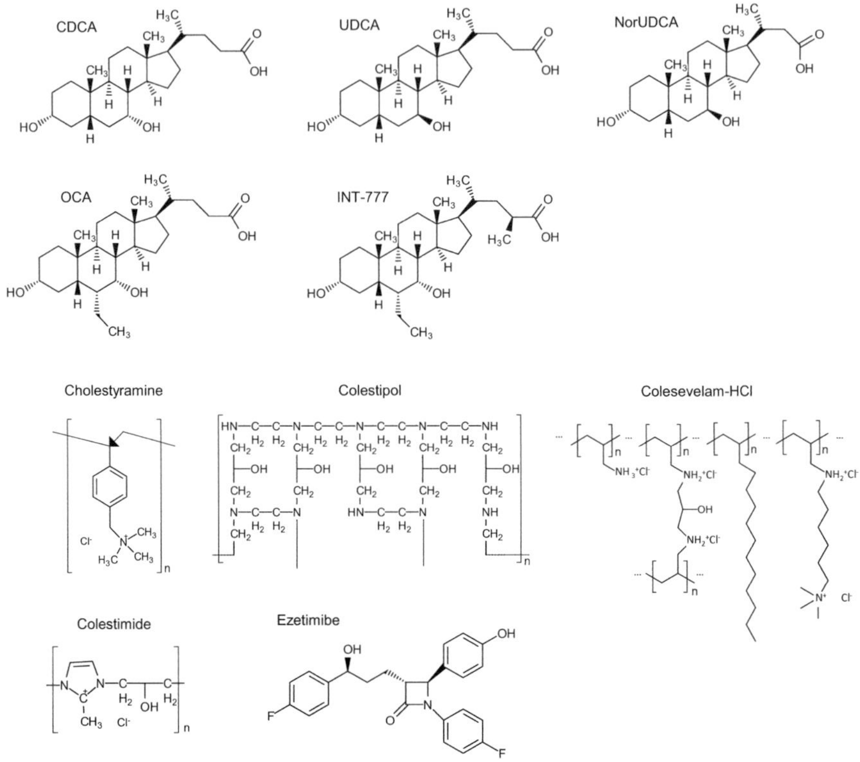

Fig. 5.1 Molecular diagram of chenodeoxycholic acid (*CDCA*), ursodeoxycholic acid (*UDCA*), nor-ursodeoxycholic acid (*NorUDCA*), obeticholic acid (*OCA*), INT-777, cholestyramine, colestipol, colesevelam-HCl, colestimide, and ezetimibe

liver. In humans, major primary bile acids are cholic acid (CA) and chenodeoxycholic acid (CDCA). Most of these bile acids are conjugated to glycine or taurine in the liver and negatively charged at the physiological pH range [1]. Conjugated as well as unconjugated bile acids are then actively secreted into the bile by bile salt export pump (BSEP; ATP-binding cassette (ABC) transporter subfamily B member 11 (ABCB11)) [2, 3]. On the other hand, secondary bile acids are synthesized from primary bile acids by enteric bacteria. Major secondary bile acids are deoxycholic acid (DCA), lithocholic acid (LCA), and ursodeoxycholic acid (UDCA). DCA and LCA are synthesized by the 7α-dehydroxylation of CA and CDCA, respectively [1]. UDCA is synthesized by the epimerization of the 7α-OH from CDCA [4] (Fig. 5.1). Secondary bile acids are also conjugated to glycine or taurine as well as primary bile acids.

Approximately 90–95% of bile acids (except for LCA) in the intestine are reabsorbed in the ilium by apical sodium-dependent bile acid transporter (ASBT; solute carrier (SLC) family 10 member 2 (SLC10A2)) [5, 6], followed by basolateral secretion to the portal blood by a heterodimer of organic solute

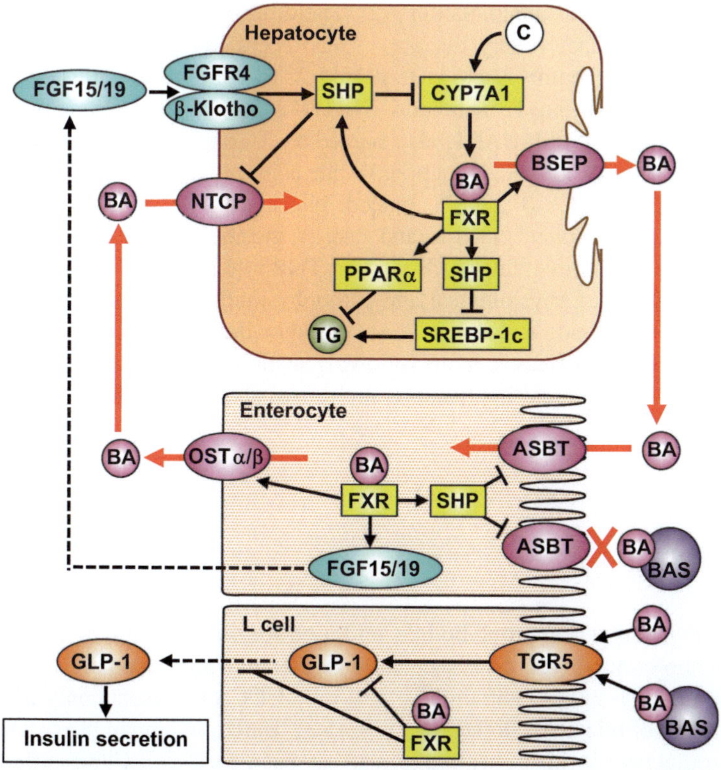

Fig. 5.2 Schematic overview of the enterohepatic circulation of bile acids and bile acid signaling in the liver and intestine. *BA* bile acid, *C* cholesterol, *TG* triglyceride

transporter α and β (OSTα/β; SLC51A/B) [7, 8] (Fig. 5.2). Bile acids in the portal blood are taken up by hepatocytes via Na^+-taurocholate cotransporting polypeptide (NTCP; SLC10A1) [9, 10] and, again, secreted into the bile by BSEP (Fig. 5.2). This continuous enterohepatic circulation acts as a recycling system of bile acids and plays an important role in bile acid metabolism and homeostasis. The remaining bile acids (5–10%) escape intestinal reabsorption and are excreted in feces. This loss of bile acids is replenished by de novo bile acid synthesis from cholesterol in the liver to maintain bile acid homeostasis. In humans, about 500 mg bile acids are synthesized per day from cholesterol in the liver, which is one of the important cholesterol elimination processes in our body [11].

To date, a number of physiological functions of bile acids have been clarified. Bile acids are known to form mixed micelles together with phospholipids and cholesterol. In the intestine, the mixed micelles play an important role in the solubilization of lipophilic compounds such as dietary lipids and fat-soluble vitamins and, thus, regulate their intestinal absorption [11, 12]. Although the detergent property of bile acids is essential to form mixed micelles and to solubilize lipophilic compounds, this property also induces cytotoxicity that promotes cellular apoptosis/necrosis and inflammation [12]. Therefore, bile acids at high concentrations can cause hepatobiliary diseases [13]. Recent findings that bile acids can activate several receptors such as farnesoid X receptor (FXR; nuclear receptor (NR) subfamily 1 group H member 4 (NR1H4)) [14, 15] and G-protein-coupled bile acid receptor 1 (GP-BAR1, also named as TGR5) [16] have provided new insights into the physiological functions of bile acids not only as detergents but also as signaling molecules (Fig. 5.2). Indeed, bile acids regulate several metabolic processes such as lipids, glucose, and energy metabolism via the activation of signaling cascades involving FXR and/or TGR5 [12, 13, 17]. These findings indicate a variety of physiological and pathophysiological functions of bile acids and provide a rationale to target bile acids and/or their related molecules for the treatment of several diseases. In the following sections, we summarized the current knowledge about clinical applications and pharmacological effects of bile acid-related drugs.

5.2 UDCA

UDCA (Fig. 5.1) is a hydrophilic bile acid used for the treatment of gallstone and various cholestatic liver diseases. Normally, endogenous human bile contains UDCA, although its concentration is very low. UDCA represents only 3% of the total amount of bile acids in the body (Fig. 5.3). Unlike in human bile, UDCA is a major component in black bears bile that has been used as a Chinese traditional medicine (Yutan) for the treatment of liver diseases [18–20]. In 1927, UDCA was first isolated and crystalized from Yutan [21]. More than 30 years after its isolation, the first report on UDCA pharmacological effects in humans was published by Japanese researchers [22]. An improvement was observed in tests of liver function

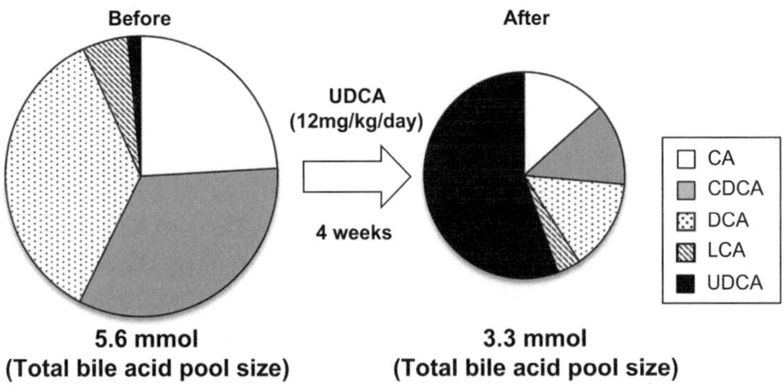

Fig. 5.3 Effects of ursodeoxycholic acid treatment on pool sizes of bile acids. The pool sizes of the major bile acids in humans were quantified before and after ursodeoxycholic acid (*UDCA*) treatment (Data from Roda et al. [31]. *CA* cholic acid, *CDCA* chenodeoxycholic acid, *DCA* deoxycholic acid, *LCA* lithocholic acid)

after UDCA administration in patients with chronic hepatitis. Since then, a variety of clinical and preclinical studies have been conducted worldwide and demonstrated UDCA beneficial effects for several diseases as described in the following sections.

5.2.1 UDCA as a Therapeutic Agent for Gallstone

In the 1970s, the first prospective study of UDCA in patients with gallbladder gallstones demonstrated that UDCA could promote the dissolution of gallstones [23]. It has been recognized that UDCA detergent property might be directly involved in the solubilization of cholesterol from the gallstone surface [20]. In addition, a unique property of UDCA, which promotes the formation of a liquid crystal mesophase of phospholipids and cholesterol, has been thought to facilitate cholesterol solubilization from gallstone [24]. Notably, such a liquid crystal can form even in the bile saturated with cholesterol, which may account for the observation that UDCA can dissolve gallstones even in the cholesterol-saturated bile. Moreover, UDCA has been reported to reduce the cholesterol saturation of the bile by decreasing the biliary excretion of cholesterol [25, 26]. Biliary cholesterol excretion is mediated by a heterodimer of ATP-binding cassette transporter subfamily G members 5 and 8 (ABCG5/G8) [27, 28]. Several studies demonstrated that micellar composition affects the cholesterol efflux activity of ABCG5/G8 [29, 30]. In particular, there is a positive correlation between the concentration of micellar bile acids and the cholesterol efflux activity of ABCG5/G8 [29, 30]. It has been reported that UDCA therapy decreases pool sizes of CA, CDCA, and DCA while increasing that of UDCA (Fig. 5.3) [31], likely because the excess of exogenous UDCA increases fecal loss of endogenous bile acids by competing for ASBT-mediated reabsorption in the intestine [32]. Thus, an altered composition and/or a reduced concentration of biliary bile acids by UDCA therapy may attenuate the cholesterol efflux activity of ABCG5/G8 and, thus, the biliary cholesterol excretion decrease.

Until the 1980s, CDCA (Fig. 5.1) was also used for gallstone therapy because it can solubilize cholesterol from gallstone as UDCA does and even better than UDCA [33, 34]. However, several clinical trials revealed that UDCA is more effective than CDCA for decreasing biliary cholesterol saturation [35, 36]. In addition, diarrhea was observed with high frequency in patients receiving CDCA therapy due to CDCA cytotoxicity to colorectal epithelial cells, while no obvious adverse effects were observed in patients receiving UDCA therapy [37]. Based on these evidences, UDCA rather than CDCA is commonly used for pharmacotherapy of gallstone today.

5.2.2 UDCA as a Therapeutic Agent for Cholestasis

In the 1990s, a number of clinical trials demonstrated UDCA beneficial effects for chronic cholestatic liver diseases such as primary biliary cirrhosis (PBC) [38, 39], intrahepatic cholestasis of pregnancy (ICP) [40], and chronic hepatitis C (CHC) [41, 42]. Currently, UDCA is the only drug approved by the US Food and Drug administration (FDA) for the treatment of PBC. The underlying mechanisms by which UDCA relieves symptoms of these cholestatic liver diseases have not been fully defined. However, a variety of recent studies indicated that at least three pharmacological activities of UDCA might be involved in its beneficial effects: (1) its cytoprotective and antiapoptotic activity, (2) the stimulation of hepatobiliary secretion of bile acids and endogenous toxic compounds, and (3) its immunomodulatory activity. Details of these pharmacological activities are described in the following sections.

5.2.2.1 UDCA Cytoprotective and Antiapoptotic Activity

Detergent properties of bile acids are important for micelle formation and lipid solubillization. However, higher concentrations of bile acids beyond physiological levels disrupt the phospholipid bilayer of the plasma membrane, resulting in damage to hepatocytes and to biliary epithelial cells. Since the detergent effects of bile acids are positively correlated with their hydrophobicity [43], hydrophobic bile acids such as CDCA, DCA, and LCA are more cytotoxic than hydrophilic bile acids such as UDCA (Table 5.1) [44]. In addition, UDCA has been reported to exert cytoprotective effects by stabilizing cellular membranes [45]. Therefore, UDCA treatment, which promotes the replacement of hydrophobic and toxic bile acids with cytoprotective UDCA, could help improving hepatobiliary injury (Fig. 5.3).

Excessive hepatic apoptosis is known to cause both acute and chronic liver injury [46]. In vitro studies demonstrated that hydrophobic bile acids such as the glycine conjugate of CDCA (GCDCA) can directly induce apoptosis in rat hepatocytes through the activation of the Fas death receptor and subsequent activation of caspase-8 [47]. In addition, GCDCA and the glycine conjugate of DCA (GDCA) increase mitochondrial membrane permeability, which triggers mitochondrial cytochrome C release with subsequent activation of the caspase-9-dependent apoptotic cascade [48, 49]. In contrast, UDCA inhibits apoptosis by decreasing the cytochrome C release through stabilization of the mitochondrial membrane [48, 49]. Moreover, UDCA activates cell survival signals, which, in part, may account for the antiapoptotic effect of UDCA. Indeed, the taurine conjugate of UDCA (TUDCA) can inhibit GCDCA-induced apoptosis in rat primary hepatocytes by activating survival signaling pathways mediated by mitogen-activated kinase (MAPK) and phosphoinositide-3 kinase (PI3K) [50]. However, since these antiapoptotic activities of UDCA have been demonstrated mainly in vitro, further in vivo studies will be necessary to demonstrate the physiological involvement of

Table 5.1 Hydrophobicity indices of individual bile acids

	Taurine conjugated	Glycine conjugated	Unconjugated	
Ursodeoxycholic acid	−0.47	−0.43	−0.31	
Cholic acid	0.00	+0.07	+0.13	
Chenodeoxycholic acid	+0.46	+0.51	+0.59	
Deoxycholic acid	+0.59	+0.65	+0.72	
Lithocholic acid	+1.00	+1.05	NA	
				More hydrophobic

Data from Heuman et al. [44]. Hydrophobicity indices of individual bile acids were determined by measuring the retention of each bile acid in reversed-phase liquid chromatography. A taurine-conjugated cholic acid was used as a standard. *NA* not available

UDCA antiapoptotic activity on its beneficial effect against cholestatic liver diseases.

5.2.2.2 Stimulation of Hepatobiliary Excretion of Bile Acids and Endogenous Toxic Compounds by UDCA

Impairment of bile flow causes the hepatic accumulation of hydrophobic bile acids and other endogenous toxic compounds such as bilirubin glucuronides and glutathione conjugates, which results in the exacerbation of liver injury with further cholestasis. In rats, UDCA stimulates biliary excretion of these endogenous toxic compounds and, thus, inhibits the progression of cholestasis [51, 52]. Consistent with the results of animal models, in humans with cholestasis, long-term treatment with UDCA stimulates biliary excretion of bile acids and bilirubin glucuronides, which results in decreasing the elevated serum levels of these compounds [39, 53, 54].

Biliary excretion of bile acids and organic anions including glucuronides and glutathione conjugates is mainly mediated by BSEP and multidrug resistance-associated protein 2 (Mrp2; ABCC2), respectively [2, 3, 55, 56]. In humans, mutations of the gene encoding BSEP cause progressive familial intrahepatic cholestasis type 2 (PFIC2) [2, 3], whereas mutations of the gene encoding MRP2 are causative of Dubin-Johnson syndrome (DJS) characterized by hyperbilirubinemia [55], indicating the physiological importance of these transporters in the liver. In the cholestatic rat liver, TUDCA significantly increases the insertion of BSEP and MRP2 on the canalicular membrane of hepatocytes, resulting in the stimulation of biliary secretion of bile acids and organic anions [51, 57]. The enhanced membrane localization of these transporters might be accounted for by the activity of TUDCA to increase cellular levels of a variety of second messengers such as intracellular Ca^{2+}, conventional protein kinase C (PKC), and cAMP, which promote the exocytic insertion of the membrane transporters [20]. In addition, correct developmental formation of bile canalicular structures is also essential for hepatobiliary excretion of bile acids and endogenous toxic compounds. Interestingly, UDCA, but not CA or CDCA, has the distinctive ability to accelerate bile canalicular formation in cultured cells and rat primary hepatocytes [58]. Consistent with the in vitro observations, UDCA can regenerate bile canalicular structures in rats with chemical-induced liver injury. The effects were dependent on the conventional PKC and p38MAPK signaling molecules in cultured cells and partially dependent on p38MAPK, MAPK/ERK, and conventional PKC in rat primary hepatocytes. Collectively, although the direct molecular target of UDCA remains to be identified, these observations indicate that UDCA stimulates biliary excretion of toxic compounds via multiple signaling pathways.

5.2.2.3 UDCA Immunomodulatory Activity

In autoimmune cholestatic liver diseases such as PBC, humoral and cellular immune responses are exacerbated by bile acids via the following mechanisms [59]. Autoantigen-presenting cells (APCs) stimulate $CD4^+$ helper T lymphocytes (HTLs) to produce and release proinflammatory cytokines such as interleukin (IL)-2, tumor necrosis factor α (TNFα), and interferon-γ (IFN-γ), followed by the activation of B lymphocytes (BLs) and $CD8^+$ cytotoxic T lymphocytes (CTLs) for humoral and cellular response, respectively. The activated BLs produce autoantibodies, while the activated CTLs attack both hepatocytes and cholangiocytes, which induce cellular death by necro-apoptosis. The binding of CTLs to hepatocytes is facilitated by the major histocompatibility complex (MHC) class I, whose expression is induced by the accumulation of bile acids (mainly CDCA) during the cholestatic process. In cholangiocytes, CDCA also induces overexpression of MHC class II, which locally facilitates sequential activation of HTLs and CTLs, resulting in cholangiocyte damages.

In contrast to CDCA, UDCA suppresses the activation of BLs and CTLs. Clinically, UDCA treatment decreased the severity and progression of PBC with reducing biomarkers of autoimmunity such as serum levels of IgM and IgG and antimitochondrial antibody titers [60]. The immunosuppressive effect of UDCA may be, in part, due to the inhibition of the production and release of proinflammatory cytokines such as IL-2, IL-6, and IFN-γ from blood mononuclear cells [61]. Besides the inhibition of cytokine release, UDCA can also inhibit the aberrant overexpression of MHCs in cholestasis. Indeed, UDCA treatment inhibits the overexpression of MHC class I in the liver of patients with PBC [62, 63]. In addition, in vitro studies demonstrated that UDCA inhibited IFN-γ-inducible overexpression of MHC class II via a glucocorticoid receptor (GR; NR3C1)-dependent pathway [64]. Taken together, these findings indicate that UDCA can suppress autoimmune activation in patients with PBC via the inhibition of proinflammatory cytokine release and reversal of the aberrant expression of MHCs. However, it should be noted that the immunomodulatory effect of UDCA observed in patients with PBC was not consistently observed in patients with other inflammatory hepatobiliary diseases. For example, UDCA therapy failed to improve the autoimmune response in patients with primary sclerosing cholangitis (PSC) [65]. Therefore, the immunosuppressive effect of UDCA should be evaluated in the context of each disease and disease pathogenesis.

5.2.3 UDCA as a Therapeutic Agent for NASH

Nonalcoholic steatohepatitis (NASH) is a progressive liver disease characterized by hepatic steatosis, inflammation, and fibrosis. Currently, there is no approved therapy for NASH, and thus, effective agents for the treatment of this disease are highly desired. In this context, UDCA has attracted the attention as a potential therapeutic agent for NASH because of its multiple hepatoprotective activities. To date, several prospective, placebo-controlled clinical trials have been conducted to test the therapeutic effect of UDCA for NASH [66, 67]. These studies demonstrated that UDCA monotherapy at a standard dose (13–15 mg/kg/day) had no positive effect on serum concentrations of liver enzymes in patients with NASH, indicating that UDCA at a standard dose hardly improves hepatic function in NASH. Meanwhile, high dose of UDCA (at 25–30 mg/kg/day) could improve biochemical parameters in patients with NASH [68, 69]. However, histological features of NASH, including liver steatosis, inflammation, and fibrosis, were hardly improved even by treatment with high doses of UDCA. Based on these clinical findings, UDCA monotherapy is no longer recommended for the treatment of NASH [70]. Nevertheless, considering that the pathogenesis of NASH is associated with multiple disease conditions such as obesity, steatosis, insulin resistance, and chronic inflammation, combined therapies using UDCA with other drugs to prevent metabolic and inflammatory disorders might be effective options for the treatment of NASH.

5.2.4 UDCA as a Therapeutic Agent for Colon Cancer

A high-fat diet is a major risk factor of colon cancer. Continuous intake of high-fat foods leads to an increase in colorectal hydrophobic bile acids. These are thought to be major diet-related carcinogenic substances in the colon. Indeed, it has been reported that increased serum and/or fecal concentrations of the hydrophobic bile acid, DCA in particular, are associated with increased adenomas and colon cancer risk in humans [71]. Recent studies demonstrated that DCA increases oxidative DNA damage and causes genomic instability that, in turn, may lead to colorectal carcinogenesis [72]. In addition, DCA activates the EGFR/MAPK pathway. Overactivation of this pathway causes upregulation of various oncogenes such as RAS, RAF, extracellular signal-regulated kinase (ERK) 1/2, and proto-oncogene activator protein 1 (AP-1) as well as EGFR itself [71, 73, 74].

Conversely, UDCA suppresses the development of colon tumor. Several preclinical studies with rats demonstrated that UDCA significantly decreases the size and number of colon tumors induced by chemical carcinogens such as N-methylnitrosourea or azoxymethane [75–77]. This antitumor effect of UDCA may be associated with a reduction of colorectal and/or fecal DCA by UDCA therapy [78]. In addition, UDCA itself, which can block the EGFR/MAPK signaling pathway, may directly contribute to its antitumor effect [73, 74].

Consistent with results in animal models, retrospective clinical studies demonstrated a significant decrease in polyp size, decreased adenoma prevalence, and decreased probability of adenoma recurrence in patients treated with UDCA [79, 80]. In addition, a prospective, placebo-controlled, phase III clinical trial was also conducted to examine the tumor-suppressive effect of UDCA [81]. In this study, UDCA was randomly administered orally to 1,285 patients who underwent surgery to remove colorectal adenomas within 6 months prior to the trial. This study indicated a significant decrease in the recurrence of colorectal adenomas in patients who received UDCA [81]. These results strongly indicate that UDCA is a promising agent for colon cancer. Interestingly, further elucidation of the data from the phase III clinical trial revealed that there is a gender difference in the tumor-suppressive effect of UDCA [82]. UDCA caused an overall reduction in the development of adenoma in men, but led to a significantly higher risk of adenoma development in women who were younger (age <65 years), obese (body mass index ≥ 30 kg/m^2), or with high-dietary fat intake (≥ 56.2 g/day). These findings suggest that there might be some unknown mechanisms underlying the tumor-suppressive effect of UDCA and that further investigations would be necessary to clarify the appropriate population for UDCA therapy against colon cancer.

5.3 Nor-ursodeoxycholic Acid

Nor-ursodeoxycholic acid (NorUDCA) is a side-chain shortened derivate of UDCA (Fig. 5.1). NorUDCA is resistant to conjugation to taurine and glycine [83]. Unconjugated NorUDCA is secreted into the bile and reabsorbed by cholangiocytes to return to the liver. Such a cholehepatic shunt of NorUDCA stimulates bicarbonate secretion into the bile, which results in hypercholeresis [84]. In addition, the cholehepatic shunting helps NorUDCA to target injured bile ducts and, thereby, may facilitate ductal healing by direct antiproliferative, anti-inflammatory, and anti-fibrotic effects. Therapeutic effects of NorUDCA have been reported in the multidrug resistance protein 3 (Mdr3; Abcb4) knockout mouse, which is widely used as a model of cholangiopathy [85, 86]. Mdr3 is predominantly expressed on the canalicular membrane of hepatocytes and acts as a phospholipid translocater involved in biliary excretion of phosphatidylcholine [87]. Phosphatidylcholine in bile facilitates micellar formation of bile acids to reduce their toxicity. Therefore, the absence of biliary phosphatidylcholine promotes bile acid-induced injury to the biliary epithelium, resulting in cholangiopathy. In humans, defects in

MDR3 are the cause of progressive familial intrahepatic cholestasis type 3 (PFIC3), an autosomal recessive liver disorder with early-onset cholestasis [88]. In vivo pharmacological studies with *Mdr3* knockout mice demonstrated that NorUDCA reversed sclerosing cholangitis [85], while UDCA worsened, rather than improved, the bile infarcts in cholestatic conditions with biliary obstruction [86]. These results suggest that the therapeutic effect of NorUDCA against cholangiocellular cholestasis would be greater than that of UDCA. However, in a model of taurolithocholate-induced hepatocellular cholestasis, NorUDCA failed to counteract cholestasis and hepatocyte apoptosis, while the taurine conjugate of UDCA did [89]. Taken together with the fact that hepatobiliary disorders progressed not only by cholangiocyte but also by hepatocyte dysfunction, these results suggest that combination therapy of NorUDCA with UDCA may be more beneficial than either monotherapy. Currently, a randomized, placebo-controlled phase II clinical trial of NorUDCA in the treatment of PSC is ongoing [83]. Results of this clinical trial will reveal the pharmacological effects of NorUDCA in humans and provide further aspects of the therapeutic potential of NorUDCA.

5.4 Bile Acid Mimetics as FXR and TGR5 Agonists

The discovery of FXR, a nuclear hormone receptor recognizing bile acids as endogenous ligands, gave rise to the idea that bile acids are signaling molecules. In particular, it has been revealed that CDCA, DCA, LCA, and CA, but not UDCA or NorUDCA, present ligand's ability to activate FXR signaling with the following order of potency: CDCA>DCA>LCA>>CA [17]. FXR is highly expressed in the liver and intestine and plays a key role in bile acid homeostasis. In the liver, binding of bile acids to FXR induces the expression of small heterodimer partner (SHP), which is a transcriptional repressor interfering with the transcription of cholesterol 7α-hydroxyrase (CYP7A1) (Fig. 5.2) [12]. CYP7A1 is a rate-limiting enzyme involved in the conversion of cholesterol to primary bile acids. The expression of CYP7A1 is also negatively regulated via an endocrine mechanism mediated by fibroblast growth factor 19 (FGF19) (human homologue of Fgf15 in rodents), which is secreted from the ileum into the portal circulation in response to the activation of intestinal FXR by bile acids [90] (Fig. 5.2). In the liver, FGF19 activates fibroblast growth factor receptor 4 (FGFR4) with its co-receptor β-Klotho. The FGFR4/β-Klotho signaling cascade then induces the expression of SHP, which, in turn, results in a decrease in CYP7A1 expression [91] (Fig. 5.2). This negative regulation of CYP7A1 expression by bile acids via FXR and FGFR/β-Klotho signaling pathways plays a key role in the feedback regulation of bile acid synthesis. In addition to the CYP7A1 expression, FXR signaling also regulates the expression of bile acid transporters involved in the enterohepatic circulation to maintain bile acid homeostasis [92, 93] (Fig. 5.2). Recent studies indicated that FXR regulates multiple metabolic pathways involved in lipogenesis, gluconeogenesis, tumor suppression, liver regeneration, and liver inflammation as well as bile acid homeostasis, indicating that FXR is a potential therapeutic target for a variety of diseases [1].

Besides FXR, TGR5 acts as a bile acid receptor. TGR5 is a cell surface receptor, abundantly expressed in the liver, bile duct, gallbladder, brown adipose tissue, muscle, and intestine (enteroendocrine L cells, in particular) [17]. In the liver, TGR5 is expressed in Kupffer cells, but not in hepatocytes [94]. Similar to FXR, TGR5 is activated by most endogenous bile acids, including LCA, DCA, CDCA, and CA, but not UDCA, with the following order of potency: LCA>DCA>CDCA>CA [17]. Upon bile acid binding to TGR5, the adenylate cyclase is stimulated, and cellular cAMP levels increase, leading to further downstream signaling events [12]. For example, in enteroendocrine L cells, TGR5 activation stimulates the secretion of glucagon-like peptide 1 (GLP-1), which enhances insulin secretion from the pancreas and improves insulin sensitivity [95, 96] (Fig. 5.2). In Kupffer cells and macrophages, TGR5 activation inhibits lipopolysaccharide-induced production and secretion of proinflammatory cytokines such as IL-1β, IL-6, IFN-γ, and TNFα [94]. In addition, in the brown adipose tissue and skeletal muscle, TGR5 regulates energy homeostasis by activating cAMP-dependent iodothyronine deiodinase 2, an enzyme responsible for the conversion of inactive thyroxine (T4) to active thyroid hormone (T3) [97]. Since T3 is a positive regulator of the basal metabolic rate and energy consumption, TGR5 activation in the muscle and brown adipose tissue results in an increase in energy expenditure. Collectively, these findings indicate that TGR5 and FXR agonists are potential therapeutic agents for several diseases such as diabetes, inflammatory liver diseases, and obesity.

Several mimetics of bile acids have been developed as agonists of these bile acid receptors for the treatment of liver diseases such as PBC, PSC, and NASH [17]. For example, obeticholic acid (OCA) (6α-ethyl-chenodeoxycholic acid) and INT-777 (6α-ethyl-23(S)-methyl-cholic acid) have been developed [98, 99] (Fig. 5.1). Although OCA was developed as a potent and selective FXR agonist, a recent study indicates that it also activates TGR5 with an EC50 value comparable to those of endogenous bile acids [100]. Meanwhile, INT-777 is a highly selective TGR5 agonist with little ability to activate FXR [99, 100]. OCA has been under investigation in clinical trials to examine its beneficial effects for the treatment of PBC. In a phase II clinical trial, OCA monotherapy markedly improved liver functions and inflammation in patients with PBC [101]. However, unexpectedly, this therapy also induced dose-dependent pruritus as a common but serious adverse effect, which results in the discontinuation of the treatment in more than 35% of the patients. For this adverse effect, a phase III clinical trial of OCA has been conducted in a limited number of patients with PBC with inadequate response to standard UDCA therapy [102]. A clinical trial of OCA in NASH patients has also been conducted and demonstrated that OCA treatment improves NASH histological features, although patients developed pruritus with a high frequency [103]. Regarding the selective TGR5 agonist INT-777, preclinical studies revealed that INT-777 administration improves insulin sensitivity and prevents obesity and hepatic steatosis in mice fed a high-fat diet, suggesting multiple pharmacological activities of INT-777

[95]. However, considering the recent finding that bile acid-induced itch may be caused, in part, by the activation of TGR5 [104], it is highly possible that pruritus will be observed with the INT-777 therapy as well as with the OCA therapy. Since bile acids are ligands for multiple receptors, including GR, vitamin D receptor (VDR; NR1I1), and pregnane X receptor (PXR; NR1I2) besides FXR and TGR5 [64, 105, 106], and have multiple biochemical activities, a comprehensive understanding of signaling pathways involving bile acids would be necessary to predict their pharmacological effects accurately.

5.5 Bile Acid Sequestrants

Bile acid sequestrants (BAS) have been used for more than 50 years for the treatment of hypercholesterolemia. Besides such a classical usage, recent advances in understanding multiple physiological functions of bile acid shed light on new medicinal applications of BAS for several metabolic diseases. In this section, we summarized BAS pharmacological activities for the treatment of dyslipidemia and type 2 diabetes mellitus (T2DM).

5.5.1 BAS as Therapeutic Agents for Dyslipidemia

BAS are non-absorbed positively charged resins that can bind to negatively charged bile acids in the intestine. Currently four BAS are available on the market: colestipol (first-generation BAS), cholestyramine, colestimide (available only in Japan), and colesevelam-HCl (Fig. 5.1). Among them, colesevelam-HCl has been specifically engineered to contain long hydrophobic side chains, which increases the affinity and specificity to bind bile acids compared to other traditional BAS [107]. Due to this property, colesevelam-HCl can be used at lower doses compared to other BAS (Table 5.2). Clinically, the efficacy of BAS monotherapies has been proven. BAS decrease total cholesterol levels (by 3–17%) and low-density lipoprotein cholesterol (LDL-C) levels (by 5–26%) without changing or only inducing a little increase in high-density lipoprotein cholesterol (HDL-C) levels (by 0–8%) in a dose-dependent manner (Table. 5.2). The aim of most of cholesterol-lowering therapies is to reduce the risk of atherosclerosis and cardiovascular diseases such as coronary heart disease (CHD). It has been reported that, compared with placebo, cholestyramine as monotherapy and colestipol in combination with lovastatin decrease the percentage of patients with CHD progression and also increase the percentage of patients with CHD regression (Table. 5.2). These results indicate that BAS (either as monotherapy or in combination with other cholesterol-lowering drugs) can reduce the risk of CHD besides improving plasma lipid profiles.

The underlying mechanism by which BAS reduce plasma cholesterol levels involves the disruption of the enterohepatic circulation of bile acids. Since bile

Table 5.2 Effects of bile acid sequestrant therapy on plasma lipid profile

Terms	Number of patients	Drugs	% Change from base line (baseline: mM) TC	LDL-C	HDL-C	TG	CHD risk (%)	Ref
As monotherapy								
7.4 years	1900	Placebo	−1% (7.2)	−3% (5.3)	2% (1.1)	13% (2.0)	Death by CHD: 2.0	[134]
							Death by MI: 8.3	
	1906	Cholestyramine (24 g/day)	−8%* (7.3)	−15%* (5.3)	5% (1.1)	17% (2.1)	Death by CHD: 1.6	
							Death by MI: 6.8	
5 years	57	Placebo	−1% (7.6)	−5%* (5.9)	2% (1.0)	26%* (1.5)	Progression: 33	[135]
							Regression: 10	
	59	Cholestyramine (24 g/day)	−17%* (8.0)	−26%* (6.3)	8%* (1.0)	28%* (1.8)	Progression: 12	
							Regression: 12	
8 weeks	38	Placebo	1% (6.9)	0% (4.9)	0% (1.3)	11%* (1.7)	NA	[136]
	38	Colestipol (2 g/day)	−3%* (7.0)	−5%* (4.8)	−1% (1.4)	15%* (1.7)	NA	
	37	Colestipol (4 g/day)	−7%* (7.0)	−11%* (4.9)	0% (1.3)	10%* (1.6)	NA	
	40	Colestipol (8 g/day)	−13%* (6.8)	−20%* (4.7)	−1% (1.3)	12%* (1.6)	NA	
	40	Colestipol (16 g/day)	−17%* (7.0)	−26%* (4.9)	−1% (1.3)	15%* (1.8)	NA	
24 weeks	88	Placebo	1% (6.3)	0% (4.0)	0% (1.3)	2% (1.9)	NA	[137]
	99	Colesevelam-HCl (2.3 g/day)	−4%* (6.3)	−9 %* (4.2)	4%* (1.3)	7%* (1.7)	NA	
	91	Colesevelam-HCl (3.0 g/day)	−6%* (6.3)	−12%* (4.1)	4%* (1.2)	4% (1.8)	NA	
	95	Colesevelam-HCl (3.8 g/day)	−7%* (6.3)	−15%* (4.1)	4%* (1.2)	9%* (1.9)	NA	
	94	Colesevelam-HCl (4.5 g/day)	−10%* (6.2)	−18%* (4.0)	4%* (1.2)	7%* (1.8)	NA	

In combination with other cholesterol-lowering drugs							
12 weeks	26	Cholestyramine (8 g/day)	−7%* (6.2)	−13%* (4.5)	3% (1.1)	15% (0.7)	NA	[138]
	26	Cholestyramine (8 g/day) + Lovastatin (5 mg/day)	−13%* (6.2)	−25%* (4.5)	5% (1.1)	28%* (0.7)	NA	
	26	Lovastatin (20 mg/day)	−13%* (6.2)	−21%* (4.5)	8% (1.1)	−5% (0.7)	NA	
12 weeks	21	Pravastatin (5-10 mg/day)	−7%* (5.4)	−4%* (2.9)	0% (1.4)	−14%* (1.5)	NA	[139]
	19	Colestimide (3 g/day) + Pravastatin (5–10 mg/day)	−12%* (5.3)	−20%* (2.9)	11%* (1.4)	27%* (1.5)	NA	
2.5 years	46	Placebo	−3% (6.8)	−7%* (4.5)	6%* (1.1)	15% (2.6)	Progression: 46	[140]
							Regression: 11	
	38	Colestipol (30 g/day) + Lovastatin (40 mg/day)	−33%* (7.1)	−45%* (5.1)	20%* (1.0)	−9% (2.3)	Progression: 21	
							Regression: 32	
4 weeks	19	Placebo	4% (6.8)	3% (4.8)	4%* (1.2)	9% (1.7)	NA	[141]
	16	Colesevelam-HCl (3.8 g/day)	−6%* (7.0)	−12%* (4.8)	3%* (1.2)	10% (1.9)	NA	
	18	Atorvastatin (10 mg/day)	−27%* (6.9)	−38%* (4.7)	8%* (1.3)	−24%* (2.0)	NA	
	18	Colesevelam-HCl (3.8 g/day) + Atorvastatin (10 mg/day)	−31%* (7.0)	−48%* (4.8)	11%* (1.2)	−1% (1.7)	NA	
	20	Atorvastatin (80 mg/day)	−39%* (6.9)	−53%* (4.7)	5%* (1.2)	−33%* (1.7)	NA	
4 weeks	26	Placebo	1% (6.6)	1% (4.4)	1% (1.3)	2% (1.9)	NA	[142]
	29	Colesevelam-HCl (2.3 g/day)	−3% (6.6)	−7%* (4.4)	4%* (1.3)	14%* (2.0)	NA	
	26	Lovastatin (10 mg/day)	−15%* (6.5)	−22%* (4.3)	3% (1.3)	5% (2.0)	NA	
	27	Colesevelam-HCl (2.3 g/day) + Lovastatin (10 mg/day)	−21%* (6.7)	−34%* (4.5)	3% (1.3)	9% (2.0)	NA	

(continued)

Table 5.2 (continued)

Terms	Number of patients	Drugs	% Change from base line (baseline: mM)					Ref
			TC	LDL-C	HDL-C	TG	CHD risk (%)	
6 weeks	33	Placebo	−2% (6.9)	−4%* (4.8)	3% (1.2)	6% (2.1)	NA	[143]
	37	Colesevelam-HCl (3.8 g/day)	−9%* (7.3)	−16%* (5.1)	2% (1.3)	11%* (1.9)	NA	
	35	Simvastatin (10 mg/day)	−19%* (6.9)	−26%* (4.7)	3%* (1.3)	−17%* (1.7)	NA	
	34	Colesevelam-HCl (3.8 g/day) + Simvastatin (10 mg/day)	−28%* (7.1)	−42%* (5.1)	10%* (1.4)	−12% (1.5)	NA	
	36	Colesevelam-HCl (2.3 g/day)	−4%* (7.0)	−8%* (4.8)	3%* (1.3)	11% (1.8)	NA	
	39	Simvastatin (20 mg/day)	−23%* (6.8)	−34%* (4.7)	7%* (1.3)	−12%* (1.7)	NA	
	37	Colesevelam-HCl (2.3 g/day) + Simvastatin (20 mg/day)	−29%* (7.1)	−42%* (4.9)	4%* (1.3)	−12%* (1.9)	NA	
6 weeks	41	Ezetimibe (10 mg/day)	−14%* (6.7)	−21%* (4.5)	3% (1.5)	−3% (1.3)	NA	[144]
	43	Colesevelam-HCl (3.8 g/day) + Ezetimibe (10 mg/day)	−20%* (6.8)	−32%* (4.6)	3% (1.5)	5% (1.5)	NA	
6 weeks	65	Fenofibrate (160 mg/day)	−10%* (6.5)	−6%* (4.1)	10% (1.2)	−37%* (2.4)	NA	[145]
	64	Colesevelam-HCl (3.8 g/day) + Fenofibrate (160 mg/day)	−15%* (6.6)	−17%* (4.1)	12% (1.2)	−32%* (2.6)	NA	

TC total cholesterol, *LDL-C* low-density lipoprotein cholesterol, *HDL-C* high-density lipoprotein cholesterol, *TG* triglyceride, *CHD* coronary heart disease, *MI* myocardial infarction, *NA* not available, *Ref* reference

*$p < 0.05$ compared to baseline

acids bound to BAS are not reabsorbed by ASBT in the ileum, fecal elimination of bile acid is increased up to more than three times during BAS therapy [108, 109]. Such a disruption of the enterohepatic circulation of bile acid causes a reduction in the bile acid pool in our body and, thereby, increases the hepatic conversion of cholesterol to primary bile acids (CA in particular), leading to intracellular cholesterol depletion in the liver. In response to the cholesterol depletion, sterol regulatory element-binding protein 2 (SREBP-2), which is a transcriptional factor regulating the expression of genes involved in cholesterol homeostasis [110], increases the hepatic expression of LDL receptor (LDLR) to enhance the uptake of LDL-C from plasma [111]. Consequently, BAS treatment decreases the plasma concentration of cholesterol, LDL-C in particular. BAS treatment also increases the expression of HMG-CoA reductase, a rate-limiting enzyme for cholesterol synthesis, via the activation of SREBP-2 and, thus, enhances de novo cholesterol synthesis in the liver [111]. Therefore, it makes sense to use BAS in combination with statin, an HMG-CoA reductase inhibitor, for the treatment of hypercholesterolemia. Indeed, several clinical studies demonstrated that combination therapies of BAS and statin showed greater decreases in plasma total cholesterol levels and LDL-C levels compared with either monotherapy (Table 5.2).

Impaired intestinal cholesterol absorption may also be associated with BAS cholesterol-lowering effect. Considering that micellar solubilization is crucial for lipid absorption in the intestine and that the bile acids are essential to form micelles, alterations in the micellar concentration and/or composition of bile acids by BAS treatment may affect cholesterol absorption in the intestine. Intestinal cholesterol absorption was for a long time thought to occur by passive diffusion through the luminal membrane of enterocytes. However, the discovery of ezetimibe, a potent intestinal cholesterol absorption inhibitor, indicates that this process is mediated by a specific transport system [112]. In 2004, it was reported that intestinal cholesterol absorption in Niemann-Pick C1-like 1 (NPC1L1) knockout mice was significantly reduced to about 30% of that in wild-type mice and the degree of this reduction was almost the same as that observed in ezetimibe-treated wild-type mice [113]. In addition, ezetimibe hardly affected the remaining cholesterol absorption in NPC1L1 knockout mice. These results, together with the fact that NPC1L1 is expressed on the apical membrane of the intestine, particularly of the jejunum, where most sterol absorption occurs [113], suggest that NPC1L1 is involved in the intestinal cholesterol absorption and is a molecular target of ezetimibe. Interestingly, in vitro studies with NPC1L1-overexpressing cells demonstrated that NPC1L1-mediated cholesterol uptake was positively regulated by the micellar concentration of bile acids [114]. Taken together with the fact that BAS can remove bile acids from micelles [115], this observation suggests that NPC1L1-mediated intestinal cholesterol absorption might be impaired by BAS treatment due to the reduction of micellar bile acids.

5.5.2 BAS as Therapeutic Agents for T2DM

In 1994, it was reported for the first time that cholestylamine treatment achieved an about 10% reduction in fasting plasma glucose in patients with T2DM [116]. Since then, the efficacy of BAS alone or in combination with other antidiabetic drugs (e.g., insulin, sulfonylurea, and metformin) on glucose homeostasis and insulin sensitivity has been examined in several clinical studies (Table 5.3). For example, monotherapy with colesevelam-HCl has been shown to reduce fasting plasma glucose and HbA1c levels by 4% and 2%, respectively, in adults with untreated prediabetes [117]. In addition, several combination therapies of colesevelam-HCl with other antidiabetic drugs achieved additive reductions in fasting plasma glucose and HbA1c of around 10% (Table 5.3). Based on these results, in 2008, the FDA approved colesevelam-HCl to control hyperglycemia in patients with T2DM. Colestimide has also been shown to reduce fasting plasma glucose and HbA1c in patients with T2DM with other antidiabetic or insulin treatment [118]. Currently, colesevelam-HCl is the only approved drug for the treatment of T2DM in the USA, even though colestimide is under clinical trials in Japan to expand its indication to T2DM.

The mechanism underlying how BAS improve glycemic control has not been fully defined. However, it has been suggested that GLP-1, a potent glucose-lowering hormone, might be involved in BAS-mediated improvement of glycemic control. Several studies revealed that BAS therapy enhances GLP-1 secretion from enteroendocrine L cells [119–121]. Indeed, BAS treatment significantly increases glucose-stimulated GLP-1 and insulin release in rat diabetic models [119, 120]. In addition, patients with T2DM treated with colestimide showed increased postprandial plasma GLP-1 levels, whereas their plasma glucose levels decreased [121].

The mechanism by which BAS stimulate GLP-1 secretion has been extensively studied. One of the plausible mechanisms is associated with the activation of TGR5, which upregulates the production and secretion of GLP-1 in enteroendocrine L cells [95, 96] (Fig. 5.2). The inhibition of bile acid reabsorption by BAS would increase bile acids in the distal intestine (ileum), where enteroendocrine L cells are highly enriched. Since bile acids, even though they are bound to BAS, are able to activate TGR5 [122], the increase in ileal bile acids by BAS treatment may stimulate GLP-1 production and secretion in enteroendocrine L cells. In addition to the TGR5 activation, FXR deactivation may also be involved in the stimulation of GLP-1 secretion. It has been reported that whole-body FXR-deficient mice are protected against obesity and present an improved glucose metabolism [123]. Interestingly, similar phenotypes were observed in intestine-specific, but not in liver-specific, FXR-deficient mice [123–125]. These results indicate that, in the intestine, FXR plays an important role in energy expenditure and glucose metabolism. A recent study demonstrated that FXR is expressed in enteroendocrine L cells and downregulates the production of GLP-1 by decreasing the expression of proglucagon, a precursor of GLP-1 (Fig. 5.2). In addition, FXR activation decreases ATP production by inhibiting glycolysis, which, in turn, suppresses GLP-1

Table 5.3 Effects of bile acid sequestrant therapy on glycemic control

Patients	Terms	Number of patients	Drugs	% Change from baseline				Ref
				LDL-C	HDL-C	HbA1c	FPG	
As monotherapy								
Untreated prediabetic patients	16 weeks	108	Placebo	2%	4%	0%	−2%	[146]
		108	Colesevelam-HCl (3.8 g/day)	−14%*	4%	−2%*	−4%*	
In combination with other antidiabetic drugs								
Patients with glyburide and/or insulin treatment	21 weeks	21	Placebo	−2%	0%	−4%	4%	[147]
		21	Cholestyramine (16 g/day)	−29%*	3%	−10%	−11%*	
Patients with antidiabetic or insulin treatment	12 weeks	35	Pravastatin (10 mg/day)	−16%*	−6%	0%	0%	[118]
		35	Colestimide (3 g/day)	−23%*	−6%	−12%*	−9%*	
Patients with metformin and/or oral antidiabetic	26 weeks	157	Placebo	3%	0%	2%	7%*	[148]
		159	Colesevelam-HCl (3.8 g/day)	−13%*	0%	−5%*	−3%	
Patients with sulfonylurea and/or oral antidiabetic	26 weeks	231	Placebo	1%	0%	2%	4%	[149]
		230	Colesevelam-HCl (3.8 g/day)	−16%*	1%	−5%*	−3%	

LDL-C low-density lipoprotein cholesterol, *HDL-C* high-density lipoprotein cholesterol, *HbA1c* glycosylated hemoglobin, *FPG* fasting plasma glucose, *Ref* reference

*$p < 0.05$ compared to baseline

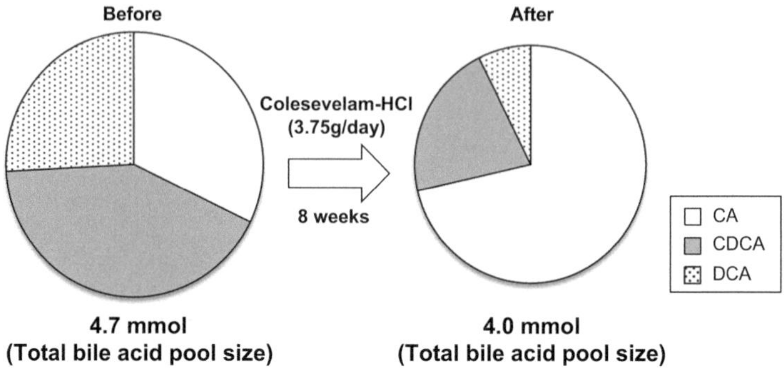

Fig. 5.4 Effects of colesevelam-HCl treatment on pool sizes of bile acids. The pool sizes of the major bile acids in humans were quantified before and after colesevelam-HCl treatment (Data from Brufau et al. [133]. *CA* cholic acid, *CDCA* chenodeoxycholic acid, *DCA* deoxycholic acid)

secretion. Furthermore, the beneficial effect on glucose tolerance in FXR-deficient mice is abolished by the administration of a GLP-1 receptor antagonist. Collectively, these findings suggest that intestinal FXR negatively regulates glucose tolerance through the downregulation of GLP-1 [126]. Considering that BAS have the potential to deactivate FXR through an alteration in bile acid composition, pool sizes of bile acids such as CDCA and DCA with higher FXR ligand abilities are reduced due to the disruption of enterohepatic circulation, whereas the pool size of CA with the lowest FXR ligand ability is increased by an enhanced CA synthesis to compensate for the increased fecal loss of bile acids (Fig. 5.4), the BAS-mediated deactivation of FXR in enteroendocrine L cells might be involved in the increase in GLP-1 secretion.

5.5.3 *BAS Adverse Effects*

Major adverse effects of BAS are gastrointestinal complaints such as constipation, abdominal pain, and nausea, which often result in the discontinuation of BAS therapy. In addition, long-term treatment with BAS leads to deficiency of fat-soluble vitamins (vitamin A, D, E, and K). This deficiency is accounted for by malabsorption of these vitamins as well as cholesterol, which is likely caused by the reduction of micellar bile acids and/or nonspecific binding to BAS. Similarly, intestinal absorption of several drugs such as warfarin, cyclosporine, and digoxin is also inhibited by BAS due to nonspecific binding. Therefore, patients should be advised to take concomitant medications at least 1 h before or 4 h after BAS intake. In contrast to BAS, ezetimibe had been thought to be a selective inhibitor of cholesterol absorption, which should hardly affect the intestinal absorption of other nutrients and drugs. This was one of the superior features of ezetimibe compared with BAS. However, recent studies demonstrated that NPC1L1 has the ability to import vitamin E and vitamin K_1 as well as cholesterol. Additionally, ezetimibe can inhibit the intestinal absorption of these vitamins in mice and rats [127–129]. These findings suggest that malabsorption of vitamin E and vitamin K_1 should be considered even in ezetimibe therapy as well as BAS therapy.

Unlike other cholesterol-lowering drugs, BAS increase plasma triglyceride (TG) levels (Table 5.2). Therefore, the use of BAS as a monotherapy in patients with hypertriglyceridemia is limited. The increase in plasma TG levels by BAS treatment appears to be associated with the BAS-induced deactivation of FXR. FXR activation in the liver causes reduction in the hepatic expression of SREBP-1c, a transcriptional factor promoting the expression of genes involved in TG biosynthesis [130] (Fig. 5.2). Additionally, in humans, FXR activation can induce the expression of peroxisome proliferator-activated receptor α (PPARα; NR1C1), leading to the suppression of TG production in the liver [131] (Fig. 5.2). Taken together with these facts, FXR deactivation by BAS would enhance TG biosynthesis in the liver, and thereby, TG hepatic secretion into the plasma increases. Notably, the increase in plasma TG levels by BAS can be attenuated by the coadministration of other drugs for dyslipidemia. In the case of combination therapy of BAS with fenofibrate, a clinically used PPARα agonist for dyslipidemia, plasma TG levels were significantly decreased even in patients receiving colesevelam-HCl (Table 5.2). Considering that the appropriate control of plasma TG levels as well as cholesterol levels is important to inhibit cardiovascular diseases, combination therapies of BAS with fibrates might be an attractive option for the treatment of dyslipidemia.

5.6 Conclusions and Future Perspectives

Bile acids are involved in a variety of physiological processes and cellular signaling such as intestinal lipid absorption, lipid metabolism, bile secretion, cell toxicity, inflammation, carcinogenesis, and glucose metabolism. Thus, bile acids and/or bile acid-related molecules are promising pharmacological targets against several diseases. However, considering the complexity of the regulatory mechanisms of bile acid homeostasis, involving many transporters and nuclear receptors (Fig. 5.2) and given the fact that a variety of signaling pathways involving bile acids exert not only beneficial but also adverse effects on the human body, the "one-size-fits-all" therapy with bile acid-related drugs will not be successful. To obtain maximum beneficial effects of bile acid-related drugs, it is necessary to use these drugs for the appropriate patient at the appropriate time (disease stage). In addition, combination with other drugs would be a key to a successful therapy. To identify the suitable patients, timing, and concomitant drugs, comprehensive and quantitative understanding of molecular pathways involving bile acids would be helpful. In line with this idea, systems biology approaches such as computational and mathematical modeling to understand complex biological systems will become increasingly important and useful [132]. A quantitative integration of segmentalized knowledge about bile acid signaling by using systems biology approaches will enable us to predict, with high accuracy, the cellular, tissue, and in vivo responses to bile acid-related drugs. In addition, it will ease the development of more effective bile acid therapies.

References

1. Lefebvre P, Cariou B, Lien F, Kuipers F, Staels B. Role of bile acids and bile acid receptors in metabolic regulation. Physiol Rev. 2009;89(1):147–91. doi:10.1152/physrev.00010.2008.
2. Strautnieks SS, Bull LN, Knisely AS, Kocoshis SA, Dahl N, Arnell H, et al. A gene encoding a liver-specific ABC transporter is mutated in progressive familial intrahepatic cholestasis. Nat Genet. 1998;20(3):233–8. doi:10.1038/3034.
3. Hayashi H, Takada T, Suzuki H, Akita H, Sugiyama Y. Two common PFIC2 mutations are associated with the impaired membrane trafficking of BSEP/ABCB11. Hepatology. 2005;41 (4):916–24. doi:10.1002/hep.20627.
4. Edenharder R, Knaflic T. Epimerization of chenodeoxycholic acid to ursodeoxycholic acid by human intestinal lecithinase-lipase-negative Clostridia. J Lipid Res. 1981;22(4):652–8.
5. Wong MH, Oelkers P, Craddock AL, Dawson PA. Expression cloning and characterization of the hamster ileal sodium-dependent bile acid transporter. J Biol Chem. 1994;269(2):1340–7.
6. Wong MH, Oelkers P, Dawson PA. Identification of a mutation in the ileal sodium-dependent bile acid transporter gene that abolishes transport activity. J Biol Chem. 1995;270 (45):27228–34.
7. Dawson PA, Hubbert M, Haywood J, Craddock AL, Zerangue N, Christian WV, et al. The heteromeric organic solute transporter alpha-beta, Ostalpha-Ostbeta, is an ileal basolateral bile acid transporter. J Biol Chem. 2005;280(8):6960–8. doi:10.1074/jbc.M412752200.
8. Ballatori N, Christian WV, Lee JY, Dawson PA, Soroka CJ, Boyer JL, et al. OSTalpha-OSTbeta: a major basolateral bile acid and steroid transporter in human intestinal, renal, and biliary epithelia. Hepatology. 2005;42(6):1270–9. doi:10.1002/hep.20961.
9. Hagenbuch B, Stieger B, Foguet M, Lubbert H, Meier PJ. Functional expression cloning and characterization of the hepatocyte Na+/bile acid cotransport system. Proc Natl Acad Sci U S A. 1991;88(23):10629–33.
10. Hagenbuch B, Meier PJ. Molecular cloning, chromosomal localization, and functional characterization of a human liver Na+/bile acid cotransporter. J Clin Invest. 1994;93 (3):1326–31. doi:10.1172/JCI117091.
11. Meier PJ, Stieger B. Bile salt transporters. Annu Rev Physiol. 2002;64:635–61. doi:10.1146/annurev.physiol.64.082201.100300.
12. Kuipers F, Bloks VW, Groen AK. Beyond intestinal soap – bile acids in metabolic control. Nat Rev Endocrinol. 2014;10(8):488–98. doi:10.1038/nrendo.2014.60.
13. Li T, Chiang JY. Bile acid signaling in metabolic disease and drug therapy. Pharmacol Rev. 2014;66(4):948–83. doi:10.1124/pr.113.008201.
14. Makishima M, Okamoto AY, Repa JJ, Tu H, Learned RM, Luk A, et al. Identification of a nuclear receptor for bile acids. Science. 1999;284(5418):1362–5.
15. Parks DJ, Blanchard SG, Bledsoe RK, Chandra G, Consler TG, Kliewer SA, et al. Bile acids: natural ligands for an orphan nuclear receptor. Science. 1999;284(5418):1365–8.
16. Maruyama T, Miyamoto Y, Nakamura T, Tamai Y, Okada H, Sugiyama E, et al. Identification of membrane-type receptor for bile acids (M-BAR). Biochem Biophys Res Commun. 2002;298(5):714–9.
17. de Aguiar Vallim TQ, Tarling EJ, Edwards PA. Pleiotropic roles of bile acids in metabolism. Cell Metab. 2013;17(5):657–69. doi:10.1016/j.cmet.2013.03.013.

18. Paumgartner G, Beuers U. Ursodeoxycholic acid in cholestatic liver disease: mechanisms of action and therapeutic use revisited. Hepatology. 2002;36(3):525–31. doi:10.1053/jhep.2002.36088.
19. Hagey LR, Crombie DL, Espinosa E, Carey MC, Igimi H, Hofmann AF. Ursodeoxycholic acid in the Ursidae: biliary bile acids of bears, pandas, and related carnivores. J Lipid Res. 1993;34(11):1911–7.
20. Ikegami T, Matsuzaki Y. Ursodeoxycholic acid: mechanism of action and novel clinical applications. Hepatol Res. 2008;38(2):123–31. doi:10.1111/j.1872-034X.2007.00297.x.
21. Shoda M. Über die Ursodesoxycholsäure aus Bärengallen und ihre physiologische Wirkung. J Biochem. 1927;7(3):505–17.
22. Ichida F. Clinical experience with ursodeoxycholic acid (S-Urso) for chronic hepatitis. Sindan-to-tiryou. 1961;49:388–92.
23. Makino I, Shinozaki K, Yoshino K, Nakagawa S. Dissolution of cholesterol gallstones by long-term administration of ursodeoxycholic acid. Nihon Shokakibyo Gakkai Zasshi. 1975;72(6):690–702.
24. Corrigan OI, Su CC, Higuchi WI, Hofmann AF. Mesophase formation during cholesterol dissolution in ursodeoxycholate-lecithin solutions: new mechanism for gallstone dissolution in humans. J Pharm Sci. 1980;69(7):869–71.
25. Nilsell K, Angelin B, Leijd B, Einarsson K. Comparative effects of ursodeoxycholic acid and chenodeoxycholic acid on bile acid kinetics and biliary lipid secretion in humans. Evidence for different modes of action on bile acid synthesis. Gastroenterology. 1983;85(6):1248–56.
26. von Bergmann K, Epple-Gutsfeld M, Leiss O. Differences in the effects of chenodeoxycholic and ursodeoxycholic acid on biliary lipid secretion and bile acid synthesis in patients with gallstones. Gastroenterology. 1984;87(1):136–43.
27. Berge KE, Tian H, Graf GA, Yu L, Grishin NV, Schultz J, et al. Accumulation of dietary cholesterol in sitosterolemia caused by mutations in adjacent ABC transporters. Science. 2000;290(5497):1771–5.
28. Yu L, Hammer RE, Li-Hawkins J, Von Bergmann K, Lutjohann D, Cohen JC, et al. Disruption of Abcg5 and Abcg8 in mice reveals their crucial role in biliary cholesterol secretion. Proc Natl Acad Sci USA. 2002;99(25):16237–42. doi:10.1073/pnas.252582399.
29. Vrins C, Vink E, Vandenberghe KE, Frijters R, Seppen J, Groen AK. The sterol transporting heterodimer ABCG5/ABCG8 requires bile salts to mediate cholesterol efflux. FEBS Lett. 2007;581(24):4616–20. doi:10.1016/j.febslet.2007.08.052.
30. Yamanashi Y, Takada T, Yoshikado T, Shoda J, Suzuki H. NPC2 regulates biliary cholesterol secretion via stimulation of ABCG5/G8-mediated cholesterol transport. Gastroenterology. 2011;140(5):1664–74. doi:10.1053/j.gastro.2011.01.050.
31. Roda E, Roda A, Sama C, Festi D, Mazzella G, Aldini R, et al. Effect of ursodeoxycholic acid administration on biliary lipid composition and bile acid kinetics in cholesterol gallstone patients. Dig Dis Sci. 1979;24(2):123–8.
32. Salvioli G, Salati R. Faecal bile acid loss and bile acid pool size during short-term treatment with ursodeoxycholic and chenodeoxycholic acid in patients with radiolucent gallstones. Gut. 1979;20(8):698–704.
33. Bell GD, Whitney B, Dowling RH. Gallstone dissolution in man using chenodeoxycholic acid. Lancet. 1972;2(7789):1213–6.
34. Danzinger RG, Hofmann AF, Schoenfield LJ, Thistle JL. Dissolution of cholesterol gallstones by chenodeoxycholic acid. N Engl J Med. 1972;286(1):1–8. doi:10.1056/NEJM197201062860101.
35. Stiehl A, Raedsch R, Czygan P, Gotz R, Manner C, Walker S, et al. Effects of biliary bile acid composition on biliary cholesterol saturation in gallstone patients treated with chenodeoxycholic acid and/or ursodeoxycholic acid. Gastroenterology. 1980;79(6):1192–8.
36. Stiehl A, Czygan P, Kommerell B, Weis HJ, Holtermuller KH. Ursodeoxycholic acid versus chenodeoxycholic acid. Comparison of their effects on bile acid and bile lipid composition in patients with cholesterol gallstones. Gastroenterology. 1978;75(6):1016–20.

37. Mok HY, Bell GD, Dowling RH. Effect of different doses of chenodeoxycholic acid on bile-lipid composition and on frequency of side-effects in patients with gallstones. Lancet. 1974;2 (7875):253–7.
38. Poupon RE, Balkau B, Eschwege E, Poupon R. A multicenter, controlled trial of ursodiol for the treatment of primary biliary cirrhosis. UDCA-PBC Study Group. N Engl J Med. 1991;324 (22):1548–54. doi:10.1056/NEJM199105303242204.
39. Lindor KD, Dickson ER, Baldus WP, Jorgensen RA, Ludwig J, Murtaugh PA, et al. Ursodeoxycholic acid in the treatment of primary biliary cirrhosis. Gastroenterology. 1994;106(5):1284–90.
40. Palma J, Reyes H, Ribalta J, Hernandez I, Sandoval L, Almuna R, et al. Ursodeoxycholic acid in the treatment of cholestasis of pregnancy: a randomized, double-blind study controlled with placebo. J Hepatol. 1997;27(6):1022–8.
41. Puoti C, Pannullo A, Annovazzi G, Filippi T, Magrini A. Ursodeoxycholic acid and chronic hepatitis C infection. Lancet. 1993;341(8857):1413–4.
42. Takano S, Ito Y, Yokosuka O, Ohto M, Uchiumi K, Hirota K, et al. A multicenter randomized controlled dose study of ursodeoxycholic acid for chronic hepatitis C. Hepatology. 1994;20 (3):558–64.
43. Attili AF, Angelico M, Cantafora A, Alvaro D, Capocaccia L. Bile acid-induced liver toxicity: relation to the hydrophobic-hydrophilic balance of bile acids. Med Hypotheses. 1986;19(1):57–69.
44. Heuman DM. Quantitative estimation of the hydrophilic-hydrophobic balance of mixed bile salt solutions. J Lipid Res. 1989;30(5):719–30.
45. Guldutuna S, Zimmer G, Imhof M, Bhatti S, You T, Leuschner U. Molecular aspects of membrane stabilization by ursodeoxycholate [see comment]. Gastroenterology. 1993;104 (6):1736–44.
46. Guicciardi ME, Gores GJ. Apoptosis: a mechanism of acute and chronic liver injury. Gut. 2005;54(7):1024–33. doi:10.1136/gut.2004.053850.
47. Faubion WA, Guicciardi ME, Miyoshi H, Bronk SF, Roberts PJ, Svingen PA, et al. Toxic bile salts induce rodent hepatocyte apoptosis via direct activation of Fas. J Clin Invest. 1999;103 (1):137–45. doi:10.1172/JCI4765.
48. Rodrigues CM, Fan G, Wong PY, Kren BT, Steer CJ. Ursodeoxycholic acid may inhibit deoxycholic acid-induced apoptosis by modulating mitochondrial transmembrane potential and reactive oxygen species production. Mol Med. 1998;4(3):165–78.
49. Botla R, Spivey JR, Aguilar H, Bronk SF, Gores GJ. Ursodeoxycholate (UDCA) inhibits the mitochondrial membrane permeability transition induced by glycochenodeoxycholate: a mechanism of UDCA cytoprotection. J Pharmacol Exp Ther. 1995;272(2):930–8.
50. Schoemaker MH, Conde de la Rosa L, Buist-Homan M, Vrenken TE, Havinga R, Poelstra K, et al. Tauroursodeoxycholic acid protects rat hepatocytes from bile acid-induced apoptosis via activation of survival pathways. Hepatology. 2004;39(6):1563–73. doi:10.1002/hep.20246.
51. Beuers U, Bilzer M, Chittattu A, Kullak-Ublick GA, Keppler D, Paumgartner G, et al. Tauroursodeoxycholic acid inserts the apical conjugate export pump, Mrp2, into canalicular membranes and stimulates organic anion secretion by protein kinase C-dependent mechanisms in cholestatic rat liver. Hepatology. 2001;33(5):1206–16. doi:10.1053/jhep.2001.24034.
52. Kitani K, Ohta M, Kanai S. Tauroursodeoxycholate prevents biliary protein excretion induced by other bile salts in the rat. Am J Physiol. 1985;248(4 Pt 1):G407–17.
53. Jazrawi RP, de Caestecker JS, Goggin PM, Britten AJ, Joseph AE, Maxwell JD, et al. Kinetics of hepatic bile acid handling in cholestatic liver disease: effect of ursodeoxycholic acid. Gastroenterology. 1994;106(1):134–42.
54. Poupon RE, Chretien Y, Poupon R, Paumgartner G. Serum bile acids in primary biliary cirrhosis: effect of ursodeoxycholic acid therapy. Hepatology. 1993;17(4):599–604.

55. Paulusma CC, Bosma PJ, Zaman GJ, Bakker CT, Otter M, Scheffer GL, et al. Congenital jaundice in rats with a mutation in a multidrug resistance-associated protein gene. Science. 1996;271(5252):1126–8.
56. Ito K, Suzuki H, Hirohashi T, Kume K, Shimizu T, Sugiyama Y. Functional analysis of a canalicular multispecific organic anion transporter cloned from rat liver. J Biol Chem. 1998;273(3):1684–8.
57. Dombrowski F, Stieger B, Beuers U. Tauroursodeoxycholic acid inserts the bile salt export pump into canalicular membranes of cholestatic rat liver. Lab Invest J Tech Methods Pathol. 2006;86(2):166–74. doi:10.1038/labinvest.3700371.
58. Ikebuchi Y, Shimizu H, Ito K, Yoshikado T, Yamanashi Y, Takada T, et al. Ursodeoxycholic acid stimulates the formation of the bile canalicular network. Biochem Pharmacol. 2012;84 (7):925–35. doi:10.1016/j.bcp.2012.07.008.
59. Roma MG, Toledo FD, Boaglio AC, Basiglio CL, Crocenzi FA, Sanchez Pozzi EJ. Ursodeoxycholic acid in cholestasis: linking action mechanisms to therapeutic applications. Clin Sci. 2011;121(12):523–44. doi:10.1042/CS20110184.
60. Poupon RE, Poupon R, Balkau B. Ursodiol for the long-term treatment of primary biliary cirrhosis. The UDCA-PBC Study Group. N Engl J Med. 1994;330(19):1342–7. doi:10.1056/NEJM199405123301903.
61. Yoshikawa M, Tsujii T, Matsumura K, Yamao J, Matsumura Y, Kubo R, et al. Immunomodulatory effects of ursodeoxycholic acid on immune responses. Hepatology. 1992;16 (2):358–64.
62. Terasaki S, Nakanuma Y, Ogino H, Unoura M, Kobayashi K. Hepatocellular and biliary expression of HLA antigens in primary biliary cirrhosis before and after ursodeoxycholic acid therapy. Am J Gastroenterol. 1991;86(9):1194–9.
63. Calmus Y, Gane P, Rouger P, Poupon R. Hepatic expression of class I and class II major histocompatibility complex molecules in primary biliary cirrhosis: effect of ursodeoxycholic acid. Hepatology. 1990;11(1):12–5.
64. Tanaka H, Makino Y, Miura T, Hirano F, Okamoto K, Komura K, et al. Ligand-independent activation of the glucocorticoid receptor by ursodeoxycholic acid. Repression of IFN-gamma-induced MHC class II gene expression via a glucocorticoid receptor-dependent pathway. J Immunol. 1996;156(4):1601–8.
65. van Milligen de Wit AW, Kuiper H, Camoglio L, van Bracht J, Jones EA, Tytgat GN, et al. Does ursodeoxycholic acid mediate immunomodulatory and anti-inflammatory effects in patients with primary sclerosing cholangitis? Eur J Gastroenterol Hepatol. 1999;11 (2):129–36.
66. Lindor KD, Kowdley KV, Heathcote EJ, Harrison ME, Jorgensen R, Angulo P, et al. Ursodeoxycholic acid for treatment of nonalcoholic steatohepatitis: results of a randomized trial. Hepatology. 2004;39(3):770–8. doi:10.1002/hep.20092.
67. Dufour JF, Oneta CM, Gonvers JJ, Bihl F, Cerny A, Cereda JM, et al. Randomized placebo-controlled trial of ursodeoxycholic acid with vitamin e in nonalcoholic steatohepatitis. Clin Gastroenterol Hepatol. 2006;4(12):1537–43. doi:10.1016/j.cgh.2006.09.025.
68. Leuschner UF, Lindenthal B, Herrmann G, Arnold JC, Rossle M, Cordes HJ, et al. High-dose ursodeoxycholic acid therapy for nonalcoholic steatohepatitis: a double-blind, randomized, placebo-controlled trial. Hepatology. 2010;52(2):472–9. doi:10.1002/hep.23727.
69. Ratziu V, de Ledinghen V, Oberti F, Mathurin P, Wartelle-Bladou C, Renou C, et al. A randomized controlled trial of high-dose ursodesoxycholic acid for nonalcoholic steatohepatitis. J Hepatol. 2011;54(5):1011–9. doi:10.1016/j.jhep.2010.08.030.
70. Namisaki T, Noguchi R, Moriya K, Kitade M, Aihara Y, Douhara A, et al. Beneficial effects of combined ursodeoxycholic acid and angiotensin-II type 1 receptor blocker on hepatic fibrogenesis in a rat model of nonalcoholic steatohepatitis. J Gastroenterol. 2015; doi:10.1007/s00535-015-1104-x.

71. Centuori SM, Martinez JD. Differential regulation of EGFR-MAPK signaling by deoxycholic acid (DCA) and ursodeoxycholic acid (UDCA) in colon cancer. Dig Dis Sci. 2014;59 (10):2367–80. doi:10.1007/s10620-014-3190-7.
72. Payne CM, Crowley-Skillicorn C, Bernstein C, Holubec H, Moyer MP, Bernstein H. Hydrophobic bile acid-induced micronuclei formation, mitotic perturbations, and decreases in spindle checkpoint proteins: relevance to genomic instability in colon carcinogenesis. Nutr Cancer. 2010;62(6):825–40. doi:10.1080/01635581003695756.
73. Qiao D, Stratagouleas ED, Martinez JD. Activation and role of mitogen-activated protein kinases in deoxycholic acid-induced apoptosis. Carcinogenesis. 2001;22(1):35–41.
74. Im E, Martinez JD. Ursodeoxycholic acid (UDCA) can inhibit deoxycholic acid (DCA)-induced apoptosis via modulation of EGFR/Raf-1/ERK signaling in human colon cancer cells. J Nutr. 2004;134(2):483–6.
75. Earnest DL, Holubec H, Wali RK, Jolley CS, Bissonette M, Bhattacharyya AK, et al. Chemoprevention of azoxymethane-induced colonic carcinogenesis by supplemental dietary ursodeoxycholic acid. Cancer Res. 1994;54(19):5071–4.
76. Ikegami T, Matsuzaki Y, Shoda J, Kano M, Hirabayashi N, Tanaka N. The chemopreventive role of ursodeoxycholic acid in azoxymethane-treated rats: suppressive effects on enhanced group II phospholipase A2 expression in colonic tissue. Cancer Lett. 1998;134(2):129–39.
77. Narisawa T, Fukaura Y, Terada K, Sekiguchi H. Inhibitory effects of ursodeoxycholic acid on N-methylnitrosourea-induced colon carcinogenesis and colonic mucosal telomerase activity in F344 rats. J Exp Clin Cancer Res: CR. 1999;18(2):259–66.
78. Kurtz WJ, Guldutuna S, Leuschner U. Differing effect of chenodeoxycholic acid and ursodeoxycholic acid on bile acids in rat colonic wall and contents. Tokai J Exp Clin Med. 1988;13(2):91–7.
79. Serfaty L, De Leusse A, Rosmorduc O, Desaint B, Flejou JF, Chazouilleres O, et al. Ursodeoxycholic acid therapy and the risk of colorectal adenoma in patients with primary biliary cirrhosis: an observational study. Hepatology. 2003;38(1):203–9. doi:10.1053/jhep.2003.50311.
80. Pardi DS, Loftus Jr EV, Kremers WK, Keach J, Lindor KD. Ursodeoxycholic acid as a chemopreventive agent in patients with ulcerative colitis and primary sclerosing cholangitis. Gastroenterology. 2003;124(4):889–93. doi:10.1053/gast.2003.50156.
81. Alberts DS, Martinez ME, Hess LM, Einspahr JG, Green SB, Bhattacharyya AK, et al. Phase III trial of ursodeoxycholic acid to prevent colorectal adenoma recurrence. J Natl Cancer Inst. 2005;97(11):846–53. doi:10.1093/jnci/dji144.
82. Thompson PA, Wertheim BC, Roe DJ, Ashbeck EL, Jacobs ET, Lance P, et al. Gender modifies the effect of ursodeoxycholic acid in a randomized controlled trial in colorectal adenoma patients. Cancer Prev Res. 2009;2(12):1023–30. doi:10.1158/1940-6207.CAPR-09-0234.
83. Trauner M, Halilbasic E, Claudel T, Steinacher D, Fuchs C, Moustafa T, et al. Potential of nor-ursodeoxycholic acid in cholestatic and metabolic disorders. Dig Dis. 2015;33(3):433–9. doi:10.1159/000371904.
84. Hofmann AF, Zakko SF, Lira M, Clerici C, Hagey LR, Lambert KK, et al. Novel biotransformation and physiological properties of norursodeoxycholic acid in humans. Hepatology. 2005;42(6):1391–8. doi:10.1002/hep.20943.
85. Fickert P, Wagner M, Marschall HU, Fuchsbichler A, Zollner G, Tsybrovskyy O, et al. 24-norUrsodeoxycholic acid is superior to ursodeoxycholic acid in the treatment of sclerosing cholangitis in Mdr2 (Abcb4) knockout mice. Gastroenterology. 2006;130(2):465–81. doi:10.1053/j.gastro.2005.10.018.
86. Fickert P, Pollheimer MJ, Silbert D, Moustafa T, Halilbasic E, Krones E, et al. Differential effects of norUDCA and UDCA in obstructive cholestasis in mice. J Hepatol. 2013;58 (6):1201–8. doi:10.1016/j.jhep.2013.01.026.
87. Ruetz S, Gros P. Phosphatidylcholine translocase: a physiological role for the mdr2 gene. Cell. 1994;77(7):1071–81.

88. Deleuze JF, Jacquemin E, Dubuisson C, Cresteil D, Dumont M, Erlinger S, et al. Defect of multidrug-resistance 3 gene expression in a subtype of progressive familial intrahepatic cholestasis. Hepatology. 1996;23(4):904–8. doi:10.1002/hep.510230435.
89. Denk GU, Maitz S, Wimmer R, Rust C, Invernizzi P, Ferdinandusse S, et al. Conjugation is essential for the anticholestatic effect of NorUrsodeoxycholic acid in taurolithocholic acid-induced cholestasis in rat liver. Hepatology. 2010;52(5):1758–68. doi:10.1002/hep.23911.
90. Inagaki T, Choi M, Moschetta A, Peng L, Cummins CL, McDonald JG, et al. Fibroblast growth factor 15 functions as an enterohepatic signal to regulate bile acid homeostasis. Cell Metab. 2005;2(4):217–25. doi:10.1016/j.cmet.2005.09.001.
91. Kurosu H, Choi M, Ogawa Y, Dickson AS, Goetz R, Eliseenkova AV, et al. Tissue-specific expression of beta Klotho and fibroblast growth factor (FGF) receptor Isoforms determines metabolic activity of FGF19 and FGF21. J Biol Chem. 2007;282(37):26687–95. doi:10.1074/jbc.M704165200.
92. Okuwaki M, Takada T, Iwayanagi Y, Koh S, Kariya Y, Fujii H, et al. LXR alpha transactivates mouse organic solute transporter alpha and beta via IR-1 elements shared with FXR. Pharm Res. 2007;24(2):390–8. doi:10.1007/s11095-006-9163-6.
93. Calkin AC, Tontonoz P. Transcriptional integration of metabolism by the nuclear sterol-activated receptors LXR and FXR. Nat Rev Mol Cell Biol. 2012;13(4):213–24. doi:10.1038/nrm3312.
94. Keitel V, Donner M, Winandy S, Kubitz R, Haussinger D. Expression and function of the bile acid receptor TGR5 in Kupffer cells. Biochem Biophys Res Commun. 2008;372(1):78–84. doi:10.1016/j.bbrc.2008.04.171.
95. Thomas C, Gioiello A, Noriega L, Strehle A, Oury J, Rizzo G, et al. TGR5-mediated bile acid sensing controls glucose homeostasis. Cell Metab. 2009;10(3):167–77. doi:10.1016/j.cmet.2009.08.001.
96. Katsuma S, Hirasawa A, Tsujimoto G. Bile acids promote glucagon-like peptide-1 secretion through TGR5 in a murine enteroendocrine cell line STC-1. Biochem Biophys Res Commun. 2005;329(1):386–90. doi:10.1016/j.bbrc.2005.01.0139.
97. Watanabe M, Houten SM, Mataki C, Christoffolete MA, Kim BW, Sato H, et al. Bile acids induce energy expenditure by promoting intracellular thyroid hormone activation. Nature. 2006;439(7075):484–9. doi:10.1038/nature04330.
98. Pellicciari R, Fiorucci S, Camaioni E, Clerici C, Costantino G, Maloney PR, et al. 6 alpha-ethyl-chenodeoxycholic acid (6-ECDCA), a potent and selective FXR agonist endowed with anticholestatic activity. J Med Chem. 2002;45(17):3569–72. doi:Unsp Jm025529g doi:10.1021/Jm025529g.
99. Pellicciari R, Gioiello A, Macchiarulo A, Thomas C, Rosatelli E, Natalini B, et al. Discovery of 6 alpha-Ethyl-23(S)-methylcholic acid (S-EMCA, INT-777) as a potent and selective agonist for the TGR5 receptor, a novel target for diabesity. J Med Chem. 2009;52(24):7958–61. doi:10.1021/jm901390p.
100. Rizzo G, Passeri D, De Franco F, Ciaccioli G, Donadio L, Rizzo G, et al. Functional characterization of the semisynthetic bile acid derivative INT-767, a dual farnesoid X receptor and TGR5 agonist. Mol Pharmacol. 2010;78(4):617–30. doi:10.1124/mol.110.064501.
101. Fiorucci S, Distrutti E, Ricci P, Giuliano V, Donini A, Baldelli F. Targeting FXR in cholestasis: hype or hope. Expert Opin Ther Targets. 2014;18(12):1449–59. doi:10.1517/14728222.2014.956087.
102. Hirschfield GM, Mason A, Luketic V, Lindor K, Gordon SC, Mayo M, et al. Efficacy of obeticholic acid in patients with primary biliary cirrhosis and inadequate response to ursodeoxycholic acid. Gastroenterology. 2015;148(4):751–U347. doi:10.1053/j.gastro.2014.12.005.
103. Neuschwander-Tetri BA, Loomba R, Sanyal AJ, Lavine JE, Van Natta ML, Abdelmalek MF, et al. Farnesoid X nuclear receptor ligand obeticholic acid for non-cirrhotic, non-alcoholic

steatohepatitis (FLINT): a multicentre, randomised, placebo-controlled trial. Lancet. 2015;385(9972):956–65. doi:10.1016/S0140-6736(14)61933-4.

104. Alemi F, Kwon E, Poole DP, Lieu T, Lyo V, Cattaruzza F, et al. The TGR5 receptor mediates bile acid-induced itch and analgesia. J Clin Investig. 2013;123(4):1513–30. doi:10.1172/JCI64551.
105. Makishima M, Lu TT, Xie W, Whitfield GK, Domoto H, Evans RM, et al. Vitamin D receptor as an intestinal bile acid sensor. Science. 2002;296(5571):1313–6. doi:10.1126/science.1070477.
106. Staudinger JL, Goodwin B, Jones SA, Hawkins-Brown D, MacKenzie KI, LaTour A, et al. The nuclear receptor PXR is a lithocholic acid sensor that protects against liver toxicity. Proc Natl Acad Sci USA. 2001;98(6):3369–74. doi:10.1073/pnas.051551698.
107. Out C, Groen AK, Brufau G. Bile acid sequestrants: more than simple resins. Curr Opin Lipidol. 2012;23(1):43–55. doi:10.1097/MOL.0b013e32834f0ef3.
108. Grundy SM, Ahrens EH, Salen G. Interruption of enterohepatic circulation of bile acids in man – comparative effects of cholestyramine and ileal exclusion on cholesterol metabolism. J Lab Clin Med. 1971;78(1):94.
109. Herrema H, Meissner M, van Dijk TH, Brufau G, Boverhof R, Oosterveer MH, et al. Bile salt sequestration induces hepatic de novo lipogenesis through farnesoid X receptor- and liver X receptor alpha-controlled metabolic pathways in mice. Hepatology. 2010;51(3):806–16. doi:10.1002/hep.23408.
110. Sato R. Sterol metabolism and SREBP activation. Arch Biochem Biophys. 2010;501(2):177–81. doi:10.1016/j.abb.2010.06.004.
111. Couture P, Lamarche B. Ezetimibe and bile acid sequestrants: impact on lipoprotein metabolism and beyond. Curr Opin Lipidol. 2013;24(3):227–32. doi:10.1097/MOL.0b013e3283613a55.
112. Rosenblum SB, Huynh T, Afonso A, Davis HR, Yumibe N, Clader JW, et al. Discovery of 1-(4-fluorophenyl)-(3R)-[3-(4-fluorophenyl)-(3S)-hydroxypropyl]-(4S)-(4-hydroxyphenyl)-2-azetidinone (SCH 58235): a designed, potent, orally active inhibitor of cholesterol absorption. J Med Chem. 1998;41(6):973–80. doi:10.1021/Jm970701f.
113. Altmann SW, Davis HR, Zhu LJ, Yao XR, Hoos LM, Tetzloff G, et al. Niemann-Pick C1 like 1 protein is critical for intestinal cholesterol absorption. Science. 2004;303(5661):1201–4. doi:10.1126/Science.1093131.
114. Yamanashi Y, Takada T, Suzuki H. Niemann-Pick C1-like 1 overexpression facilitates ezetimibe-sensitive cholesterol and beta-sitosterol uptake in CaCo-2 cells. J Pharmacol Exp Ther. 2007;320(2):559–64. doi:10.1124/jpet.106.114181.
115. Ventimiglia JB, Levesque MC, Chang TY. Preparation and characterization of unilamellar vesicles from cholate phospholipid micelle treated with cholestyramine. Anal Biochem. 1986;157(2):323–30. doi:10.1016/0003-2697(86)90633-0.
116. Garg A, Grundy SM. Cholestyramine therapy for dyslipidemia in non-insulin-dependent diabetes-mellitus – a short-term, double-blind. Crossover Trial Ann Intern Med. 1994;121(6):416–22.
117. Handelsman Y, Goldberg RB, Garvey WT, Fonseca VA, Rosenstock J, Jones MR, et al. Colesevelam hydrochloride to treat hypercholesterolemia and improve glycemia in prediabetes: a randomized. Prospect Study Endocrinol Pract. 2010;16(4):617–28. doi:10.4158/EP10129.OR.
118. Yamakawa T, Takano T, Utsunomiya H, Kadonosono K, Okamura A. Effect of colestimide therapy for glycemic control in type 2 diabetes mellitus with hypercholesterolemia. Endocr J. 2007;54(1):53–8. doi:10.1507/Endocrj.K05-098.
119. Chen LH, McNulty J, Anderson D, Liu YP, Nystrom C, Bullard S, et al. Cholestyramine reverses hyperglycemia and enhances glucose-stimulated glucagon-like peptide 1 release in Zucker diabetic fatty rats. J Pharmacol Exp Ther. 2010;334(1):164–70. doi:10.1124/jpet.110.166892.

120. Shang Q, Saumoy M, Holst JJ, Salen G, Xu GR. Colesevelam improves insulin resistance in a diet-induced obesity (F-DIO) rat model by increasing the release of GLP-1. Am J Physiol-Gastrointest Liver. 2010;298(3):G419–G24. doi:10.1152/ajpgi.00362.2009.
121. Suzuki T, Oba K, Igari Y, Matsumura N, Watanabe K, Futami-Suda S, et al. Colestimide lowers plasma glucose levels and increases plasma glucagon-like PEPTIDE-1 (7-36) levels in patients with type 2 diabetes mellitus complicated by hypercholesterolemia. J Nippon Med Sch Nippon Ika Daigaku Zasshi. 2007;74(5):338–43.
122. Harach T, Pols TWH, Nomura M, Maida A, Watanabe M, Auwerx J et al. TGR5 potentiates GLP-1 secretion in response to anionic exchange resins. Sci Rep-Uk. 2012;2. doi:Artn 430, 10.1038/Srep00430.
123. Prawitt J, Abdelkarim M, Stroeve JHM, Popescu I, Duez H, Velagapudi VR, et al. Farnesoid X receptor deficiency improves glucose homeostasis in mouse models of obesity. Diabetes. 2011;60(7):1861–71. doi:10.2337/db11-0030.
124. Li F, Jiang CT, Krausz KW, Li YF, Albert I, Hao HP et al. Microbiome remodelling leads to inhibition of intestinal farnesoid X receptor signalling and decreased obesity. Nat Commun. 2013;4. doi:Artn 2384, 10.1038/Ncomms3384.
125. Fang S, Suh JM, Reilly SM, Yu E, Osborn O, Lackey D, et al. Intestinal FXR agonism promotes adipose tissue browning and reduces obesity and insulin resistance. Nat Med. 2015;21(2):71–7. doi:10.1038/nm.3760.
126. Trabelsi MS, Daoudi M, Prawitt J, Ducastel S, Touche V, Sayin SI et al. Farnesoid X receptor inhibits glucagon-like peptide-1 production by enteroendocrine L cells. Nat Commun. 2015;6. doi:Artn 7629, 10.1038/Ncomms8629.
127. Narushima K, Takada T, Yamanashi Y, Suzuki H. Niemann-pick C1-like 1 mediates alpha-tocopherol transport. Mol Pharmacol. 2008;74(1):42–9. doi:10.1124/mol.107.043034.
128. Takada T, Suzuki H. Molecular mechanisms of membrane transport of vitamin E. Mol Nutr Food Res. 2010;54(5):616–22. doi:10.1002/mnfr.200900481.
129. Takada T, Yamanashi Y, Konishi K, Yamamoto T, Toyoda Y, Masuo Y, et al. NPC1L1 is a key regulator of intestinal vitamin K absorption and a modulator of warfarin therapy. Sci Transl Med. 2015;7(275):275ra23. doi:10.1126/scitranslmed.3010329.
130. Watanabe M, Houten SM, Wang L, Moschetta A, Mangelsdorf DJ, Heyman RA, et al. Bile acids lower triglyceride levels via a pathway involving FXR, SHP, and SREBP-1c. J Clin Invest. 2004;113(10):1408–18. doi:10.1172/JCI21025.
131. Pineda Torra I, Claudel T, Duval C, Kosykh V, Fruchart JC, Staels B. Bile acids induce the expression of the human peroxisome proliferator-activated receptor alpha gene via activation of the farnesoid X receptor. Mol Endocrinol. 2003;17(2):259–72. doi:10.1210/me.2002-0120.
132. Kariya Y, Honma M, Suzuki H. Systems-based understanding of pharmacological responses with combinations of multidisciplinary methodologies. Biopharm Drug Dispos. 2013;34 (9):489–507. doi:10.1002/bdd.1865.
133. Brufau G, Stellaard F, Prado K, Bloks VW, Jonkers E, Boverhof R, et al. Improved glycemic control with colesevelam treatment in patients with type 2 diabetes is not directly associated with changes in bile acid metabolism. Hepatology. 2010;52(4):1455–64. doi:10.1002/hep.23831.
134. The Lipid Research Clinics Coronary Primary Prevention Trial results. I. Reduction in incidence of coronary heart disease. Jama. 1984;251(3):351–64.
135. Brensike JF, Levy RI, Kelsey SF, Passamani ER, Richardson JM, Loh IK, et al. Effects of therapy with cholestyramine on progression of coronary arteriosclerosis: results of the NHLBI Type II Coronary Intervention Study. Circulation. 1984;69(2):313–24.
136. Hunninghake DB, Stein EA, Bremner WF, Greenland P, Demke DM, Oliphant TH. Dose – response study of colestipol tablets in patients with moderate hypercholesterolemia. Am J Ther. 1995;2(3):180–9.
137. Insull Jr W, Toth P, Mullican W, Hunninghake D, Burke S, Donovan JM, et al. Effectiveness of colesevelam hydrochloride in decreasing LDL cholesterol in patients with primary

hypercholesterolemia: a 24-week randomized controlled trial. Mayo Clin Proc. 2001;76 (10):971–82. doi:10.4065/76.10.971.
138. Denke MA, Grundy SM. Efficacy of low-dose cholesterol-lowering drug therapy in men with moderate hypercholesterolemia. Arch Intern Med. 1995;155(4):393–9.
139. Suzuki T, Oba K, Igari Y, Watanabe K, Matsumura N, Futami-Suda S, et al. Effects of bile-acid-binding resin (colestimide) on blood glucose and visceral fat in Japanese patients with type 2 diabetes mellitus and hypercholesterolemia: an open-label, randomized, case-control, crossover study. J Diabetes Complicat. 2012;26(1):34–9. doi:10.1016/j.jdiacomp.2011.11.008.
140. Brown G, Albers JJ, Fisher LD, Schaefer SM, Lin JT, Kaplan C, et al. Regression of coronary artery disease as a result of intensive lipid-lowering therapy in men with high levels of apolipoprotein B. N Engl J Med. 1990;323(19):1289–98. doi:10.1056/NEJM199011083231901.
141. Hunninghake D, Insull Jr W, Toth P, Davidson D, Donovan JM, Burke SK. Coadministration of colesevelam hydrochloride with atorvastatin lowers LDL cholesterol additively. Atherosclerosis. 2001;158(2):407–16.
142. Davidson MH, Toth P, Weiss S, McKenney J, Hunninghake D, Isaacsohn J, et al. Low-dose combination therapy with colesevelam hydrochloride and lovastatin effectively decreases low-density lipoprotein cholesterol in patients with primary hypercholesterolemia. Clin Cardiol. 2001;24(6):467–74.
143. Knapp HH, Schrott H, Ma P, Knopp R, Chin B, Gaziano JM, et al. Efficacy and safety of combination simvastatin and colesevelam in patients with primary hypercholesterolemia. Am J Med. 2001;110(5):352–60.
144. Bays H, Rhyne J, Abby S, Lai YL, Jones M. Lipid-lowering effects of colesevelam HCl in combination with ezetimibe. Curr Med Res Opin. 2006;22(11):2191–200. doi:10.1185/030079906X148436.
145. McKenney J, Jones M, Abby S. Safety and efficacy of colesevelam hydrochloride in combination with fenofibrate for the treatment of mixed hyperlipidemia. Curr Med Res Opin. 2005;21(9):1403–12. doi:10.1185/030079905X59157.
146. Handelsman Y, Goldberg RB, Garvey WT, Fonseca VA, Rosenstock J, Jones MR, et al. Colesevelam hydrochloride to treat hypercholesterolemia and improve glycemia in prediabetes: a randomized, prospective study. Endocr Pract. 2010;16(4):617–28. doi:10.4158/EP10129.OR.
147. Garg A, Grundy SM. Cholestyramine therapy for dyslipidemia in non-insulin-dependent diabetes mellitus. A short-term, double-blind, crossover trial. Ann Intern Med. 1994;121 (6):416–22.
148. Bays HE, Goldberg RB, Truitt KE, Jones MR. Colesevelam hydrochloride therapy in patients with type 2 diabetes mellitus treated with metformin: glucose and lipid effects. Arch Intern Med. 2008;168(18):1975–83. doi:10.1001/archinte.168.18.1975.
149. Fonseca VA, Rosenstock J, Wang AC, Truitt KE, Jones MR. Colesevelam HCl improves glycemic control and reduces LDL cholesterol in patients with inadequately controlled type 2 diabetes on sulfonylurea-based therapy. Diabetes Care. 2008;31(8):1479–84. doi:10.2337/dc08-0283.

Part II
Bile Acids and Diseases

Chapter 6
Bile Acids and Gallstones: Epidemiology, Pathogenesis, Diagnosis, and Management

Susumu Tazuma

Abstract Gallstone disease is a major health problem in the world. There are two major types of stones, cholesterol stones and pigment stones, classified by dominant constituents such as cholesterol and/or bilirubin. Cholesterol stones and black pigment stones are primarily formed in the gallbladder, whereas brown pigment stones are frequently formed in biliary tracts. Since bile acids are dictating the solubility of cholesterol and somehow bilirubin in bile, the gallstone pathogenesis is based, at least in part, upon the defect of bile acid metabolism. In this chapter, pathogenesis and clinical management of gallstone diseases are summarized.

Keywords Cholesterol gallstone • Pigment gallstone • Common bile stone • Bile acid • Cholesterol • Phospholipids • Bilirubin • ATP-dependent binding cassette transporters • Nuclear receptors

6.1 Introduction

Gallstone disease is a major health problem worldwide. Based upon various surveys, it is known to have an extremely high prevalence in American Indians and Northern Europeans, fairly lower in European and American whites, intermediate in Asians and black Americans, and quite low in black Africans [1, 2]. Gender dominancy varies, and a recent survey in Japan reveals the male predominance in overall prevalence, despite the female dominancy being evident in the 1990s [3]. In addition, an increased overall mortality has recently been reported in those with gallstones in the United States, and main causes of death are diabetes and cardiovascular diseases, but not cancers [4]. Another intensive interest of this report is that cholecystectomy increases the mortality as an independent risk factor. Taken together, gallstone pathogenesis is based presumably upon both immutable and

S. Tazuma (✉)
Department of General Medicine, Hiroshima University Hospital, Graduate School of Biomedical & Health Sciences, Hiroshima University, 1-2-3 Kasumi, Minami-ku, Hiroshima 734-8551, Japan
e-mail: stazuma@hiroshima-u.ac.jp

S. Tazuma, H. Takikawa (eds.), *Bile Acids in Gastroenterology*,
DOI 10.1007/978-4-431-56062-3_6

circumstantial factors, and therefore, clinical managements for gallstone diseases are to be modified in the light of update evidences including epidemiology.

6.2 Epidemiology, Risk Factors, and Classification

The prevalence of gallstone diseases has recently been defined in population surveys [1, 2]. The highest prevalence occurs in North American Indians such as Pima Indians with a gender distribution of 60% in women. Such a high prevalence is also evident in Europe, especially in Norway and Germany, with a female predominance, but intermediate prevalence rates occur in Asian populations. In this regard, the recent report of a nationwide survey in Japan provides the male predominance [3], and, thus, circumstantial factors are to be involved into ethnicity. Certain risk factors for gallstones are immutable, female gender, increasing age, and ethnicity/family, whereas modifiable factors are obesity, rapid weight loss, drugs, and certain diseases: liver cirrhosis, inflammatory bowel disease, and, further, total parenteral nutrition (TPN)-associated gallbladder stasis [1]. Gallstone diseases are associated with metabolic disorders and/or inappropriate nutrition and seemingly share risk factors with metabolic syndrome such as obesity and dyslipidemias [5].

Gallstone pathogenesis is multifactorial. Risk factors identified are ethnicity, genetics, advancing age, and female gender as unmodifiable. In addition, diet, physical activity, rapid weight loss, and obesity are other modifiable factors [6–13]. Gallstones are primarily classified into cholesterol stone and pigment stone according to the major constituents. Thus, defects of hepatic metabolism of lipids and organic anions lead to gallstone formation. Pigment stones appear in two major forms, "black" and "brown." Black pigment stones consist dominantly of calcium bilirubinate polymer, overproduced under hemolysis, whereas brown pigment stones are associated with biliary infections [11–13]. Cholesterol stone and black pigment stone are found frequently in the gallbladder, whereas brown pigment stones are mostly found in common bile ducts (Table 6.1). Gallstone pathogenesis is in a complex interaction of genetic and environmental risk factors.

6.3 Cholesterol Gallstone Pathogenesis

Cholesterol gallstone formation is processed by two major steps: (1) *metabolic abnormalities*, genetics and defects of lipid metabolism, and (2) *physical-chemical events*, bile cholesterol supersaturation, cholesterol crystal nucleation, and crystal growth to macroscopic stones (Table 6.2). The gallbladder and intestines play a role in these processes.

Table 6.1 Classification of gallstones based on biochemical structure

	Gallbladder stones	CBD stones
Cholesterol stone (%)	58.3	31.1
Bilirubin stone		
Black pigment stone (%)	23.7	11.8
Brown pigment stone (%)	15.9	54.3
Others (%)	2.1	2.8

Table 6.2 Cholesterol gallstone pathogenesis

Genetics and defects of lipid metabolism
↓
Bile cholesterol supersaturation
↓
Cholesterol crystal nucleation
↓
Crystal growth to macroscopic stones
↓
(Clinical symptoms)

6.3.1 Metabolic Abnormalities

Cholesterol gallstone formation is based primarily upon the defect of cholesterol homeostasis mainly in the hepatobiliary system [5–13]. Cholesterol is an insoluble molecule that is eliminated from the liver into bile through ATP-binding cassette transporter (ABC) G5/G8, and, similarly, biliary secretion of phospholipids and bile acids is mediated by ABCB4 (MDR3) and ABCB11 (BSEP), respectively (Fig. 6.1). Bile cholesterol is predominantly originated from high-density lipoprotein (HDL) fraction, and the hepatic uptake of HDL cholesterol is mediated through scavenger receptor class B type 1 (SRB1), a receptor for HDL [14–22]. Under physiological circumstances, cholesterol in bile is a solubilized bile salt micelle, which is physicochemically stabilized. Once metabolic defects occur, bile becomes metastable due to cholesterol supersaturation to promote cholesterol crystallization, the so-called nucleation, an initial step for cholesterol gallstone formation.

Bile acids are capable for solubilizing bile cholesterol by forming micelles, and such a cholesterol solubility is based upon a relative composition of cholesterol to bile acid and phospholipids. Especially, the bile acid composition in an enterohepatic circulation pool is a crucial factor to dictate potential to solubilize cholesterol. In this regard, deoxycholate, a secondary bile acid, is increased in enterohepatic circulation pool in cholesterol gallstone disease [23]. Since deoxycholate suppresses hepatic de novo synthesis of primary bile salt, biliary cholesterol secretion relatively increases to enhance bile cholesterol saturation [24]. Intestinal hypomotility induces prolonged intestinal transit times to prolong exposure time of primary bile salt, cholate, to gut microbiota to produce deoxycholate, and, therefore, this eventually attributes gallstone formation [25, 26].

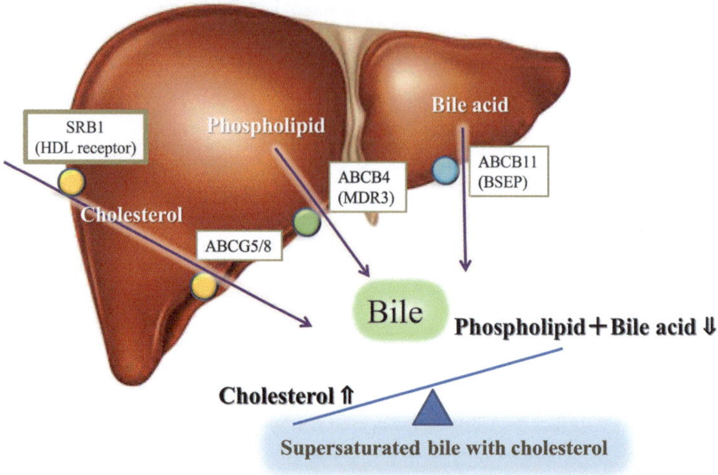

Fig. 6.1 Formation of bile supersaturated with cholesterol (Reused with permission from Ref. [87]). Bile cholesterol is predominantly originated from HDL and secreted through ABCG5/ABCG8. Excess cholesterol leads to bile supersaturation, with a relatively high ratio to phospholipids and bile acid

6.3.2 *Cholesterol Crystal Nucleation and Growth to Macroscopic Gallstones*

The cholesterol crystal nucleation process is accelerated by mucins produced and secreted by the gallbladder wall, and such a gallbladder function is mediated through arachidonate-prostanoid pathway (Fig. 6.2). The gallbladder epithelium absorbs lipids from bile in a different manner for cholesterol, phospholipid, and bile salts to reduce bile cholesterol saturation, and its impairment leads to formation of metastable bile [27, 28]. Thus, gallbladder dysfunction in motility plays a role in cholesterol gallstone formation process [28, 29], and contractility defects associated with cholesterol gallstones are attributable to excess membrane accumulation in gallbladder smooth muscle cells of bile cholesterol [30–32]. Further, increases in mucin synthesis and secretion of the gallbladder, mediated by arachidonate-prostanoid pathway, accelerate cholesterol crystallization and growth, and eventually macroscopic gallstones form in the gallbladder cavity.

Studies in model and native bile have suggested the presence of two distinct mechanisms for cholesterol crystallization [33]. In bile with relatively high phosphatidylcholine contents, aggregation and fusion of cholesterol-rich vesicles result in the formation of multilamellar vesicles, which give rise to cholesterol monohydrate crystals [34, 35] as summarized in Fig. 6.3. At lower phosphatidylcholine contents, vesicles may become unstable and spawn anhydrous cholesterol crystals. This occurs similarly with increasing of cholesterol in composition. Such a microscopic event of cholesterol crystal nucleation in in vitro study using the

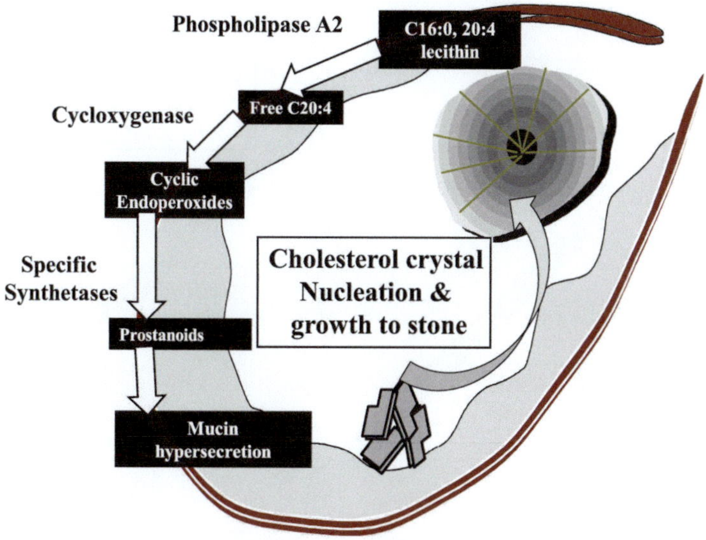

Fig. 6.2 Events for cholesterol gallstone formation process in the gallbladder (Reused with permission from Ref. [87]). Cholesterol crystal nucleation and growth are promoted by mucin hypersecretion mediated through arachidonate-prostanoid pathway

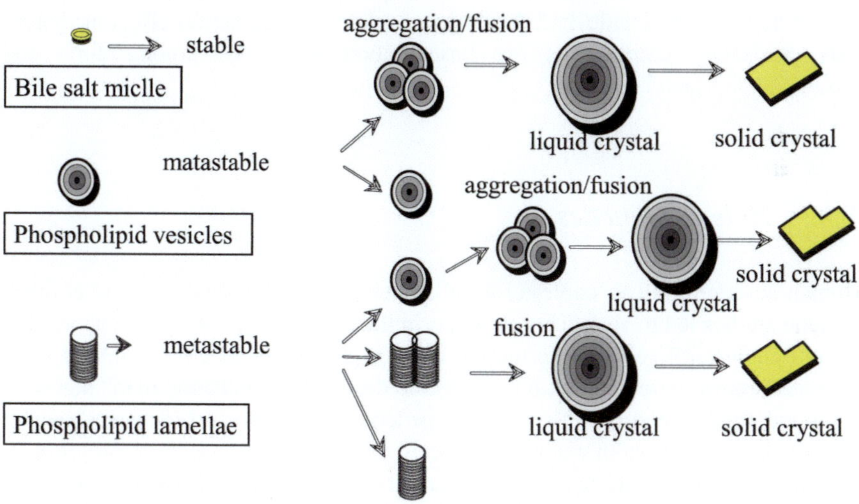

Fig. 6.3 Bile lipid particulate species and cholesterol crystallization (Reused with permission from Ref. [11])

supersaturated model bile solution is shown in Fig. 6.4. Cholesterol crystal nucleation is dictated in a balance of nucleation-effecter substances of promoters and inhibitors and protein and non-protein components [36]. Meanwhile, concanavalin Λ-binding fraction has been reported to promote cholesterol crystallization in bile

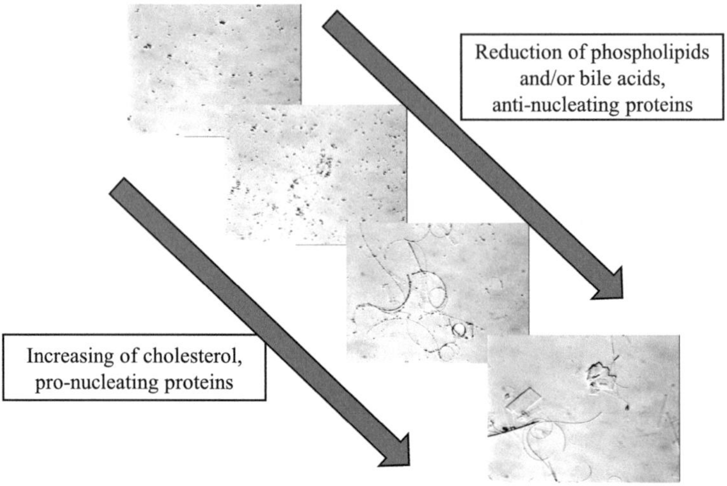

Fig. 6.4 Cholesterol crystallization in cholesterol-supersaturated bile

[37] and, thereafter, demonstrated to contain pronase-resistant glycoprotein component of the low-density protein-lipid complex, the carcinoembryonic antigen-related adhesion molecule 1 [38]. Taken together, crystallization-effecting potentials of biliary components are based upon imbalance among anti- and pro-nucleating factors.

6.3.3 Role of Genetics

Human susceptibility to cholesterol gallstones is partially under genetic control. Genetic studies led to significant progress in the characterization of *Lith* genes that control cholesterol gallstone formation in mice [39]. Only specific strains of mice form gallstones by feeding with a lithogenic diet, and a "gallstone map" has been compiled to the relationships between genetic loci, such as *Lith* genes, which control the regulation of nucleating factor expression [40]. Recent progress in genetics provides the susceptibility of heredity contribution to gallstone formation for apolipoproteins E and B and cholesterol 7alpha-hydroxylase genes [41–46]. Further, based upon understanding of the role of ABCG5 and ABCG8 in digestive systems, liver and intestine, the association of polymorphism of ABCG8 with gallstone diseases has been published [47–58]. The most studied loci are D19H, T400K, and Y54C, and a meta-analysis of the association between each locus and gallstone disease shows the strong association of D19H polymorphism with gallstone disease. T400K and Y54C polymorphism are less associated [56]. Taken together, the role of disease genetics is still to be elucidated.

6.4 Pigment Gallstone Pathogenesis

Pigment stones are divided into two major types, black pigment stone and brown pigment stone. Black pigment stones consist dominantly of calcium bilirubinate, produced increasingly under hemolysis. Black pigment gallstones are composed mostly of polymerized shape of calcium bilirubinate and formed in noninfectious gallbladder. In contrast, brown pigment stones are formed, following biliary infection of anaerobic bacteria [59]. In principle, the risk factor is biliary secretion of excess bilirubin conjugates, resulting from hemolysis, ineffective erythropoiesis, or induced enterohepatic cycling of unconjugated bilirubin in association with gallbladder hypomotility caused by diabetes mellitus, total parenteral nutrition, and truncal vagotomy [60–63].

Black pigment stones consist of calcium phosphate and/or carbonate, whereas brown pigment stones are composed of amorphous calcium salts of long-chain saturated fatty acids. In addition, cholesterol is present in both types, with a higher proportion for brown pigment stones [64], especially intrahepatic stones [7]. Also, a mixed mucin glycoprotein matrix secreted by biliary epithelial cells promotes both types of pigment gallstones on the basis of biliary hypersecretion of bilirubin conjugates and endogenous biliary β-glucuronidase hydrolysis of bilirubin conjugates in gallbladder bile to precipitate as insoluble calcium salts. Further, reactive oxygen species, secreted by gallbladder mucosa when inflamed, promote precipitation of calcium bilirubinate polymers, and, therefore, its suppression is to be of therapeutic benefit in pigment gallstone treatment.

6.5 Clinical Managements

Gallstones cause certain typical symptoms: abdominal or back pain, fever, nausea and/or vomiting, and jaundice. Colic pain at the right upper quadrant is less frequent, and considerable cases remain asymptomatic. The typical history is to be as follows: a hypochondrial pain at the right side starts following oily meal, radiating to the right scapula or shoulder, and thereafter reaches a peak level within several hour. Usually gallstone-associated pain is improved by stone moving back to original position or passing through physiological strictures, but most patients find recurrent pain within 10 years after the first attack [65]. According to the Japanese Society of Gastroenterology Practice Guidelines for gallstone diseases 2009, asymptomatic gallstone patients are not recommended to undergo therapeutics, but recommended to a conservative follow-up (Fig. 6.5) [66]. Nevertheless, cases with gallbladder wall thickness or nonfunctioning, or hard condition for image assessment, can be subjected to prophylactic cholecystectomy. Patients with increased risk for gallbladder cancer, with large stones of diameter of >3 cm, and with chronic cholecystitis such as "porcelain gallbladder" are recommended to prophylactic cholecystectomy [67, 68].

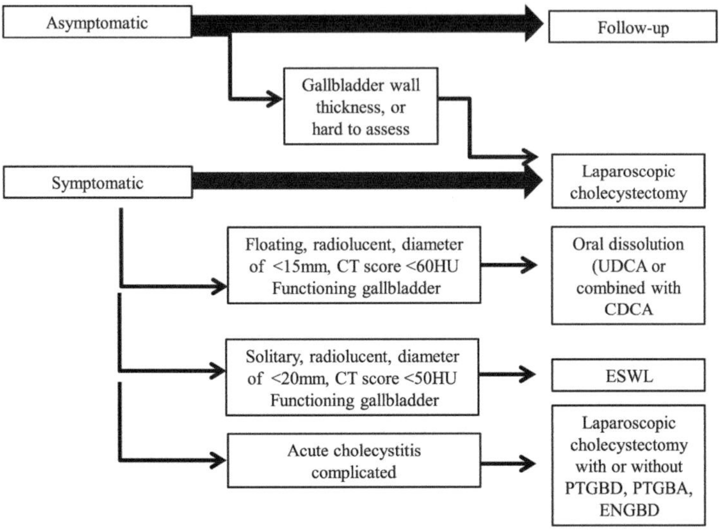

Fig. 6.5 Flowchart of therapeutic managements [66]

Symptomatic gallstone patients need treatment, and laparoscopic cholecystectomy is to be a standard modality. The US National Institutes of Health consensus conference concluded that laparoscopic cholecystectomy is safe and cost-effective compared with open cholecystectomy [69]. For cases not indicated to surgery, optional treatments are oral dissolution for cholesterol gallstones; the indication is to be floating, radiolucent, diameter of <15 mm, CT score <60 HU, and functioning gallbladder [70–74]. A representative case is successfully treated by a combination of ursodeoxycholic acid (400 mg per day) and chenodeoxycholic acid (200 mg per day) that is shown in Fig. 6.6. UDCA monotherapy is also effective in mixed-type cholesterol gallstone dissolution as shown in Fig. 6.7. The underlying mechanism(s) of such an action of bile acids is understood as the enhancement of micelle formation by CDCA and liquid formation to dissolve cholesterol by UDCA (Fig. 6.8) [75, 76]. Extracorporeal shock wave lithotripsy (ESWL) can be considered for cholesterol gallstone, solitary, radiolucent, diameter of <20 mm, CT score <50 HU, and functioning gallbladder. Of the nonsurgical treatment, gallstone recurrence after treatment together with cost-benefit analysis is the weakness with less priority compared to laparoscopic cholecystectomy [77]. Bile acid adjuvant therapy is recommended for this technique in order to shorten a treatment period. On the other hand, cases complicated with acute cholecystitis are managed according to severity, periods after onset, and physical status; laparoscopic cholecystectomy with or without biliary drainage such as percutaneous transhepatic gallbladder drainage (PTGBD), percutaneous transhepatic gallbladder aspiration (PTGBA), endoscopic nasal gallbladder drainage (ENGBD) [78–86].

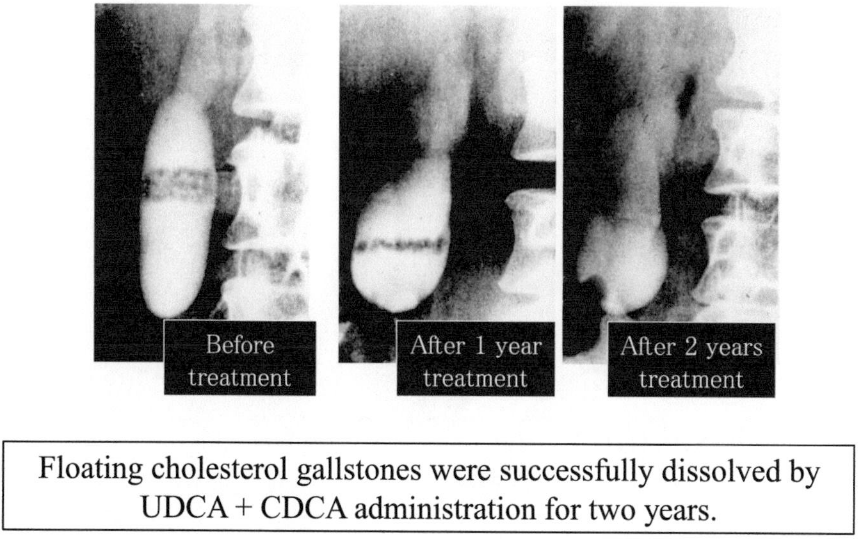

Fig. 6.6 Bile acid treatment of floating cholesterol gallstones (UDCA + CDCA combination therapy)

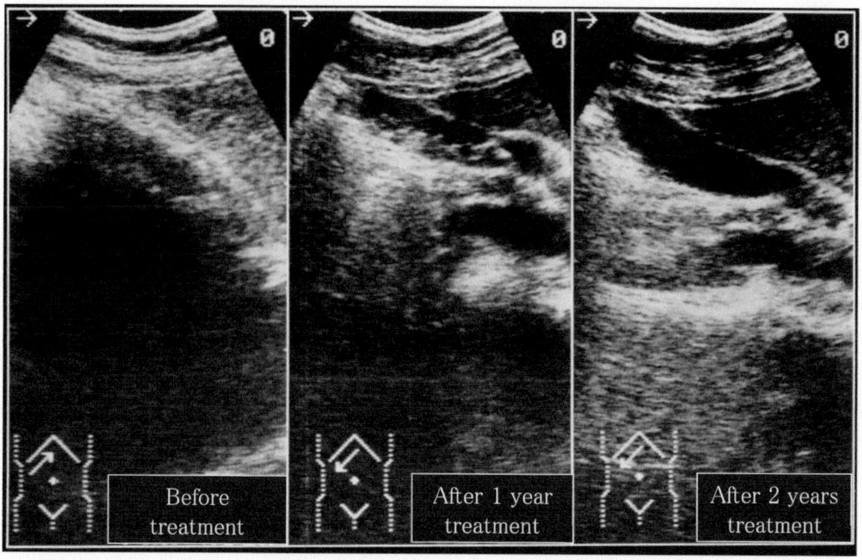

Fig. 6.7 Bile acid treatment of mixed-type cholesterol gallstones (UDCA monotherapy)

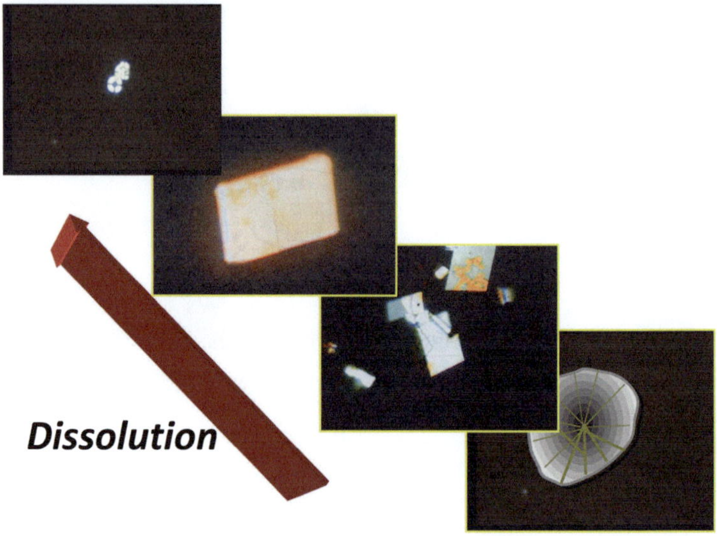

Fig. 6.8 Mechanism(s) of action of UDCA: liquid crystal formation by UDCA leads to cholesterol gallstone dissolution

6.6 Future Direction

Recent investigations provide evidences to understand underlying mechanism(s) of gallstone formation process in the aspects of physiology, physical chemistry, molecular biology, and genetics of biliary lipid metabolism, supplying ideas of future strategies for prevention and/or nonsurgical therapeutics, instead for cholecystectomy. Based upon epidemiological studies that reveal an increased overall mortality of gallstone patients in association with diabetes and cardiovascular diseases, but not cancers, this field should be shifted to handling metabolic disorders for lipids, bile acids, and other nutrients.

Acknowledgments This work was supported in part by the Health and Labour Sciences Research Grant for intrahepatic gallstones awarded to S.T.

Conflict of Interest Statement None declared.

References

1. Shaffer EA. Gallstone disease: epidemiology of gallbladder stone disease. Best Pract Res Clin Gastroenterol. 2006;20(6):981–96.
2. Stinton LM, Shaffer EA. Epidemiology of gallbladder disease: cholelithiasis and cancer. Gut Liver. 2012;6:172–87.

3. Tazuma S, Kanno K, Kubota K, Tsuyuguchi T, Kamisawa T, Isayama H, Nakagohri T, Inui K, Academic Committee of the Japan Biliary Association. Report on the 2013 national cholelithiasis survey in Japan. J Hepato-Biliary-Pancreat Sci. 2015;22(5):392–5. doi:10.1002/jhbp.206. Epub 2015 Jan 18
4. Ruhl CE, Everhart JE. Gallstone disease is associated with increased mortality in the United States. Gastroenterology. 2011;140(2):508–16.
5. Tazuma S, Kanno K, Sugiyama A, Kishikawa N. Nutritional factors (nutritional aspects) in biliary disorders: bile acid and lipid metabolism in gallstone diseases and pancreaticobiliary maljunction. J Gastroenterol Hepatol. 2013;28(Suppl 4):103–7.
6. Stinton LM, Shaffer EA. Epidemiology of gallbladder disease: cholelithiasis and cancer. Gut Liver. 2012;6(2):172–87.
7. Tazuma S. Gallstone disease: epidemiology, pathogenesis, and classification of biliary stones (common bile duct and intrahepatic). Best Pract Res Clin Gastroenterol. 2006;20(6):1075–83.
8. Shaffer EA, Small DM. Biliary lipid secretion in cholesterol gallstone disease. The effect of cholecystectomy and obesity. J Clin Invest. 1977;59:828–40.
9. Reuben A, Maton PN, Murphy GM, et al. Bile lipid secretion in obese and non-obese individuals with and without gallstones. Clin Sci. 1985;69:71–9.
10. Diehl AK. Epidemiology and natural history of gallstone disease. In: Cooper AD, editor. Gastroenterology clinics of North America. Philadelphia: W.B. Saunders; 1991. p. 1–19.
11. Tazuma S. Recent understanding of cholesterol gallstone pathogenesis: implication to non-surgical therapeutic strategy. Clin J Gastroenterol. 2008;1(3):87–92.
12. Carey MC. Pathogenesis of gallstones. Am J Surg. 1993;165:410–9.
13. Portincasa P, Moschetta A, Palasciano G. Cholesterol gallstone disease. Lancet. 2006;368 (9531):230–9.
14. Elferink RP, Groen AK. The mechanism of biliary lipid secretion and its defects. Gastroenterol Clin N Am. 1999;28:59–74.
15. de Vree JM, Jacquemin E, Sturm E, et al. Mutations in the MDR3 gene cause progressive familial intrahepatic cholestasis. Proc Natl Acad Sci U S A. 1998;95:282–7.
16. Wu JE, Basso F, Shamburek RD, et al. Hepatic ABCG5 and ABCG8 overexpression increases hepatobiliary sterol transport but does not alter aortic atherosclerosis in transgenic mice. J Biol Chem. 2004;279:22913–25.
17. Rothblat GH, de la Llera-Moya M, Atger V, et al. Cell cholesterol efflux: integration of new and old observations provides new insights. J Lipid Res. 1999;40:781–96.
18. Oram JF, Lawn RM, ABCA. The gatekeeper for eliminating excess tissue cholesterol. J Lipid Res. 2001;42:1173–9.
19. Ikemoto M, Arai H, Feng D, et al. Identification of a PDZ-domain-containing protein that interacts with the scavenger receptor class B type I. Proc Natl Acad Sci U S A. 2000;97:6538–43.
20. Silver DL, Nan W, Xiao X, et al. HDL particle uptake mediated by SR-BI results in selective sorting of HDL cholesterol from protein and polarized cholesterol secretion. J Biol Chem. 2001;276:25287–93.
21. Groen AK, Bloks VW, Bandsma RH, et al. Hepatobiliary cholesterol transport is not impaired in Abca1-null mice lacking HDL. J Clin Invest. 2001;108:843–50.
22. Drobnik W, Lindenthal B, Lieser B, et al. ATP-binding cassette transporter A1 (ABCA1) affects total body sterol metabolism. Gastroenterology. 2001;120:1203–11.
23. Marcus SN, Heaton KW. Deoxycholic acid and the pathogenesis of gall stones. Gut. 1988;29:522–33.
24. Einarsson C, Hillebrant CG, Axelson M. Effects of treatment with deoxycholic acid and chenodeoxycholic acid on the hepatic synthesis of cholesterol and bile acids in healthy subjects. Hepatology. 2001;33:1189–93.
25. Dowling RH. Review: pathogenesis of gallstones. Aliment Pharmacol Ther. 2000;14(Suppl 2):39–47.

26. Thomas LA, Veysey MJ, Bathgate T, et al. Mechanism for the transit-induced increase in colonic deoxycholic acid formation in cholesterol cholelithiasis. Gastroenterology. 2000;119:806–15.
27. Ginanni Corradini S, Ripani C, Della Guardia P, et al. The human gallbladder increases cholesterol solubility in bile by differential lipid absorption: a study using a new in vitro model of isolated intra-arterially perfused gallbladder. Hepatology. 1998;28:314–22.
28. Corradini SG, Elisei W, Giovannelli L, et al. Impaired human gallbladder lipid absorption in cholesterol gallstone disease and its effect on cholesterol solubility in bile. Gastroenterology. 2000;118:912–20.
29. Pellegrini CA, Ryan T, Broderick W, et al. Gallbladder filling and emptying during cholesterol gallstone formation in the prairie dog. A cholescintigraphic study. Gastroenterology. 1986;90:143–9.
30. Jazrawi RP, Pazzi P, Petroni ML, et al. Postprandial gallbladder motor function: refilling and turnover of bile in health and in cholelithiasis. Gastroenterology. 1995;109:582–91.
31. Chen Q, Amaral J, Biancani P, et al. Excess membrane cholesterol alters human gallbladder muscle contractility and membrane fluidity. Gastroenterology. 1999;116:678–85.
32. Chen Q, Amaral J, Oh S, et al. Gallbladder relaxation in patients with pigment and cholesterol stones. Gastroenterology. 1997;113:930–7.
33. Carey MC. Formation and growth of cholesterol gallstones: the new synthesis. In: Fromm H, Leuschner U, editors. Bile acids-cholestasis-gallstones. Dordrecht: Kluwer; 1996. p. 147–75.
34. Konikoff FM, Danino D, Weihs D, et al. Microstructural evolution of lipid aggregates in nucleating model and human biles visualized by cryogenic transmission electron microscopy. Hepatology. 2000;31:261–8.
35. Ochi H, Tazuma S, Kajiyama G. Lecithin hydrophobicity modulates the process of cholesterol crystal nucleation and growth in supersaturated model bile systems. Biochem J. 1996;318:139–44.
36. Nishioka T, Tazuma S, Yamashita G, et al. Quantitative assessment on comparative potencies of cholesterol crystal promoting factors: relation to mechanistic characterization. Biochem J. 1998;332:343–50.
37. Miquel JF, Van Der Putten J, Pimentel F, et al. Increased activity in the biliary Con A-binding fraction accounts for the difference in crystallization behavior in bile from Chilean gallstone patients compared with Dutch gallstone patients. Hepatology. 2001;33:328–32.
38. Jirsa M, Muchova L, Draberova L, et al. Carcinoembryonic antigen-related cell adhesion molecule 1 is the 85-kilodalton pronase-resistant biliary glycoprotein in the cholesterol crystallization promoting low density protein-lipid complex. Hepatology. 2001;34:1075–82.
39. Paigen K. A miracle enough: the power of mice. Nat Med. 1995;1:215–20.
40. Lammert F, Carey MC, Paigen B. Chromosomal organization of candidate genes involved in cholesterol gallstone formation: a murine gallstone map. Gastroenterology. 2001;120:221–38.
41. Marschall HU, Katsika D, Rudling M, Einarsson C. The genetic background of gallstone formation: an update. Biochem Biophys Res Commun. 2010;396:58–62.
42. Katsika D, Grjibovski A, Einarsson C, Lammert F, Lichtenstein P, et al. Genetic and environmental influences on symptomatic gallstone disease: a Swedish study of 43,141 twin pairs. Hepatology. 2005;41:1138–43.
43. Bertomeu A, Ros E, Zambon D, Vela M, Perez-Ayuso RM, et al. Apolipoprotein E polymorphism and gallstones. Gastroenterology. 1996;111:1603–10.
44. Xue P, Niu WQ, Jiang ZY, Zheng MH, Fei J. A Meta-analysis of apolipoprotein E gene epsilon2/epsilon3/epsilon4 polymorphism for gallbladder stone disease. PLoS ONE. 2012;7:e45849.
45. Jiang ZY, Han TQ, Suo GJ, Feng DX, Chen S, et al. Polymorphisms at cholesterol 7alpha-hydroxylase, apolipoproteins B and E and low density lipoprotein receptor genes in patients with gallbladder stone disease. World J Gastroenterol. 2004;10:1508–12.

46. Sanchez-Cuen J, Aguilar-Medina M, Arambula-Meraz E, Romero-Navarro J, Granados J, et al. ApoB-100, ApoE and CYP7A1 gene polymorphisms in Mexican patients with cholesterol gallstone disease. World J Gastroenterol. 2010;16:4685–90.
47. Yu L, Li-Hawkins J, Hammer RE, Berge KE, Horton JD, et al. Overexpression of ABCG5 and ABCG8 promotes biliary cholesterol secretion and reduces fractional absorption of dietary cholesterol. J Clin Invest. 2002;110:671–80.
48. Stender S, Frikke-Schmidt R, Nordestgaard BG, Tybjaerg-Hansen A. Sterol transporter adenosine triphosphate-binding cassette transporter G8, gallstones, and biliary cancer in 62,000 individuals from the general population. Hepatology. 2011;53:640–8.
49. Xu HL, Cheng JR, Andreotti G, Gao YT, Rashid A, et al. Cholesterol metabolism gene polymorphisms and the risk of biliary tract cancers and stones: a population-based case-control study in Shanghai, China. Carcinogenesis. 2011;32:58–62.
50. Srivastava A, Srivastava A, Srivastava K, Choudhuri G, Mittal B. Role of ABCG8 D19H (rs11887534) variant in gallstone susceptibility in northern India. J Gastroenterol Hepatol. 2010;25:1758–62.
51. Siddapuram SP, Mahurkar S, Duvvuru NR, Mitnala S, Guduru VR, et al. Hepatic cholesterol transporter ABCG8 polymorphisms in gallstone disease in an Indian population. J Gastroenterol Hepatol. 2010;25:1093–8.
52. Kuo KK, Shin SJ, Chen ZC, Yang YH, Yang JF, et al. Significant association of ABCG5 604Q and ABCG8 D19H polymorphisms with gallstone disease. Br J Surg. 2008;95:1005–11.
53. Buch S, Schafmayer C, Volzke H, Becker C, Franke A, et al. A genome-wide association scan identifies the hepatic cholesterol transporter ABCG8 as a susceptibility factor for human gallstone disease. Nat Genet. 2007;39:995–9.
54. Grunhage F, Acalovschi M, Tirziu S, Walier M, Wienker TF, et al. Increased gallstone risk in humans conferred by common variant of hepatic ATP-binding cassette transporter for cholesterol. Hepatology. 2007;46:793–801.
55. Wang Y, Jiang ZY, Fei J, Xin L, Cai Q, et al. ATP binding cassette G8 T400K polymorphism may affect the risk of gallstone disease among Chinese males. Clin Chim Acta. 2007;384:80–5.
56. Katsika D, Magnusson P, Krawczyk M, Grunhage F, Lichtenstein P, et al. Gallstone disease in Swedish twins: risk is associated with ABCG8 D19H genotype. J Intern Med. 2010;268:279–85.
57. von Kampen O, Buch S, Nothnagel M, Azocar L, Molina H, et al. Genetic and functional identification of the likely causative variant for cholesterol gallstone disease at the ABCG5/8 lithogenic locus. Hepatology. 2013;2013(57):2407–17.
58. Jiang Z-Y, Cai Q, Chen E-Z. Association of three common single nucleotide polymorphisms of ATP binding cassette G8 gene with gallstone disease: a meta-analysis. PLoS ONE. 2014;9(1):e87200.
59. Vítek L, Carey MC. New pathophysiological concepts underlying pathogenesis of pigment gallstones. Clin Res Hepatol Gastroenterol. 2012;36(2):122–9.
60. Schafmayer C, Hartleb J, Tepel J, Albers S, Freitag S, Volzke H, et al. Predictors of gallstone composition in 1025 symptomatic gallstones from Northern Germany. BMC Gastroenterol. 2006;6:36–44.
61. Cahalane MJ, Neubrand MW, Care MC. Physical-chemical pathogenesis of pigment gallstones. Semin Liver Dis. 1988;8:317–28.
62. Suzuki N, Nakamura Y, Kobayashi N, Sato T. On metal elements in pure pigment gallstones. Tohoku J Exp Med. 1975;116:233–40.
63. Tsunoda K, Shirai Y, Wakai T, Yokoyama N, Akazawa K, Hatakeyama K. Increased risk of cholelithiasis after esophagectomy. J Hepato-Biliary-Pancreat Surg. 2004;11:319–23.
64. Robins SJ, Fasulo JM, Patton GM. Lipids of pigment gallstones. Biochim Biophys Acta. 1982;712:21–5.

65. Tomida S, Abei M, Yamaguchi T, et al. Long-term ursodeoxycholic acid therapy is associated with reduced risk of biliary pain and acute cholecystitis in patients with gallbladder stones: a cohort analysis. Hepatology. 1999;30:6–13.
66. Japanese Society of Gastroenterology. Practice guidelines for cholelithiasis 2009 (in Japanese), Tokyo, Nankodo, 2009
67. Lowenfels AB, Walker AM, Althaus DP, Townsend G, Domellof L. Gallstone growth, size, and risk of gallbladder cancer: an interracial study. Int J Epidemiol. 1989;18:50–4.
68. Ashur H, Siegal B, Oland Y, Adam YG. Calcified gallbladder (porcelain gallbladder). Arch Surg. 1978;113:594–6.
69. National Institutes of Health Consensus Development Conference Statement on gallstones and laparoscopic cholecystectomy. Am J Surg. 1993;165:390–8
70. May GR, Sutherland LR, Shaffer EA. Efficacy of bile acid therapy for gallstone dissolution: a meta-analysis of randomized trials. Aliment Pharmacol Ther. 1993;7:139–48.
71. Podda M, Zuin M, Battezzati PM, et al. Efficacy and safety of a combination of chenodeoxycholic acid and ursodeoxycholic acid for gallstone dissolution: a comparison with ursodeoxycholic acid alone. Gastroenterology. 1989;96:222–9.
72. Grundy SM, Lan SP, Lachin J. The effects of chenodiol on biliary lipids and their association with gallstone dissolution in the National Cooperative Gallstone Study (NCGS). J Clin Invest. 1984;73:1156–66.
73. Fromm H, Roat JW, Gonzalez V, et al. Comparative efficacy and side effects of ursodeoxycholic and chenodeoxycholic acids in dissolving gallstones: a double-blind controlled study. Gastroenterology. 1983;85:1257–64.
74. Erlinger S, Le Go A, Husson JM, et al. Franco-Belgian cooperative study of ursodeoxycholic acid in the medical dissolution of gallstones: a double-blind, randomized, dose-response study, and comparison with chenodeoxycholic acid. Hepatology. 1984;4:308–14.
75. Park YH, Igimi H, Carey MC. Dissolution of human cholesterol gallstones in stimulated chenodeoxycholate-rich and ursodeoxycholate-rich biles. An in vitro study of dissolution rates and mechanisms. Gastroenterology. 1984;87:150–8.
76. Igimi H, Carey MC. Cholesterol gallstone dissolution in bile: dissolution kinetics of crystalline (anhydrate and monohydrate) cholesterol with chenodeoxycholate, ursodeoxycholate, and their glycine and taurine conjugates. J Lipid Res. 1981;22:254–70.
77. Paumgartner G, Sauter GH. Extracorporeal shock wave lithotripsy of gallstones: 20th anniversary of the first treatment. Eur J Gastroenterol Hepatol. 2005;17:525–7.
78. Yokoe M, Takada T, Strasberg SM, et al. New diagnostic criteria and severity assessment of acute cholecystitis in revised Tokyo guidelines. J Hepato-Biliary-Pancreat Sci. 2012;19:578–85.
79. Miura F, Takda T, Strasberg SM, et al. TG13 flowchart for the management of acute cholangitis and cholecystitis. J Hepato-Biliary-Pancreat Sci. 2013;20:47–54.
80. Banz V, Gsponer T, Candinas D, et al. Population-based analysis of 4113 patients with acute cholecystitis: defining the optimal time-point for laparoscopic cholecystectomy. Ann Surg. 2011;254:964–70.
81. Riall TS, Zhang D, Townsend Jr CM, et al. Failure to perform cholecystectomy for acute cholecystitis in elderly patients is associated with increased morbidity, mortality, and cost. J Am Coll Surg. 2010;210:668–77. 677–679
82. Lee SW, Yang SS, Chang CS, et al. Impact of the Tokyo guidelines on the management of patients with acute calculous cholecystitis. J Gastroenterol Hepatol. 2009;24:1857–61.
83. Moyson J, Thill V, Simoens C, et al. Laparoscopic cholecystectomy for acute cholecystitis in the elderly: a retrospective study of 100 patients. Hepato-Gastroenterology. 2008;55:1975–80.
84. Ito K, Fujita N, Noda Y, et al. Percutaneous cholecystostomy versus gallbladder aspiration for acute cholecystitis: a prospective randomized controlled trial. AJR Am J Roentgenol. 2004;183:193–6.
85. Borzellino G, de Manzoni G, Ricci F, et al. Emergency cholecystostomy and subsequent cholecystectomy for acute gallstone cholecystitis in the elderly. Br J Surg. 1999;86:1521–5.

86. Akhan O, Akinci D, Ozmen MN. Percutaneous cholecystostomy. Eur J Radiol. 2002;43:229–36.
87. Tazuma S. Statins affect gallstone diseases: Underlying mechanism(s) are to be established. Hepatol Res. 2015;45(9):939–41.

Chapter 7
Bile Acids and Cholestatic Liver Disease 1: Primary Biliary Cholangitis (PBC)

Atsushi Tanaka

Abstract Primary biliary cholangitis (PBC), formally known as primary biliary cirrhosis and recently the name was changed with keeping the abbreviation "PBC" along with a global consensus, is a chronic cholestatic liver disease, potentially resulting in liver failure. While the aspect of autoimmune disease of PBC was formally emphasized and immune reactions with lymphocytes against autoantigens were extensively investigated, the interactions between bile acids and cholangiocytes have been well clarified in this decade. Cytotoxic hydrophobic bile acids play an important role in pathogenesis of PBC via defect in the biliary HCO_3^- "umbrella." This biliary HCO_3^- "umbrella" is maintained by Cl^-/HCO_3^- exchanger (anion exchanger 2 (AE2)) located at apical surface of cholangiocytes, and accumulating evidences have indicated that lack or reduction of AE2 activities is closely associated with PBC. Treatment is targeted to cytotoxicity of hydrophobic bile acids; ursodeoxycholic acid (UDCA) exerts its effect through reduction of cytotoxicity of hydrophobic bile acids and stabilizing biliary HCO_3^- umbrella. Both bezafibrate and obeticholic acids are also capable of reducing cytotoxicity of hydrophobic bile acids. The alternative treatment is strongly awaited for patients with PBC refractory to UDCA, and targeting cytotoxicity of hydrophobic bile acids, as well as immune-based therapies, is expected to be a promising approach for new pharmacotherapy.

Keywords Ursodeoxycholic acid • Bezafibrate • Anion exchanger 2 • Obeticholic acids

7.1 Primary Biliary Cholangitis (PBC)

Primary biliary cholangitis, formally known as primary biliary cirrhosis, is a chronic and progressive cholestatic liver disease, potentially resulting in liver failure and mortality without liver transplantation [1]. PBC mainly develops in

A. Tanaka (✉)
Department of Medicine, Teikyo University School of Medicine, 2-11-1, Kaga, Itabashi-ku, Tokyo 173-8605, Japan
e-mail: a-tanaka@med.teikyo-u.ac.jp

S. Tazuma, H. Takikawa (eds.), *Bile Acids in Gastroenterology*,
DOI 10.1007/978-4-431-56062-3_7

Table 7.1 Diagnostic criteria of PBC

1. Elevated cholestatic liver enzymes (e.g., alkaline phosphatase)
2. Detectable antimitochondrial antibodies (AMA) in sera
3. The presence of chronic nonsuppurative destructive cholangitis

The diagnosis of PBC is made if two of the above three were met

middle-aged women and is characterized by elevated cholestatic liver enzymes, the presence of serum antimitochondrial antibodies (AMA), and pathologically chronic nonsuppurative destructive cholangitis [1, 2], and clinical guidelines of PBC recommend that the patient is diagnosed as having PBC if two of these three were met (Table 7.1) [1, 3, 4]. Although the precise pathophysiology of PBC remains unsolved, it is generally accepted that autoimmune reactions against bile duct epithelial cells play a critical role in PBC, and it is reasoned that indeed immune injury against small intrahepatic bile ducts would be a first step in PBC pathogenesis. Then intrahepatic cholestasis gradually occurs, leading to further insult to cholangiocytes by toxic hydrophobic bile acids. The main target of drugs currently used for PBC is this second step, i.e., reducing the toxicity of bile with replacement of hydrophobic bile acids with hydrophilic bile acids.

In this review, I would like to take a glance at autoimmunity in PBC and then discuss the role of bile acids in PBC, as both pathogenicity and therapeutic options. Besides, I would like to start with recent global agreement about name change of PBC [5].

7.2 Changing Nomenclature for PBC: From "Cirrhosis" to "Cholangitis"

It was 1949 when the term "primary biliary cirrhosis" first appeared in the literatures referring to the disease in which small intrahepatic bile ducts were destructed with massive infiltration of mononuclear cells [6]. The term "primary biliary cirrhosis" exactly reflected the disease at that time since most of PBC presenting with advanced liver disease. However, along with introduction of several biomarkers such as AMA which help physicians to diagnose the disease in much earlier stage, it is uncommon in these days that the patients are diagnosed as having PBC in advanced stage; rather, more than 70% of patients with PBC lack any symptom including variceal rupture, jaundice, and even pruritus [4].

With a global cooperative effort toward the correction of misuse, the Governing Board of European Association for the Study of the Liver (EASL), the American Association for the Study of Liver Diseases (AASLD), and the American Gastroenterological Association (AGA) approved the proposal for a name change of primary biliary cirrhosis to primary biliary "cholangitis" from 2014 to 2015, followed by publish of this statement in eight leading journals, including *Hepatology*, *J Hepatology*, and *Gastroenterology* [7–9]. At the moment of this article was written, the Japan Society of Hepatology (JSH) and Asia Pacific Association for the Study of the Liver (APASL) have not approved the name change yet, but are about to move on this direction as well. Hence, I choose the nomenclature "primary biliary "cholangitis," instead of "cirrhosis" in this review. It may be true that the name "primary biliary cholangitis" is somewhat imperfect and is a tautology. But I believe it is time to go forward to the correction of misused term, leaving endless debates behind which term would be the best for describing the pathogenesis of this disease.

7.3 Autoimmunity and PBC

Although the precise pathophysiology of PBC remains unsolved, it is generally accepted that autoimmune reactions against bile duct epithelial cells play a critical role, mainly because of the followings. First, AMA, autoantibodies directed to mitochondrial autoantigens, are detected in more than 90% of patients with PBC. By contrast, AMA is scarcely seropositive in other autoimmune diseases, and therefore AMA is a hallmark of PBC. Major targeted autoantigens of AMA are E2 component of pyruvate dehydrogenase complex (PDC-E2), branched-chain 2-oxo acid dehydrogenase complex (BCOADC-E2), and 2-oxoglutarate dehydrogenase complex (OGDC-E2), all located in the inner membrane of the mitochondria [10]. It remains unsolved why these ubiquitous proteins are targeted by AMA which are highly disease-specific autoantibodies in PBC. Second, numerous mononuclear cells are accumulating around small damaged interlobular bile ductules, establishing PBC-specific histopathological features called chronic nonsuppurative destructive cholangitis (CNSDC) [11]. Among these inflammatory infiltrates, PDC-E2-specific T and B lymphocytes are detected, and obviously these autoantigen-specific lymphocytes are crucial for pathogenesis of PBC. In addition, recent studies revealed an important role of innate immunity for etiopathogenesis of PBC [12–14]. Indeed, NK cells as well as NKT cells increase in the periphery and liver of PBC [15], and innate immunity is supposed to operate as machinery attacking bile ducts before adaptive immunity [16]. Third, it is not uncommon that patients with PBC develop other autoimmune diseases as comorbidities, such as rheumatoid arthritis, Sjogren's syndrome, and chronic thyroiditis (Hashimoto's disease), suggesting for long that genetic backgrounds are identical in part among these autoimmune diseases and PBC [4]. Recent evidences with genome-wide association studies (GWAS) clearly support this hypothesis; a number of susceptible genes in PBC are shared with other autoimmune diseases including Crohn's disease, multiple sclerosis, rheumatoid arthritis, and autoimmune thyroid disease [17], and it is also notable that most of these shared genes are related to immune pathways. The identification of shared susceptible genes between PBC and other autoimmune diseases is also confirmed in Japanese PBC patients [18].

7.4 Bile Acids as Pathogenesis in PBC

In the past, cholangiocytes were believed to be "innocent victims" in PBC pathogenesis. Deteriorated immune reactions, both innate and adaptive, against intrahepatic small biliary ductules result in destruction of bile ducts, and biliary epithelial cells were supposed to be unilaterally damaged. Recent findings, however, have revealed that cholangiocytes are not "innocent victims" anymore but are "actively participating" in this process, and bile acids are important players in pathogenesis of PBC as well.

The cholangiocytes are physiologically exposed to hydrophobic bile acids, which are potentially toxic to cholangiocytes. Indeed, in acidic condition glycine conjugates of bile acids will be protonated and easily pass cell membranes by simple diffusion. It was also shown that bile acids at pH 4.0, but not pH 7.4, induce oxidative stress and DNA damage in human esophageal epithelial cells [19]. Additionally, acidification of bile at the apical membrane may damage cell membranes and mitochondria, leading to leakage of cytochrome c out of mitochondria and apoptosis [20].

To survive in this hazardous environment, the apical surface of cholangiocytes is covered and protected by dense layer of HCO_3^- secreted from cholangiocytes, which keeps luminal pH at alkaline level, resulting in deprotonation of apolar hydrophobic bile acids and preventing them from permeation into the cholangiocytes [20]. This biliary HCO_3^- "umbrella" is maintained by Cl^-/HCO_3^- exchanger (anion exchanger 2 (AE2)) located at apical surface of cholangiocytes (Fig. 7.1).

Accumulating evidences have indicated that damaged biliary HCO_3^- "umbrella" through lack or reduction of AE2 activities is closely associated with cholangiopathies and PBC. Defects of the biliary $HCO3^-$ umbrella due to inadequate AE2 expression may lead to the development of chronic cholangiopathies [21]. Mice lacking AE2 genes (Ae2a, b) related to the replacement of two anions including $HCO3^-$ and Cl^- inside and outside the cells indicate the pathology similar to that of PBC [22]. In human, immunostaining demonstrated that expression of AE2 was decreased in PBC livers [23]. PBC cholangiocytes exhibit a widespread failure in the regulation of carriers involved in transepithelial HCO_3^- transport [24]. Genetic analysis revealed that allelic variations in AE2 were associated with disease susceptibility and progression of under UDCA therapy [25]. Finally, recent studies revealed that microRNA (miR-506) was upregulated in cholangiocytes from PBC patients and was directly associated with diminished AE2 expression through binding the 30UTR region of AE2 mRNA [26]. Taken together, destabilization of biliary $HCO3^-$ umbrella over the apical membrane with the reduced expression and inadequate function of AE2 may expose cholangiocytes to apolar hydrophobic bile acids, thereby contributing to the development and progression on PBC [20].

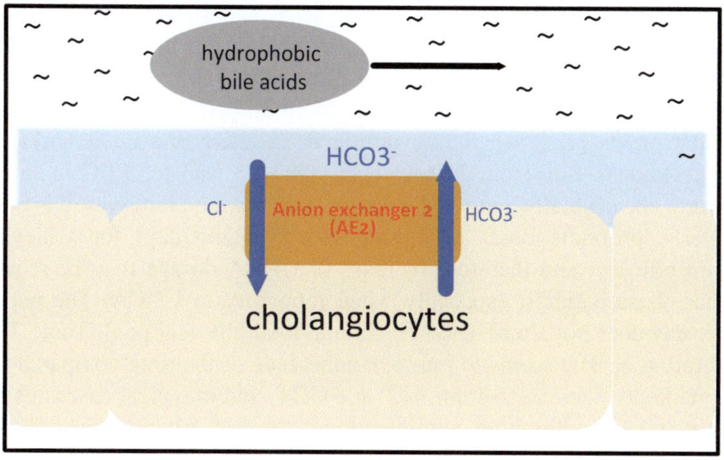

Fig. 7.1 Biliary HCO_3^- umbrella. Cl^-/HCO_3^- exchanger (anion exchanger 2, AE2) is located at apical surface of cholangiocytes and maintains the biliary HCO_3^- umbrella, which is crucial for keeping cholangiocytes intact against hydrophobic bile acids

7.5 Bile Acids as Therapeutic Options in PBC

For the moment, ursodeoxycholic acid (UDCA) is the only drug officially approved for the use in PBC. Besides, although not bile acids, bezafibrate (BF) is frequently used in patients with PBC refractory to UDCA, yet has not been officially approved in Japan. The third drug, obeticholic acid (OCA), is now under development and is expected to be another therapeutic option. All these three are able to diminish toxicity of hydrophobic bile acids with replacement to hydrophilic bile acids, stabilizing the biliary HCO_3^- umbrella and reducing de novo bile acid synthesis, and help to keep cholangiocytes intact.

7.5.1 Ursodeoxycholic Acid (UDCA)

UDCA is a naturally occurring hydrophilic bile acid, the 7-β-epimer of the primary bile acid chenodeoxycholic acid, normally consisting of <5% of the bile acid pool, while UDCA fraction in bile is enriched up to 50–70% with administration at recommended dosage, given at 13–15 mg/kg/day (Table 7.1). Since the first report from Japan indicating the therapeutic effect of UDCA for PBC in 1987 [27], several lines of evidences including placebo-controlled trials demonstrate that UDCA is effective for improvement of long-term prognosis of patients with PBC, and currently UDCA is the only accepted first-line treatment for PBC in several clinical guidelines [1, 4, 28]. UDCA exerts its effect through reduction of cytotoxicity of hydrophobic bile acids by upregulation of hepatic transporters BSEP and MDR3 and by replacement with hydrophilic bile acids and stabilizing biliary HCO_3^- umbrella with upregulation of AE2 [29], in addition to inhibition of bile acid-induced hepatocyte and cholangiocyte apoptosis [30, 31].

UDCA 13–15 mg/kg/day is recommended for all patients with PBC, except for intolerant patients [1, 3, 4]. Safety profile is excellent and no remarkable side effects are known. Since the dosage in the phase 3 trial for PBC in Japan was 600 mg/day, the officially approved dosage is 600 mg/day; however, it is crucial to administer appropriate doses of UDCA (13–15 mg/kg/day) for achieving the maximum efficacy, and therefore increase of UDCA dosage may be required in somewhat obese patients, especially when refractory to UDCA. The number of times per day does not alter UDCA fraction in total bile acid pool (Table 7.2), and administration at BID seems to improve adherence of the drug compared to TID. UDCA markedly decreases serum ALP and GGT, and in typical cases this decline is evident 6–12 months after administration. Several criteria using blood tests 6–12 months after commencement of UDCA have been proposed to suggest optimal responses to UDCA resulting in favorable prognosis (Table 7.3) [32–37]. Very recently, the consortium from Europe and North America as well as the UK reported other criteria to predict outcomes of patients with PBC with employing more than 2,000 PBC patients, called GLOBE score and UK-PBC risk score, respectively (Table 7.4) [38, 39]. These scores are expected to be used as surrogate endpoints for clinical studies in the very near future.

On the other hand, there are up to 40% of patients who exhibit suboptimal response to UDCA treatment [40], and the outcomes of these patients have been reported to be significantly worse compared to general population [33, 35, 37]. Therefore, the second-line treatment regimens for nonresponders to UDCA are strongly warranted in clinical setting. Furthermore, UDCA has little effect on symptoms of PBC including fatigue and pruritus and also on late-stage PBC.

7.5.2 *Bezafibrate (BF)*

BF is a fibrate drug that is currently approved for the treatment of hypertriglyceridemia in Japan. Like the other fibrates, BF is an agonist of peroxisome proliferator-activated receptors (PPARs), and BF is supposed to exert anti-cholestatic activity through formation of mixed micelles of bile salts and phospholipids with induction of MDR3 and also through inhibition of CYP7A1, being linked to decrease de novo bile acid synthesis [41]. Additionally, and probably more importantly, BF works as a pregnane X receptor (PXR) agonist as well, leading to upregulation of CYP3A4 and detoxification of toxic bile acids, including lithocholic acid [41]. In this manner, cytotoxicity of hydrophobic bile acids is attenuated with administration of BF. It is of note that agonistic function of PXR is exclusively observed in BF, not in UDCA, and therefore BF administration additively works for biochemical improvement in PBC with UDCA.

Table 7.2 The proportion of each bile acid fraction depending on prescription* [46]

	QD	BID	TID
UDCA (%)	42 ± 27	69 ± 6	56 ± 25
Glyco-UDCA (%)	23 ± 16	40 ± 15	41 ± 20
Tauro-UDCA (%)	1 ± 5	3 ± 3	3 ± 4
Free UDCA (%)	18 ± 20	26 ± 15	12 ± 22
CA (%)	3 ± 3	5 ± 3	7 ± 7
CDCA (%)	49 ± 30	24 ± 6	28 ± 21
DCA (%)	5 ± 5	3 ± 5	8 ± 5
LCA (%)	1 ± 1	1 ± 2	1 ± 1

CA cholic acid, *CDCA* chenodeoxycholic acid, *DCA* deoxycholic acid, *LCA* lithocholic acid
* The values are expressed as mean±SD

Table 7.3 Criteria to define response to UDCA

Barcelona [37]	1 year	ALP 40% decrease from baseline or normal value
Paris-1 [33]	1 year	ALP <3 x ULN, AST <2 x sULN, and normal bilirubin
Rotterdam [35]	1 year	Normal bilirubin or albumin
Toronto [36]	2 years	ALP <1.67 x ULN
Paris-2 [34]	1 year	ALP <1.5 x ULN or AST <1.5 x ULN, and normal bilirubin
Ehime [32]	6 months	GGT <70% from baseline or normal value

Table 7.4 GLOBE score and UK-PBC score

GLOBE score	(0.044378∗age at start of UDCA therapy + 0.93982∗LN (bilirubin times the upper limit of normal (ULN) at 1-year follow-up)) + (0.335648∗LN (alkaline phosphatase times the ULN at 1-year follow-up)) –2.266708 * albumin level times the lower limit of normal (LLN) at 1-year follow-up –0.002581∗platelet count per 109/L at 1-year follow-up) + 1.216865
UK-PBC score	1-baseline survival function^exp(0.0287854∗(alp12xuln-1.722136304) – 0.0422873∗(((altast12xuln/10)^ – 1) – 8.675729006) + 1.4199∗(ln(bil12xuln/10) + 2.709607778) – 1.960303∗(albxlln-1.17673001) – 0.4161954∗(pltxlln-1.873564875))

Note: Baseline survivor function = 0. 982 (at 5 years); 0. 941 (at 10 years); 0.893 (at 15 years)

In 1999, BF was firstly reported by Iwasaki et al. to exhibit biochemical improvements in patients with PBC [42], and since then small case series and pilot study confirmed biochemical improvement of BF. Nevertheless, well-designed phase 3 trials of BF for PBC have not been done, and long-term effect of BF for prognosis of patients with PBC has not been confirmed. As a result the use of BF has not been officially approved even in Japan, despite aggressive off-label use of BF for PBC patients refractory to UDCA. A recent placebo-controlled randomized study demonstrated that while add-on of BF to UDCA significantly decreased serum ALP and Mayo score, overall survival did not significantly differ between UDCA monotherapy and BF add-on [43]. This could be partially explained by the fact that patients refractory both to UDCA and BF might be present and have poorer outcome. Indeed, our large-scale retrospective study indicated that BF in addition to UDCA itself did not improve survival as well as development of liver-related symptoms in patients with PBC but only in those who responded well to coadministration of BF and demonstrated normalization of ALT [44]. Taken together, the role of BF in patients refractory to UDCA is clearly present, yet suboptimal.

7.5.3 *Obeticholic Acid (OCA)*

OCA (6-α-ethyl-chenodeoxycholic acid, INT-747) is a semisynthetic agonist of the nuclear hormone receptor farnesoid X receptor (FXR). FXR agonist is known to inhibit CYP7A1, like PPARs, and therefore to be capable of inhibiting de novo synthesis of bile acids and promoting their secretion. The results of phase 2 clinical trial of OCA for PBC were recently published [45]. In this double-blind, placebo-controlled study, 165 PBC patients who were already treated with UDCA, yet in whom serum ALP levels were more that 1.5-fold the upper limit of normal, were included. These patients were allocated into four groups: 10 mg, 25 mg, or 50 mg doses of OCA and placebo, once daily for 3 months. The primary outcome was ALP reduction after 3 months of OCA treatment. As a result, administration of OCA achieved significant decrease of ALP compared to placebo. In addition to ALP, GGT and ALT were also found to reduce with OCA. This reduction of liver enzymes was not dose dependent and almost equal among three doses. In terms of drug safety, the most prevalent adverse effect was pruritus, which was noted in 47%, 87%, 80%, and 50% in the OCA 10 mg, 25 mg, and 50 mg and placebo, respectively. These results suggest that 10 mg of OCA for patients with PBC refractory to UDCA would be capable of reducing serum ALP and minimizing adverse effects, especially pruritus. The main concern of this drug, however, is that OCA could substantially worsen the quality of life of patients with PBC, another important outcome of this chronic and slowly progressive disease, through deterioration of pruritus. Additionally, it still remains unsolved whether reduction of ALP is really reliable as a surrogate endpoint for prediction of long-term outcomes. Currently, in Japan, clinical trial of OCA for nonalcoholic steatohepatitis (NASH) is ongoing, not for PBC.

7.6 Closing Remarks

As discussed UDCA is the only officially approved drug for PBC worldwide and is capable of improving the long-term outcome of responded patients. Besides, responses to UDCA are not favorable in up to 40% of UDCA-treated patients, and the alternative treatment is strongly awaited for those patients to avoid progression to cirrhosis and liver transplantation. So far the results of clinical trials for generalized immune-based therapies are disappointing, and targeting cytotoxicity of hydrophobic bile acids such as OCA and other drugs in clinical trials is expected to be a promising approach.

References

1. Lindor KD, Gershwin ME, Poupon R, Kaplan M, Bergasa NV, Heathcote EJ et al. Primary biliary cirrhosis. Hepatology. 2009;50(1):291–308. doi:10.1002/hep.22906 [doi].
2. Kaplan MM, Gershwin ME. Primary biliary cirrhosis. N Engl J Med. 2005;353(12):1261–73.
3. EASL Clinical Practice Guidelines: management of cholestatic liver diseases. J Hepatol. 2009;51(2):237–67. doi:S0168-8278(09)003092 [pii]10.1016/j.jhep.2009.04.009 [doi].
4. Working Subgroup for Clinical Practice Guidelines for Primary Biliary C. Guidelines for the management of primary biliary cirrhosis: the Intractable Hepatobiliary Disease Study Group supported by the Ministry of Health, Labour and Welfare of Japan. Hepatol Res. 2014;44 Suppl S1:71–90. doi:10.1111/hepr.12270 [doi].
5. Shimoda S, Tanaka A. It is time to change PBC: new nomenclature from "cirrhosis" to "cholangitis", and upcoming treatment based on unveiling pathology. Hepatol Res. 2015; doi:10.1111/hepr.12615.
6. Dauphinee JA, Sinclair JC. Primary biliary cirrhosis. Can Med Assoc J. 1949;61(1):1–6.
7. Beuers U, Gershwin ME, Gish RG, Invernizzi P, Jones DE, Lindor K, et al. Changing nomenclature for PBC: from 'cirrhosis' to 'cholangitis'. J Hepatol. 2015; doi:10.1016/j.jhep.2015.06.031.
8. Beuers U, Gershwin ME, Gish RG, Invernizzi P, Jones DE, Lindor K, et al. Changing nomenclature for PBC: from 'Cirrhosis' to 'Cholangitis'. Gastroenterology. 2015; doi:10.1053/j.gastro.2015.08.031.
9. Beuers U, Gershwin ME, Gish RG, Invernizzi P, Jones DE, Lindor K, et al. Changing nomenclature for PBC: from 'cirrhosis' to 'cholangitis'. Hepatology. 2015; doi:10.1002/hep.28140.
10. Muratori L, Granito A, Muratori P, Pappas G, Bianchi FB. Antimitochondrial antibodies and other antibodies in primary biliary cirrhosis: diagnostic and prognostic value. Clin Liver Dis 2008;12(2):261–276; vii. doi:S1089-3261(08)00025-1 [pii].
11. Rubin E, Schaffner F, Popper H. Primary biliary cirrhosis. Chronic non-suppurative destructive cholangitis. Am J Pathol. 1965;46:387–407.
12. Kikuchi K, Lian ZX, Yang GX, Ansari AA, Ikehara S, Kaplan M, et al. Bacterial CpG induces hyper-IgM production in CD27(+) memory B cells in primary biliary cirrhosis. Gastroenterology. 2005;128(2):304–12. . doi:S0016508504020013 [pii]
13. Mao T, Lian Z, Selmi C, Ichiki Y, Ashwood P, Ansari A, et al. Altered monocyte responses to defined TLR ligands in patients with primary biliary cirrhosis. Hepatology. 2005;42(4):802–8.
14. Moritoki Y, Lian Z, Wulff H, Yang G, Chuang Y, Lan R, et al. AMA production in primary biliary cirrhosis is promoted by the TLR9 ligand CpG and suppressed by potassium channel blockers. Hepatology. 2007;45(2):314–22.
15. Kita H, Naidenko OV, Kronenberg M, Ansari AA, Rogers P, He XS, et al. Quantitation and phenotypic analysis of natural killer T cells in primary biliary cirrhosis using a human CD1d tetramer. Gastroenterology. 2002;123(4):1031–43. . doi:S0016508502002081 [pii]
16. Shimoda S, Hisamoto S, Harada K, Iwasaka S, Chong Y, Nakamura M, et al. Natural killer cells regulate T cell immune responses in primary biliary cirrhosis. Hepatology. 2015; doi:10.1002/hep.28122.
17. Carbone M, Lleo A, Sandford RN, Invernizzi P. Implications of genome-wide association studies in novel therapeutics in primary biliary cirrhosis. Eur J Immunol 2014. doi:10.1002/eji.201344270 [doi].

18. Aiba Y, Yamazaki K, Nishida N, Kawashima M, Hitomi Y, Nakamura H, et al. Disease susceptibility genes shared by primary biliary cirrhosis and Crohn's disease in the Japanese population. J Hum Genet. 2015; doi:10.1038/jhg.2015.59.
19. Dvorak K, Payne CM, Chavarria M, Ramsey L, Dvorakova B, Bernstein H, et al. Bile acids in combination with low pH induce oxidative stress and oxidative DNA damage: relevance to the pathogenesis of Barrett's oesophagus. Gut. 2007;56(6):763–71. doi:10.1136/gut.2006.103697.
20. Beuers U, Hohenester S, de Buy Wenniger LJ, Kremer AE, Jansen PL, Elferink RP. The biliary HCO(3)(−) umbrella: a unifying hypothesis on pathogenetic and therapeutic aspects of fibrosing cholangiopathies. Hepatology. 2010;52(4):1489–96. doi:10.1002/hep.23810.
21. Hohenester S, Wenniger LM, Paulusma CC, van Vliet SJ, Jefferson DM, Elferink RP, et al. A biliary HCO3- umbrella constitutes a protective mechanism against bile acid-induced injury in human cholangiocytes. Hepatology. 2012;55(1):173–83. doi:10.1002/hep.24691.
22. Salas JT, Banales JM, Sarvide S, Recalde S, Ferrer A, Uriarte I et al. Ae2a,b-deficient mice develop antimitochondrial antibodies and other features resembling primary biliary cirrhosis. Gastroenterology 2008;134(5):1482–1493. doi:S0016-5085(08)00253-9 [pii] 1053/j.gastro.2008.02.020 [doi].
23. Medina JF, Martinez A, Vazquez JJ, Prieto J. Decreased anion exchanger 2 immunoreactivity in the liver of patients with primary biliary cirrhosis. Hepatology. 1997;25(1):12–7. doi:10.1002/hep.510250104.
24. Melero S, Spirli C, Zsembery A, Medina JF, Joplin RE, Duner E et al. Defective regulation of cholangiocyte Cl−/HCO3(−) and Na+/H+ exchanger activities in primary biliary cirrhosis. Hepatology 2002;35(6):1513–1521. doi:S0270913902912619 [pii] 1053/jhep.2002.33634 [doi].
25. Poupon R, Ping C, Chretien Y, Corpechot C, Chazouilleres O, Simon T et al. Genetic factors of susceptibility and of severity in primary biliary cirrhosis. J Hepatol. 2008;49(6):1038–1045. doi:S0168-8278(08)00602-8 [pii]10.1016/j.jhep.2008.07.027 [doi].
26. Banales JM, Saez E, Uriz M, Sarvide S, Urribarri AD, Splinter P et al. Up-regulation of microRNA 506 leads to decreased Cl(−) /HCO(3) (−) anion exchanger 2 expression in biliary epithelium of patients with primary biliary cirrhosis. Hepatology. 2012;56(2):687–697. doi:10.1002/hep.25691 [doi].
27. T Wada, R Kohziro, K Tanikawa. The effect of long-term administration of ursodeoxycholic acid in patients with primary biliary cirrhosis. Tokyo Tanabe Q. 1989: 39–46. [in Japanese]
28. European Association for the Study of the L. EASL Clinical Practice Guidelines: management of cholestatic liver diseases. J Hepatol 2009;51(2):237–267. doi:S0168-8278(09)00309-2 [pii] 1016/j.jhep.2009.04.009 [doi].
29. Arenas F, Hervias I, Uriz M, Joplin R, Prieto J, Medina JF. Combination of ursodeoxycholic acid and glucocorticoids upregulates the AE2 alternate promoter in human liver cells. J Clin Invest. 2008;118(2):695–709. doi:10.1172/JCI33156.
30. Carey EJ, Ali AH, Lindor KD. Primary biliary cirrhosis. Lancet. 2015; doi:10.1016/s0140-6736(15)00154-3.
31. Mousa HS, Lleo A, Invernizzi P, Bowlus CL, Gershwin ME. Advances in pharmacotherapy for primary biliary cirrhosis. Expert Opin Pharmacother. 2015;16(5):633–43. doi:10.1517/14656566.2015.998650.
32. Azemoto N, Abe M, Murata Y, Hiasa Y, Hamada M, Matsuura B, et al. Early biochemical response to ursodeoxycholic acid predicts symptom development in patients with asymptomatic primary biliary cirrhosis. J Gastroenterol. 2009;44(6):630–4. doi:10.1007/s00535-009-0051-9.
33. Corpechot C, Abenavoli L, Rabahi N, Chretien Y, Andreani T, Johanet C, et al. Biochemical response to ursodeoxycholic acid and long-term prognosis in primary biliary cirrhosis. Hepatology. 2008;48(3):871–7. doi:10.1002/hep.22428.
34. Corpechot C, Chazouilleres O, Poupon R. Early primary biliary cirrhosis: biochemical response to treatment and prediction of long-term outcome. J Hepatol 2011;55(6):1361–1367. doi:S0168-8278(11)00282-0 [pii] 1016/j.jhep.2011.02.031 [doi].

35. Kuiper EM, Hansen BE, de Vries RA, den Ouden-Muller JW, van Ditzhuijsen TJ, Haagsma EB et al. Improved prognosis of patients with primary biliary cirrhosis that have a biochemical response to ursodeoxycholic acid. Gastroenterology 2009;136(4):1281–1287. doi:S0016-5085 (09)00007-9 [pii] 1053/j.gastro.2009.01.003 [doi].
36. Kumagi T, Guindi M, Fischer SE, Arenovich T, Abdalian R, Coltescu C et al. Baseline ductopenia and treatment response predict long-term histological progression in primary biliary cirrhosis. Am J Gastroenterol 2010;105(10):2186–2194. doi: ajg2010216 [pii] 1038/ ajg.2010.216 [doi].
37. Pares A, Caballeria L, Rodes J. Excellent long-term survival in patients with primary biliary cirrhosis and biochemical response to ursodeoxycholic acid. Gastroenterology. 2006;130 (3):715–20.
38. Carbone M, Sharp SJ, Flack S, Paximadas D, Spiess K, Adgey C, et al. The UK-PBC risk scores: derivation and validation of a scoring system for long-term prediction of end-stage liver disease in primary biliary cirrhosis. Hepatology. 2015; doi:10.1002/hep.28017.
39. Lammers WJ, Hirschfield GM, Corpechot C, Nevens F, Lindor KD, Janssen HL, et al. Development and validation of a scoring system to predict outcomes of patients with primary biliary cirrhosis receiving ursodeoxycholic acid therapy. Gastroenterology. 2015; doi:10.1053/ j.gastro.2015.07.061.
40. Poupon R. Primary biliary cirrhosis: a 2010 update. J Hepatol 2010;52(5):745–758. doi:S0168-8278(10)00027-9 [pii] 1016/j.jhep.2009.11.027 [doi].
41. Honda A, Ikegami T, Nakamuta M, Miyazaki T, Iwamoto J, Hirayama T, et al. Anticholestatic effects of bezafibrate in patients with primary biliary cirrhosis treated with ursodeoxycholic acid. Hepatology. 2013;57(5):1931–41. doi:10.1002/hep.26018.
42. Iwasaki S, Tsuda K, Ueta H, Aono R, Ono M, Saibara T et al. Bezafibrate may have a beneficial effect in pre-cirrhotic primary biliary cirrhosis. Hepatol Res. 1999;16(1):12–18. doi:http://dx.doi.org/10.1016/S1386-6346(99)00033-9.
43. Hosonuma K, Sato K, Yamazaki Y, Yanagisawa M, Hashizume H, Horiguchi N, et al. A prospective randomized controlled study of long-term combination therapy using ursodeoxycholic acid and bezafibrate in patients with primary biliary cirrhosis and dyslipidemia. Am J Gastroenterol. 2015;110(3):423–31. doi:10.1038/ajg.2015.20.
44. Tanaka A, Hirohara J, Nakanuma Y, Tsubouchi H, Takikawa H. Biochemical responses to bezafibrate improve long-term outcome in asymptomatic patients with primary biliary cirrhosis refractory to UDCA. J Gastroenterol. 2015;50(6):675–82. doi:10.1007/s00535-014-0998-z.
45. Hirschfield GM, Mason A, Luketic V, Lindor K, Gordon SC, Mayo M, et al. Efficacy of obeticholic acid in patients with primary biliary cirrhosis and inadequate response to ursodeoxycholic acid. Gastroenterology. 2015;148(4):751–61. e8 doi:10.1053/j.gastro.2014. 12.005.
46. Uegaki S, Mikami M, Morisawa Y, Negoro S, Goto H, Fukami M, et al. A study on dividing doses of ursodeoxycholic acid (UDCA) for patients with chronic hepatitis C. Kanzo. 2007;48:559–61.

Chapter 8
Bile Acids and Cholestatic Liver Disease 2: Primary Sclerosing Cholangitis

Takahiro Nakazawa

Abstract Primary sclerosing cholangitis (PSC) is a chronic inflammatory disease characterized by idiopathic fibrous obstruction, leading to hepatic cirrhosis and a poor prognosis. PSC likely occurs in genetically susceptible individuals, perhaps after exposure to environmental triggers including toxic bile acids, bacterial infections, and intestinal pathogens. These could initiate a series of events that involve complex interactions between the innate and adaptive immune systems, ultimately leading to lymphocyte migration and cholangiocyte damage. Leakage of bile acids into the portal tract leads to an inflammatory response and progressive fibrosis. Therapies for PSC can be classified roughly into two categories: regulation of immunomechanisms and regulation of bile acids. The former therapies primarily target the interaction between adhesion molecules and lymphocyte recruitment to the liver. The latter aim to alter the bile acid pool composition and reduce the total serum bile acid pool by administration of ursodeoxycholic acid (UDCA) or the C23 homolog of UDCA, stimulation of farnesoid X receptors, and inhibition of apical sodium-dependent bile acid transporter.

Keywords Primary sclerosing cholangitis • PSC • Bile acid

8.1 Introduction

Primary sclerosing cholangitis (PSC) is a chronic inflammatory disease, characterized by idiopathic fibrous obstruction [1]. The fibrosis causes diffuse narrowing of the intrahepatic and extrahepatic bile ducts. The persistent biliary stasis leads to hepatic cirrhosis. Liver transplantation is the only potentially curative treatment for PSC. According to the diagnostic criteria for PSC proposed by the Mayo Clinic in 1999 [1] and 2003 [2], in addition to cholangiographic findings, the presence of inflammatory bowel disease (IBD) is important.

T. Nakazawa (✉)
Department of Gastroenterology, Japanese Red Cross Nagoya Daini Hospital,
2-9 Myoken-cho, Showa-ku, Nagoya, Aichi 466-8650, Japan
e-mail: tnakazaw@nagoya2.jrc.or.jp

S. Tazuma, H. Takikawa (eds.), *Bile Acids in Gastroenterology*,
DOI 10.1007/978-4-431-56062-3_8

8.2 Etiology of PSC

The etiology of PSC is still poorly understood. Toxic bile acids, such as lithocholate, were regarded as etiologic factors for the association between PSC and IBD [3]. However, this idea was abandoned, because no abnormal findings were seen in the composition of bile acids in bile and serum of patients with PSC and IBD [4]. Several hypotheses have emerged since then.

PSC likely occurs in genetically susceptible individuals, perhaps after exposure to environmental triggers, including toxic bile acids, bacterial infections, and intestinal pathogens (Fig. 8.1). These could initiate a series of events that involve complex interactions between the innate and adaptive immune systems, ultimately leading to lymphocyte migration, cholangiocyte damage, and progressive fibrosis. Several important observations, coupled with the strong association between certain human leukocyte antigen (HLA) haplotypes and the frequency of concurrent extrahepatic autoimmune disorders, support the concept that PSC is an immune-mediated phenomenon [5].

Three ulcerative colitis (UC) susceptibility loci associated with PSC, harboring the putative candidate genes REL, IL2, and CARD9, have been identified [6]. A study reported 12 significant genome-wide associations outside the HLA region, nine of which were new, increasing the number of known PSC risk loci to 16. Despite comorbidity with IBD in 72% of the included cases, six of the 12 loci showed significantly stronger associations with PSC than with IBD, suggesting overlapping, yet distinct, genetic mechanisms for the two diseases [7].

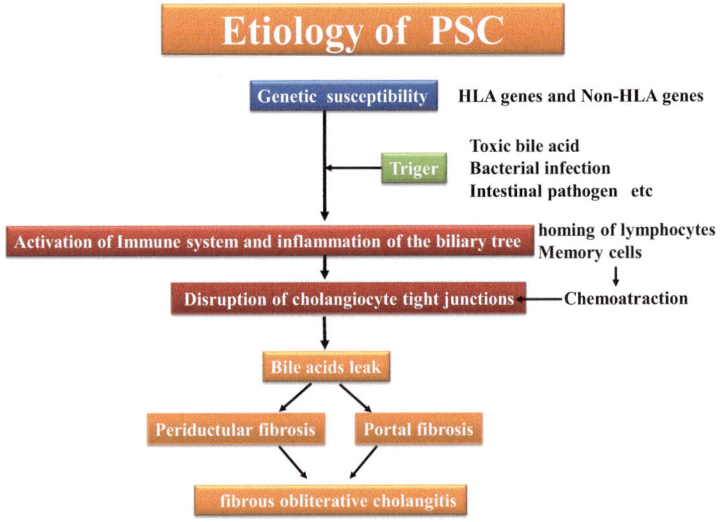

Fig. 8.1 Etiology of PSC

Translocation of microbial flora across the gut is one hypothesized mechanism for the development of PSC [8]. Small intestinal bacterial overgrowth and the introduction of bacterial antigens into the portal circulation can cause pericholangitis in animal models [9–11]. However, studies in humans have suggested that portal venous bacteremia is uncommon in UC [12]. Although some antibiotics have been shown to reduce serum alkaline phosphatase levels and Mayo risk scores, the long-term effects of antibiotics on PSC progression are unclear [13, 14]. Growing interest in the relationship between the human microbiome and chronic disease will undoubtedly lead to studies in patients with PSC.

Normally, biliary epithelial cells are exposed to common intestinal pathogen-associated molecular patterns, such as lipopolysaccharide and lipoteichoic acid. However, exposure to lipopolysaccharide may disrupt tight junctions in colonic and biliary epithelial cells, through Toll-like receptor (TLR)4-dependent mechanisms [14, 15]. Alteration of such barriers can expose cholangiocytes to a variety of substances, such as bile acids, that could promote injury and inflammation. Disruption of cholangiocyte tight junctions is an important step in the development of PSC in animal models [16, 17]. For example, mice with altered cholangiocyte tight junctions exhibit leakage of bile acids into the portal tract. This leads to an inflammatory response involving $CD8^+$ and $CD4^+$ T cells and upregulation of tumor necrosis factor (TNF)-α, transforming growth factor-β1, and interleukin (IL)1β. This inflammatory infiltrate causes myofibroblast activation and fibrosis [16].

The pathogenesis of PSC has been examined from the standpoint of PSC-IBD. Translocation of the microbial flora across an inflamed, permeable gut with subsequent activation of the immune system and inflammation of the biliary tree is another hypothesized mechanism for the development of PSC (Fig. 8.2). It appears

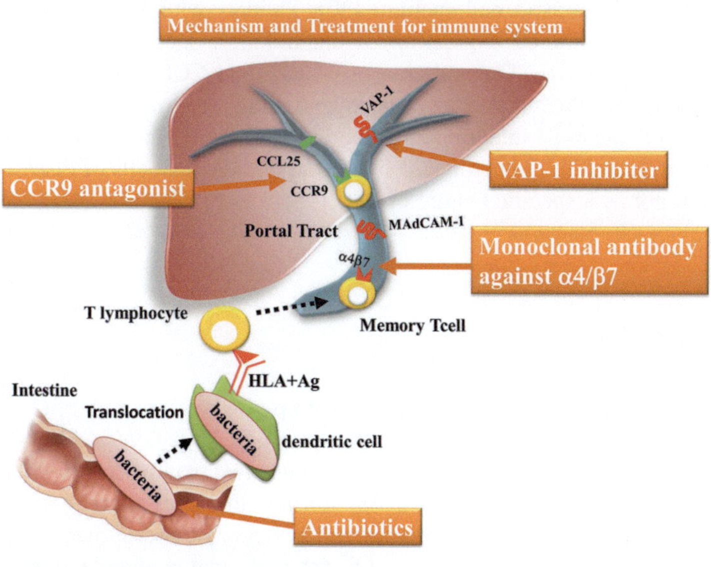

Fig. 8.2 Mechanism and treatment for immune system

that the $\alpha4\beta7^{+}CCR9^{+}CD8^{+}$ T cells that infiltrate the liver in PSC are primed by dendritic cells in the intestine. Activated intestinal lymphocytes enter the enterohepatic circulation and persist as memory cells that cause hepatic inflammation. Chemokines and adhesion molecules shared by the intestine and liver could contribute to immune cell binding at both sites [18].

The observations that PSC can develop after colectomy [19] and that IBD can develop after liver transplantation have caused some investigators to suggest that aberrant homing of lymphocytes between the intestine and liver could be involved in the pathogenesis of PSC [20]. Three studies indirectly supporting this theory have been published. Patients who received a liver transplant had lower clinical and histological IBD activities than those of the non-transplant group [21]. Marelli et al. [22] reported that progressive PSC requiring liver transplantation is associated with a milder course of UC, including reduced disease activity and use of steroids, azathioprine, and surgery. Navaneethan et al. [23] reported that severe, progressive PSC requiring liver transplantation appeared to reduce the disease activity of UC and the need for a colectomy. However, these theories cannot explain why only 2–7.5% of IBD patients develop PSC [24], whereas PSC is strongly associated with development of IBD, or why Crohn's disease is less associated with PSC. It is also unclear why immunosuppression does not improve PSC.

The involvement of adhesion molecules in lymphocyte recruitment to the liver is emerging as an important step in the pathogenesis of PSC. Inflammatory mediators appear to upregulate various adhesion molecules during the development of PSC, including intercellular adhesion molecules, vascular cell adhesion molecule-1 (VCAM-1) [25], and mucosal addressin cellular adhesion molecule 1 - (MAdCAM-1) [26] (Fig. 8.2). Typically, MAdCAM-1 is expressed in the mucosal vessels of the intestine. However, under conditions of inflammation, it can be expressed by the hepatic endothelium [27]. Patients with PSC have also been observed to have altered expression of chemokines, such as CCL25, CCL28, CXCL12, and CXCL16. Upregulation of CCL25 and CCL28 leads to activation of $\alpha4\beta7$ integrins, which increase lymphocyte binding to MAdCAM-1. CCL28 also appears to activate $\alpha4\beta1$ integrin and to increase its adhesion to VCAM-1, which is primarily expressed in the portal and sinusoidal endothelial cells of diseased liver, so it might not be a specific feature of PSC [28].

8.3 Treatment for PSC

At this time, there is no beneficial medical therapy for patients with PSC, and liver transplantation is the only potentially curative option for patients with PSC. Therapies for PSC can be classified roughly into two categories: regulation of immunomechanisms and bile acids. The former therapies mainly regulate the interaction between adhesion molecules and lymphocyte recruitment to the liver (Fig. 8.2). The latter alter the composition of the bile acid pool and reduce the total

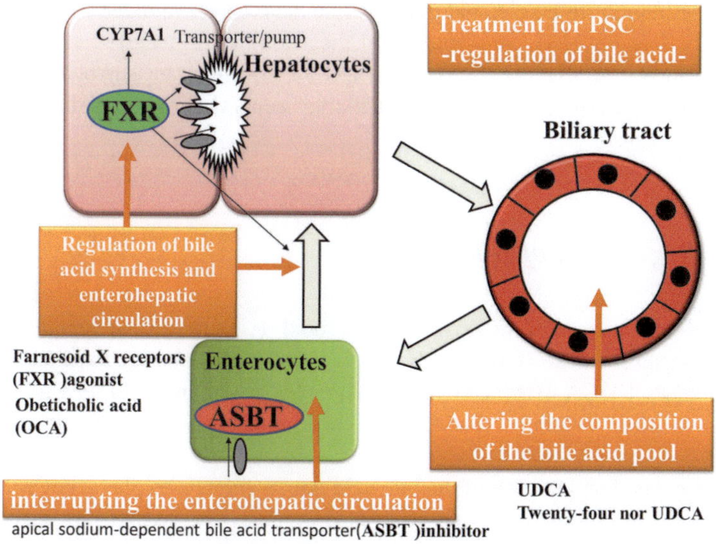

Fig. 8.3 Treatment for PSC regulation of bile acid

serum bile acid pool (Fig. 8.3). Recent trends and clinical trials of treatment for PSC are reviewed in Ali's paper [29].

8.3.1 Regulation of Immunomechanisms

Several agents including immunosuppressants and immunomodulators, such as azathioprine [30], budesonide, methotrexate [31], prednisolone, and tacrolimus, have been evaluated in PSC patients but failed to show positive results. VCAM-1 and MAdCAM-1 are expressed in the mucosal vessels of the intestine and hepatic endothelium in PSC patients [26, 27] (Fig. 8.2). Vascular adhesion protein 1 (VAP-1) has been found to induce the expression of MAdCAM-1 in the hepatic endothelial cells of human liver tissue [25]. Targeting VAP-1 and MAdCAM-1 could be beneficial in patients with PSC. A monoclonal antibody against $\alpha4\beta7$ and a VAP-1 blocking agent have been investigated [32]. Liver-infiltrating T cells recruited by aberrant expression of the gut-specific chemokine CCL25 activate $\alpha4\beta7$ binding to MAdCAM-1 on the hepatic endothelium. Targeting the CCL25-MAdCAM-1 axis could have a beneficial effect [33].

Several animal experiments have demonstrated a link between the gut microbiota and development of PSC [34]. Induction of small bowel bacterial overgrowth by ligation of the jejunum in rats resulted in the development of hepatic lesions compatible with PSC. Daily treatment with antibiotics resulted in significant improvement of these lesions, suggesting that modification of the gut microbiota could be of therapeutic benefit at least in a selected group of PSC patients.

Vancomycin, metronidazole, and minocycline have been evaluated in clinical trials in patients with PSC [35, 36]. The use of these antibiotics resulted in a significant reduction in serum alkaline phosphatase (ALP), an important surrogate marker in PSC. Thus, antibiotic therapy for PSC patients seems to be a promising tool in the treatment of PSC.

8.3.2 Regulation of Bile Acids

The synthetic bile acid ursodeoxycholic acid (UDCA) is the 7-β-epimer of chenodeoxycholic acid (CDCA). Because it has been shown to improve liver biochemistry, UDCA has been used frequently for therapy in PSC. However, there is no clear evidence that UDCA contributes to improvements in patient survival.

An abnormal composition of the bile acid pool is thought to play a key role in the pathogenesis and progression of PSC [37] (Fig. 8.3). This hypothesis was derived from several animal [38] and human studies. PSC-like lesions occur in mice devoid of the canalicular transporter Mdr2, which mediates biliary excretion of phospholipids that normally form mixed micelles with bile acids, thus protecting the liver against the detergent effects of bile acids [39]. Bile acid toxicity to the biliary epithelium could result from decreased biliary HCO_3 secretion [40]. The bile salt-sensing receptor TGR5 plays a key role in the regulation of HCO_3 secretion, and TGR5 was identified as a likely disease-susceptibility gene in a large genome-wide study of PSC [41].

Animal and in vitro studies have also suggested that UDCA may have a role as a chemopreventive agent in the prevention of colorectal neoplasia. Several mechanisms in which UDCA may act to prevent colorectal cancer have been proposed, including downregulation of cyclooxygenase-2 expression; prevention of carcinogen-induced changes in protein C; inhibition of cell proliferation by suppressing epidermal growth factor receptor, which is typically activated by deoxycholic acid (DCA); and alteration of the bile acid milieu to reduce secondary bile acid levels [42–46]. Lower doses of UDCA may have a protective role because of its potential antiapoptotic effect. For example, exposing human colon cancer cell lines to UDCA can decrease DCA-induced apoptosis [47].

Multiple human studies also have investigated the role of UDCA as a chemopreventive agent, but the results are conflicting. Two clinical studies suggested that UDCA reduces the incidence of colorectal neoplasia in patients with UC and PSC [48, 49]. Tung et al. [48] performed a retrospective review of 59 patients and found that UDCA was associated with a significant reduction in the odds ratio for colonic dysplasia development. However, after excluding cases of indefinite dysplasia, a multivariate analysis did not reveal a statistically significant association with UDCA. A secondary analysis revealed a significant association between UDCA use and the development of high-grade dysplasia only. Furthermore, in this study, the control group had a high proportion of dysplasia (72%), and 50% of those who received UDCA went on to develop dysplasia. Compared with those who did not receive UDCA, the UDCA-treated group had a shorter duration of colitis and were older at the time of diagnosis of colitis. A third study indicated that the times of cancer and dysplasia development were the same, regardless of whether subjects received UDCA [50]. Consequently, it remains unclear in clinical practice whether patients with PSC and UC should be started on UDCA for the prevention of colonic neoplasia.

Treatment with high-dose UDCA, compared with placebo, was associated with an increased rate of serious clinical events. A multicenter, placebo-controlled trial investigated the use of UDCA 28–30 mg/kg/day in patients with PSC. That study revealed an improvement in liver biochemistry, but no improvement in survival, and a higher rate of adverse events [51, 52], as well as the development of colon cancer [53] in the UDCA group. Sinakos et al. investigated the serum bile acid composition in patients in the high-dose UDCA arm and compared it with that of control group patients [54]. Long-term use of high-dose UDCA is associated with an increased risk of colorectal neoplasia in patients with UC and PSC. In total, 56 subjects were followed for a total of 235 patient years. Patients who received high-dose UDCA had a significantly higher risk of developing colorectal neoplasia (dysplasia and cancer) during the study compared with those who received placebo (hazard ratio = 4.44, 95% confidence interval = 1.30–20.10, $P = 0.02$). They concluded that bile acids may have a role in colon carcinogenesis, particularly the secondary bile acids (lithocholic acid (LCA) and DCA) [55–57]. In in vitro studies, prolonged exposure to high bile acid concentrations has been suggested to play a role in gastrointestinal cancers, leading to oxidative stress, selection of apoptosis-resistant cells, and replication of unrepaired damaged DNA [57, 58]. They reported a statistically significant increase in serum UDCA and LCA levels in the treatment group, compared with the placebo group, and an expansion of the total serum bile acid pool without significant changes in CA, DCA, or CDCA levels [54]. It is expected that a proportion of the UDCA pool would be metabolized by bacterial flora into other bile acids. UDCA can be metabolized into both LCA and CDCA by intestinal flora. CDCA is typically metabolized to LCA by bacterial flora. Both CDCA and LCA have been shown to stimulate in vitro cell invasion in a dose-dependent manner [59, 60]. Furthermore, physiological levels of CDCA and DCA can increase colon adenoma cell proliferation and reduce apoptosis [61]. The American Association for the Study of Liver Disease (AASLD) recommends against the use of UDCA in PSC patients [62].

NorUDCA is a C23 homolog of UDCA that is currently being evaluated in a phase II randomized clinical trial in patients with PSC. In a rodent model of cholestasis, the administration of norUDCA to Mdr2 knockout mice improved sclerosing cholangitis, possibly by altering the composition of the bile acid pool by displacing the toxic bile acids and increasing the hydrophilicity of the bile acids [63]. In a more recent animal model of cholestasis, norUDCA, compared with UDCA, significantly improved indices of liver injury in common bile duct-ligated mice [64].

The farnesoid X receptors (FXRs) are a group of nuclear hormone receptors expressed at high levels in tissues involved in bile acid metabolism, such as the liver, intestine, and kidney [65]. Bile acids have been identified as natural ligands of FXRs [66, 67]. FXRs play a key role in bile acid homeostasis by regulating genes involved in bile acid synthesis, secretion, conjugation, transportation, absorption, and detoxification [68–72] (Fig. 8.3). An important target of the FXRs is the gene encoding cholesterol 7α hydroxylase (CYP7A1), the rate-limiting enzyme in bile acid biosynthesis. When bound to bile acids, FXRs repress this gene [66]. Moreover, the expression of an important transport protein (cytosolic intestinal bile acid-binding protein) [73], located in the intestines, is increased as a result of activation of the FXRs [66, 74]. This protein is believed to play a key role in the regulation of the enterohepatic circulation [66, 74]. In addition to their role in bile acid homeostasis, FXRs have been found to regulate liver regeneration in liver injury [75–80].

Obeticholic acid (OCA, INT-747), a 6-ethyl derivative of the natural human bile acid CDCA, is a first-in-class selective FXR agonist, with ~100-fold greater FXR agonistic activity than that of CDCA [81–83]. In a male Wistar rat model of cholestasis, OCA protected hepatocytes against the deleterious effects caused by administration of LCA [83]. In another animal model, the administration of OCA reduced liver fibrosis and indices of hepatic damage in bile duct-ligated rats [84]. These results suggest that FXR agonists could be of therapeutic benefit in patients with cholestatic liver diseases. The safety and efficacy of OCA has been evaluated in two randomized clinical trials in patients with primary biliary cirrhosis (PBC) with promising results [85, 86]. The administration of OCA to PBC patients resulted in a significant reduction of serum ALP, an important surrogate marker in PBC [85, 86]. One important adverse event was pruritus, which was affected by OCA in a dose-dependent manner and led to discontinuation of the drug in 38% of PBC patients [85, 86].

The apical sodium-dependent bile acid transporter (ASBT), also known as the ileal bile acid transporter, is expressed predominantly in the distal ileal tissue and plays a key role in the reabsorption of bile acids from the lumen of the small intestine, which is critical for the enterohepatic circulation of the bile acids [87]. Normally, ~95% of secreted bile acids are reabsorbed from the intestine into the portal circulation and back to the liver [88]. Under this biological rationale, interrupting the enterohepatic circulation could result in a decreased bile acid load on the liver, which, in turn, could be of potential therapeutic benefit in patients with PSC (Fig. 8.3). The safety and efficacy of an ASBT inhibitor is being evaluated in patients with PSC.

8.4 Conclusion

Here, we summarized the etiology and treatment of PSC with regard to bile acids. Genetic backgrounds and immune mechanisms for PSC are becoming clarified gradually. New therapeutic strategies have also been trialed. Further studies are necessary to clarify the etiology of PSC.

Acknowledgments This work was supported by Health Labor Science Research Grants from Research on Measures for Intractable Diseases, the Intractable Hepato-biliary Diseases Study Group in Japan.

References

1. Lazaridis KN, Wiesner RH, Porayko MK, Ludwig J, LaRusso NF. Primary sclerosing cholangitis. In: Schiff ER, Sorrel MF, Maddrey WC, editors. Schiff's disease of the liver. English ed. Philadelphia: Lippincott-Raven; 1999. p. 649–78.
2. Lindor KD, LaRusso NF. Primary sclerosing cholangitis. In: Schiff L, Schiff ER, editors. Schiff's disease of the liver. 9th ed. Philadelphia: JB Lippincott; 2003. p. 673–84.
3. Carey JB. Bile acids, cirrhosis and human evolution. Gastroenterology. 1964;46:490–2.
4. Dew MJ, van Berge Henegouwen GP, Huybregts AW, Allan RN. Hepatotoxic effect of bile acids in inflammatory bowel disease. Gastroenterology. 1980;78:1393–401.
5. Pollheimer MJ, Halilbasic E, Fickert P, Trauner M. Pathogenesis of primary sclerosing cholangitis. Best practice & research. Clin Gastroenterol. 2011;25:727–39. doi:10.1016/j.bpg.2011.10.009.
6. Janse M, Lamberts LE, Franke L, Raychaudhuri S, Ellinghaus E, Muri Boberg K, et al. Three ulcerative colitis susceptibility loci are associated with primary sclerosing cholangitis and indicate a role for IL2, REL, and CARD9. Hepatology. 2011;53:1977–85. doi:10.1002/hep.24307.
7. Liu JZ, Hov JR, Folseraas T, Ellinghaus E, Rushbrook SM, Doncheva NT, et al. Dense genotyping of immune-related disease regions identifies nine new risk loci for primary sclerosing cholangitis. Nat Genet. 2013;45:670–5. doi:10.1038/ng.2616.
8. O'Mahony CA, Vierling JM. Etiopathogenesis of primary sclerosing cholangitis. Semin Liver Dis. 2006;26:3–21. doi:10.1055/s-2006-933559.
9. Lichtman SN, Sartor RB. Hepatobiliary injury associated with experimental small-bowel bacterial overgrowth in rats. Immunol Res. 1991;10:528–31. doi:10.1007/BF02919752.
10. Yamada S, Ishii M, Liang LS, Yamamoto T, Toyota T. Small duct cholangitis induced by N-formyl L-methionine L-leucine L-tyrosine in rats. J Gastroenterol. 1994;29:631–6. doi:10.1007/BF02365447.
11. Pollheimer MJ, Trauner M, Fickert P. Will we ever model PSC? – "it's hard to be a PSC model". Clin Res Hepatol Gastroenterol. 2011;35:792–804. doi:10.1016/j.clinre.2011.04.014.
12. Palmer KR, Duerden BI, Holdsworth CD. Bacteriological and endotoxin studies in cases of ulcerative colitis submitted to surgery. Gut. 1980;21:851–4. doi:10.1136/gut.21.10.851.
13. Farkkila M, Karvonen AL, Nurmi H, Nuutinen H, Taavitsainen M, Pikkarainen P, et al. Metronidazole and ursodeoxycholic acid for primary sclerosing cholangitis: a randomized placebo-controlled trial. Hepatology. 2004;40:1379–86. doi:10.1002/hep.20457.
14. Sheth P, Delos Santos N, Seth A, LaRusso NF, Rao RK. Lipopolysaccharide disrupts tight junctions in cholangiocyte monolayers by a c-Src-, TLR4-, and LBP-dependent mechanism. American journal of physiology. Gastrointest Liver Physiol 2007;293:G308–G318. doi.org/10.1152/ajpgi.00582.2006
15. Guo S, Al-Sadi R, Said HM, Ma TY. Lipopolysaccharide causes an increase in intestinal tight junction permeability in vitro and in vivo by inducing enterocyte membrane expression and localization of TLR-4 and CD14. Am J Pathol. 2013;182:375–87. doi:10.1016/j.ajpath.2012.10.014.
16. Fickert P, Fuchsbichler A, Wagner M, Marschall HU, Denk H, Trauner M. Regurgitation of bile acids from leaky bile ducts causes sclerosing cholangitis in Mdr2(Abcb4) knockout mice. Gastroenterology. 2004;127:261–74. doi:10.1053/j.gastro.2004.04.009.

17. Fickert P, Fuchsbichler A, Marschall HU, Wagner M, Zollner G, Krause R, et al. Lithocholic acid feeding induces segmental bile duct obstruction and destructive cholangitis in mice. Am J Pathol. 2006;168:410–22. doi:10.2353/ajpath.2006.050404.
18. Grant AJ, Lalor PF, Salmi M, Jalkanen S, Adams DH. Homing of mucosal lymphocytes to the liver in the pathogenesis of hepatic complications of inflammatory bowel disease. Lancet. 2002;359:150–7. doi:10.1016/S0140-6736(02)07374-9.
19. Cangemi JR, Wiesner RH, Beaver SJ, Ludwig J, MacCarty RL, Dozois RR, et al. Effect of proctocolectomy for chronic ulcerative colitis on the natural history of primary sclerosing cholangitis. Gastroenterology. 1989;96:790–4.
20. Singh S, Loftus EV, Talwalkar JA. Inflammatory bowel disease after liver transplantation for primary sclerosing cholangitis. Am J Gastroenterol. 2013;108:1417–25. doi:10.1038/ajg.2013.163.
21. Jørgensen KK, Grzyb K, Lundin KE, Clausen OP, Aamodt G, Schrumpf E, et al. Inflammatory bowel disease in patients with primary sclerosing cholangitis: clinical characterization in liver transplanted and nontransplanted patients. Inflamm Bowel Dis. 2012;18:536–45. doi:10.1002/ibd.21699.
22. Marelli L, Xirouchakis E, Kalambokis G, Cholongitas E, Hamilton MI, Burroughs AK. Does the severity of primary sclerosing cholangitis influence the clinical course of associated ulcerative colitis? Gut. 2011;60:1224–8. doi:10.1136/gut.2010.235408.
23. Navaneethan U, Venkatesh PG, Mukewar S, Lashner BA, Remzi FH, McCullough AJ, et al. Progressive primary sclerosing cholangitis requiring liver transplantation is associated with reduced need for colectomy in patients with ulcerative colitis. Clin Gastroenterol Hepatol. 2012;10:540–6. doi:10.1016//j.cgh.2012.01.006.
24. Eaton JE, Talwalkar JA, Lazaridis KN, Gores GJ, Lindor KD. Pathogenesis of primary sclerosing cholangitis and advances in diagnosis and management. Gastroenterology. 2013;145:521–36. doi:10.1053/j.gastro.2013.06.052.
25. Liaskou E, Karikoski M, Reynolds GM, Lalor PF, Weston CJ, Pullen N, et al. Regulation of mucosal addressin cell adhesion molecule 1 expression in human and mice by vascular adhesion protein 1 amine oxidase activity. Hepatology. 2011;53:661–72. doi:10.1002/hep.24085.
26. Briskin M, Winsor-Hines D, Syjan A, Cochran N, Bloom S, Wilson J, et al. Human mucosal addressin cell adhesion molecule-1 is preferentially expressed in intestinal tract and associated lymphoid tissue. Am J Pathol. 1997;151:97–110.
27. Grant AJ, Lalor PF, Hubscher SG, Brikts M, Adams DH. MAdCAM-1 expressed in chronic inflammatory liver disease supports mucosal lymphocyte adhesion to hepatic endothelium. Hepatology. 2001;33:1065–72. doi:10.1053/jhep.2001.24231.
28. Bochers AT, Shimmoda S, Bowlus C, Keen CL, Gershwin ME. Lymphocyte recruitment and homing to the liver in primary biliary cirrhosis and primary sclerosing cholangitis. Semin Immunopathol. 2009;31:309–22. doi:10.1007/s00281-009-0167-2.
29. Ali AH, Carey EJ, Lindor KD. Current research on the treatment of primary sclerosing cholangitis. Intractable Rare Dis Res. 2015;4:1–6. doi:10.5582/irdr.2014.01018.
30. Schramm C, Schirmacher P, Helmreich-Becker I, Gerken G, Zum Büschenfelde KH, Lohse AW. Combined therapy with azathioprine, prednisolone, and ursodiol in patients with primary sclerosing cholangitis. a case series. Ann Intern Med. 1999;131:943–6. doi:10.7326/0003-4819-131-12-199912210-00006.
31. Bach N, Bodian C, Bodenheimer H, Croen E, Berk PD, Thung SN, et al. Methotrexate therapy for primary biliary cirrhosis. Am J Gastroenterol. 2003;98:187–93. doi:10.1111/j.1572-0241.2003.07173.
32. Feagan BG, Rutgeerts P, Sands BE, Hanauer S, Colombel JF, Sandborn WJ, et al. Vedolizumab as induction and maintenance therapy for ulcerative colitis. N Engl J Med. 2013;369:699–710. doi:10.1056/NEJMoa1215734.

33. Eksteen B, Grant AJ, Miles A, Curbishley SM, Lalor PF, Hubscher SG, et al. Hepatic endothelial CCL25 mediates the recruitment of CCR9+ gut-homing lymphocytes to the liver in primary sclerosing cholangitis. J Exp Med. 2004;200:1511–7. doi:10.1084/jem.20041035.
34. Lichtman SN, Keku J, Clark RL, Schwab JH, Sartor RB. Biliary tract disease in rats with experimental small bowel bacterial overgrowth. Infect Immun. 1991;59:555–62. doi:10.1002/hep.1840130425.
35. Silveria MG, Torok NJ, Gossard AA, Keach JC, Jorgensen RA, Petz JL, et al. Minocycline in the treatment of patients with primary sclerosing cholangitis. Results of a pilot study. Am J Gastroenterol. 2009;104:83–8. doi:10.1038/ajg.2008.14.
36. Tabian JH, Weeding E, Jorgensen RA, Petz JL, Keach JC, Talwalkar JA, et al. Randomised clinical trial: vancomycin or metronidazole in patients with primary sclerosing cholangitis-pilot study. Aliment Pharmacol Ther. 2013;37:604–12. doi:10.1111/apt.12232.
37. Chazouilleres O. Primary sclerosing cholangitis and bile acids. Clin Res Hepatol Gastroenterol. 2012;36:S21–5. doi:10.1016/S2210-7401(12)70017-7.
38. Nakazawa T, Hoshino M, Hayakawa T, Tanaka A, Ohiwa T. Vaasopressin reduces tauro-chenodeoxycholate-induced hepatotoxicity by lowering the hepatocyte taurochenodeoxycholate content. J Hepatol. 1996;25:739–47. doi:10.1016/S0168-8278(96)80247-9.
39. Fickert P, Fuchsbicheler A, Wagener M, Zollner G, Kaser A, Tilg H, et al. Regurgitation of bile acids from leaky bile ducts causes sclerosing cholangitis in Mdr2(ABCB4) knockout mice. Gastroenterology. 2004;127:261–74. doi:10.1053/j.gastro.2004.04.009.
40. Beuers U, Honester S, de Buy Wenniger LJ, Kremer AE, Jansen PL, Elferink RP. The biliary HCO_{3-} umbrella: a unifying hypothesis on pathogenetic and therapeutic aspects of fibrosing cholangiopathies. Hepatology 2010;52:1489–1496. doi.org/10.1002/hep.23810
41. Karlsen TH, Franke A, Melum E, Kaser A, Hov JR, Balschun T, et al. Genome-wide association analysis in primary sclerosing cholangitis. Gastroenterology. 2010;138:1102–11. doi:10.1053/j.gastro.2009.11.046.
42. Khare S, Mustafi R, Cerda S, Yuan W, Jagadeeswaran S, Dougherty U, et al. Ursodeoxycholic acid suppresses Cox-2 expression in colon cancer: roles of ras, p38, and ccaat/enhancer-binding protein. Nutr Cancer. 2008;60:389–400. doi:10.1080/01635580701883003.
43. Batta AK, Salen G, Holubec H, Brasitus TA, Alberts D, Earnest DL. Enrichment of the more hydrophilic bile acid ursodeoxycholic acid in the fecal water-soluble fraction after feeding to rats with colon cancer polyps. Cancer Res. 1998;58:1684–7.
44. Wall RK, Frawley BP, Hartmann S, Roy HK, Khare S, Scaglione-Sewell BA, et al. Mechanism of action of chemo-protective ursodeoxycholate in the azoxymethane model of colon carcinogenesis: potential roles of protein kinase C-α, -βII, and-zeta. Cancer Res. 1995;55:5257–64.
45. Rodrigues CMP, Kren BT, Steer CJ, Setchell KD. The site-specific delivery of ursodeoxycholic acid to the rat colon by sulfate conjugation. Gastroenterology. 1995;9:1835–44. doi:10.1016/0016-5085(95)90750-5.
46. Im E, Martinez JD. Ursodeoxycholic acid (UDCA) can inhibit deoxycholic acid (DCA) induced apoptosis via modulation of EGFR/RAF-1/ERK signaling in human colon cancer cells. J Nutr. 2004;134:483–6.
47. Yui S, Saeki T, Kanamoto R, Iwami K. Characteristics of apoptosis in HCT116 colon cancer cells induced by deoxycholic acid. J Biochem. 2005;138:151–7. doi:10.1093/jb/mvi106.
48. Tung BY, Emond MJ, Haggitt RC, Bronner MP, Kimmey MB, Kowdley KV, et al. Ursodiol use is associated with lower prevalence of colonic neoplasia in patients with ulcerative colitis and primary sclerosing cholangitis. Ann Intern Med. 2001;134:89–95. doi:10.7326/0003-4819-134-2-200101160-00008.
49. Pardi DS, Loftus EV, Kremers WK, Keach J, Lindor KD. Ursodeoxycholic acid as a chemo-preventative agent in patients with ulcerative colitis and primary sclerosing cholangitis. Gastroenterology. 2003;124:889–93. doi:10.1053/gast.2003.50156.
50. Wolf JM, Rybicki LA, Lashner BA. The impact of ursodeoxycholic acid on cancer, dysplasia and mortality in ulcerative colitis patients with primary sclerosing cholangitis. Aliment Pharmacol Ther. 2005;22:783–8. doi:10.1111/j.1365-2036.2005.02650.

51. Lindor KD, Kowdley KV, Luketic VA, Harrison ME, MacCashland T, Befeler AS, et al. High-dose ursodeoxycholic acid for the treatment of primary sclerosing cholangitis. Hepatology. 2009;50:808–14. doi:10.1002/hep.23082.
52. Imam MH, Sinakos E, Gossard AA, Kowdely KV, Luketic VA, Edwyn Harrison M, et al. High-dose ursodeoxycholic acid increases risk of adverse outcomes in patients with early stage primary sclerosing cholangitis. Aliment Pharmacol Ther. 2011;34:1185–92. doi:10.1111/j.1365-2036.2011.04863.
53. Eaton JE, Silveira MG, Pardi DS, Sinakos E, Kowdley KV, Luketic VA, et al. High-dose ursodeoxycholic acid is associated with the development of colorectal neoplasia in patients with ulcerative colitis and primary sclerosing cholangitis. Am J Gastroenterol. 2011;106:1638–45.
54. Sinakos E, Marschall HU, Kowdley KV, Befeler A, Keach J, Lindor K, et al. Bile acid changes after high-dose ursodeoxycholic acid treatment in primary sclerosing cholangitis: relation to disease progression. Hepatology. 2010;52:197–203. doi:10.1002/hep.23631.
55. Kay RM. Effects of diet on fecal excretion and bacterial modification of acidic and neutral steroids, and implications for colon carcinogenesis. Cancer Res. 1981;41:3774–7.
56. Nagengast FM, Grubben MJ, van Munster IP. Role of bile acids in colorectal carcinogenesis. Eur J Cancer. 1995;31:1067–70. doi:10.1016/0959-8049(95)00216-6.
57. Bernstein H, Bernstein C, Payne CM, Dvorak K. Bile acids as endogenous etiologic agents in gastrointestinal cancer. World J Gastroenterol. 2009;15:3329–40. doi:10.3748/wjg.15.3329.
58. Bernstein H, Bernstein C, Payne CM, Dvorakova K, Garewal H. Bile acids as carcinogens in human gastrointestinal cancers. Mutat Res. 2005;589:47–65. doi:10.1016/j.mrrev.2004.08.001.
59. Debruyne PR, Bruynell EA, Karaguni I-M, Li X, Flatau G, Müller O, et al. Bile acids stimulate invasion and haptotaxis in human colorectal cancer cells through activation of multiple oncogenic signaling pathways. Oncogene. 2002;21:6740–50. doi:10.1038/sj.onc.1205729.
60. Baek MK, Park JS, Park JH, Kim MH, Kim HD, Bae WK, et al. Lithocholic acid upregulates uPAR and cell invasiveness via MAPK and AP-1 signaling in colon cancer cells. Cancer Lett. 2010;290:123–8. doi:10.1016/j.canlet.2009.08.030.
61. McMillan L, Butcher S, Wallis Y, Neoptolemos JP, Lord JM. Bile acids reduce the apoptosis effects of sodium butyrate on human colon adenoma (AA/C1) cells: implications for colon carcinogenesis. Biochem Biophys Res Commun. 2000;273:45–9. doi:10.1006/bbrc.2000.2899.
62. Chapman R, Fevery J, Kalloo A, Nagorney DM, Boberg KM, Schneider B, et al. Diagnosis and management of primary sclerosing cholangitis. Hepatology. 2010;51:660–78. doi:10.1002/hep.23294.
63. Fickert P, Wagner M, Marschall HU, Fuchsbichler A, Zollner G, Tsybrovskyy O, et al. 24-nor Ursodeoxycholic acid is superior to ursodeoxycholic acid in the treatment of sclerosing cholangitis in Mdr2 knockout mice. Gastroenterology. 2006;130:465–81. doi:10.1053/j.gastro.2005.10.018.
64. Fickert P, Pollheimer MJ, Silbert D, Moustafa T, Halibasic E, Krones E, et al. Differential effects of nor UDCA and UDCA in obstructive cholestasis in mice. Gastroenterology. 2006;130:465–81. doi:10.1053/j.gastro.2005.10.018.
65. Forman BM, Goode E, Chen J, Oro AE, Bradley DJ, Perlmann T. Identification of a nuclear receptor that is activated by farnesol metabolites. Cell. 1995;81:687–93. doi:10.1016/0092-8674(95)90530-8.
66. Makishima M, Okamoto AY, Repa JJ, Tu H, Learned RM, Luk A, et al. Identification of a nuclear receptor for bile acids. Science. 1999;284:1362–5. doi:10.1126/science.284.5418.1362.
67. Wang H, Chen J, Hollister K, Sowers LC, Forman BM. Endogenous bile acids are ligands for the nuclear receptor FXR/BAR. Mol Cell. 1999;3:545–53. doi:10.1016/S1097-2765(00)80348-2.

68. Cariou B, Staels B. FXR: a promising target for the pathogenesis of primary sclerosing cholangitis. Best Pract Res Clin Gastroenterol. 2011;25:727–39. doi:10.1016/j.bpg.2011.10.009.
69. Edwards PA, Kast HR, Anisfeld AM. BAREing it all: the adoption of LXR and FXR and their roles in lipid homeostasis. J Lipid Res. 2002;43:2–12.
70. Li J, Pircher PC, Schulman IG, Westin SK. Regulation of complement C3 expression by the bile acid receptor FXR. J Biol Chem. 2005;280:7427–34. doi:10.1074/jbc.M411473200.
71. Sinal CJ, Tohkin M, Miyata M, Ward JM, Lambert G, Gonzalez FJ. Targeted disruption of the nuclear receptor FXR/BAR impairs bile acid and lipid homeostasis. Cell. 2000;102:731–44. doi:10.1016/S0092-8674(00)00062-3.
72. Zhang Y, Castellani LW, Sinai CJ, Gonzalez FJ, Edwards PA. Peroxisome proliferator-activated receptor-gamma coactivator 1alpha (PGC-1alpha) regulates triglyceride metabolism by activation of the nuclear receptor FXR. Genes Dev. 2004;18:157–69. doi:10.1101/gad.1138104.
73. Kanda T, Foucand L, Nakamura Y, Niot I, Besnard P, Fujita M, et al. Regulation of expression of human intestinal bile acid binding protein in Caco-2 cells. Biochem J. 1998;330:261–5. doi:10.1042/bj3300261.
74. Gong YZ, Everett ET, Schwartz DA, Norris JS, Wilson FA. Molecular cloning, tissue distribution, and expression of a 14-kDa bile acid-binding protein from rat ileal cytosol. Proc Natl Acad Sci U S A. 1994;91:4741–5. doi:10.1073/pnas.91.11.4741.
75. Huang W, Ma K, Zhang J, Katanani M, Cuviller J, Liu J, et al. Nuclear receptor dependent bile acid signaling is required for normal liver regeneration. Science. 2006;312:233–6. doi:10.1126/science.1121435.
76. Goldfarb M. Signaling by fibroblast growth factors: the inside story. Sci STKE. 2001;2001:e37. doi:10.1101/gad.1083503.
77. Holt JA, Luo G, Billin AN, Bisi J, McNeill YY, Kozarsky KF, et al. Definition of a novel growth factor-dependent signal cascade for the suppression of bile acid biosynthesis. Genes Dev. 2003;17:1581–91. doi:10.1101/gad.1083503.
78. Ornitz DM, Itoh N. Fibroblast growth factors. Genome Biol. 2001; 2:REVIEWS3005.
79. Song KH, Ellis E, Strom S, Chiang JY. Hepatocyte growth factor signaling pathway inhibits cholesterol 7alpha-hydroxylase and bile acid synthesis in human hepatocytes. Hepatology. 2007;46:1993–2002. doi:10.1002/hep.21878.
80. Zhang L, Huang X, Meng Z, Dong B, Shiah S, DD M, et al. Significance and mechanism of CYP7a1 gene regulation during the acute phase of liver regeneration. Mol Endocrinol. 2009;23:137–45. doi:10.1210/me.2008-0198.
81. Adorini L, Pruzanski M, Shapiro D. Farnesoid X receptor targeting to treat nonalcoholic steatohepatitis. Drug Discov Today. 2012;17:988–97. doi:10.1016/j.drudis.2012.05.012.
82. Pellicciari R, Costanitino G, Camaioni E, Sadeghpour BM, Entrena A, Willson TM, et al. Bile acid derivatives as ligands of the farnesoid X receptor. Synthesis, evaluation, and structure-activity relationship of a series of body and side chain modified analogues of chenodeoxycholic acid. J Med Chem. 2004;47:4559–69. doi:10.1021/jm049904b.
83. Pellicciari R, Fiorucci S, Camaioni E, Clerici C, Costantino G, Maloney PR, et al. 6alpha-ethyl-chenodeoxycholic acid (6-ECDCA), a potent and selective FXR agonist endowed with anticholestatic activity. J Med Chem. 2002;45:3569–72. doi:10.1021/jm025529g.
84. Fiorucci S, Antonelli E, Rizzo G, Renga B, Mencarelli A, Riccardi L, et al. The nuclear receptor SHP mediates inhibition of hepatic stellate cells by FXR and protects against liver fibrosis. Gastroenterology. 2004;127:1497–512. doi:10.1053/j.gastro.2004.08.001.
85. Mason A, Luketic VA, Lindor KD, et al. Farnesoid-X receptor agonists: a new class of drugs for the treatment of PBC? An international study evaluating the addition of INT-747 to ursodeoxycholic acid. J Hepatol. 2010;52(Suppl 1):S1–2. doi:10.1016/S0168-8278(10)60004-9.
86. Kowedley KV, Jones D, Luketic V, et al. An international study evaluating the farnesoid X receptor agonist obeticholic acid as monotherapy in PBC. J Hepatol. 2011;54:S13. doi:10.1016/S0168-8278(11)60030-5.

87. Chen L, Yao X, Young A, McNulty J, Anderson D, Liu Y, et al. Inhibition of apical sodium-dependent bile acid transporter as a novel treatment for diabetes. Am J Physiol Endocrinol Metab. 2012;302:E68–76. doi:10.1152/ajpendo.00323.2011.
88. Meier PJ, Stieger B. Bile salt transporters. Annu Rev Physiol. 2002;64:635–61. doi:10.1146/annurev.physiol.64.082201.100300.

Chapter 9
Bile Acids and Cholestatic Liver Disease 3: Inborn Errors of Bile Acid Synthesis

Hiroshi Nittono, Akihiko Kimura, Hajime Takei, Takao Kurosawa, and Takashi Iida

Abstract Inborn errors of bile acid synthesis are rare genetic disorders that can present as neonatal cholestasis and fat-soluble vitamin deficiency. Though rare, these diseases account for some patients with cholestasis of unknown etiology. Seven known defects of bile acid synthesis occur in children. These defects may be categorized as deficiencies in activity of enzymes catalyzing reactions affecting the steroid nucleus or the side chain. Defects in reactions involving the steroid nucleus include cholesterol 7α-hydroxylase deficiency, 3β-hydroxysteroid-Δ^5-C_{27}-steroid dehydrogenase/isomerase deficiency, Δ^4-3-oxosteroid 5β-reductase deficiency, and oxysterol 7α-hydroxylase deficiency. Defects in reactions involving side-chain modification are sterol 27-hydroxylase deficiency, α-methyl-CoA racemase deficiency, disorders of peroxisomal β-oxidation, bile acid-CoA: amino acid N-acyltransferase deficiency, and bile acid-CoA ligase deficiency. Cholesterol 7α-hydroxylase deficiency and disorders of peroxisomal β-oxidation are not considered here, since cholesterol 7α-hydroxylase deficiency is not known to occur in children and disorders of peroxisomal β-oxidation represent disease of peroxisomes. When identified early, many patients with inborn errors of bile acid synthesis have a favorable clinical response to oral primary bile acid therapy. These inborn errors characteristically result in elevated serum bilirubin and aminotransferase concentrations but produce no abnormalities of serum γ-glutamyltransferase or of total bile acid concentrations detectable by enzymatic methods. Screening for

---

H. Nittono (✉) • H. Takei
Junshin Clinic Bile Acid Institute, 2-1-22 Haramachi, Meguro-ku, Tokyo 152-0011, Japan
e-mail: bile-res@eco.ocn.ne.jp

A. Kimura
Department of Pediatrics and Child Health, Kurume University School of Medicine, 67 Asahi-machi, Kurume 830-0011, Japan

T. Kurosawa
School of Pharmaceutical Sciences, Health Sciences University of Hokkaido, Kanazawa, Ishikari-Tobetsu, Hokkaido 061-0293, Japan

T. Iida
Department of Chemistry, College of Humanities and Sciences, Nihon University, Sakurajousui, Setagaya-ku, Tokyo 156-8550, Japan

S. Tazuma, H. Takikawa (eds.), *Bile Acids in Gastroenterology*,
DOI 10.1007/978-4-431-56062-3_9

inborn errors of bile acid synthesis using fast atom bombardment ionization mass spectrometry, gas chromatography-mass spectroscopy, and liquid chromatography-electrospray ionization tandem mass spectrometry is useful. Genetic analysis is available for a definitive diagnosis. Disorders of bile acid synthesis account for some 2–3% of screened cases of cholestatic liver disease in infants and children.

Keywords Inborn error of bile acid synthesis (IEBAS) • Cholestasis • Giant cell hepatitis • γ-Glutamyl-transpeptidase (GGT) • Oral primary bile acid therapy

9.1 Two Main Pathways from Cholesterol to Primary Bile Acids [1, 2]

The primary bile acids, cholic acid (CA) and chenodeoxycholic acid (CDCA), are synthesized by sequential enzymatic modifications to cholesterol that involve at least 14 enzymes, multiple subcellular compartments, and two complementary chemical pathways (Fig. 9.1). There are two pathways of 7α-hydroxylation that include a neutral pathway in which cholesterol is hydroxylated by cholesterol 7α-hydroxylase and an acidic pathway in which cholesterol is hydroxylated and oxidized at position 27 and then hydroxylated by oxysterol 7α-hydroxylase. Nine defects in bile acid synthesis show a phenotype of familial and progressive infantile or late-onset cholestasis or fat-soluble vitamin deficiency. In this chapter, however, cholesterol 7α-hydroxylase (CYP7A1) deficiency and disorder of peroxisomal β-oxidation are not considered, because CYP7A1 deficiency has not been found to occur in children and disorders of peroxisomal β-oxidation are disease of peroxisomes, representing a separate category.

9.2 Clinical Features and Diagnosis of Inborn Errors of Bile Acid Synthesis [3]

Although inborn errors of bile acid synthesis (IEBAS) show cholestasis, serum total bile acid (TBA) concentrations are normal when measured by enzymatic methods. Serum γ-glutamyltransferase (GGT) concentrations also are normal. Even though the patient shows obstructive jaundice, pruritus is absent. Histopathologic findings associated with defects involving reactions affecting the steroid nucleus vary with patient age and rate of disease progression. Specimens from infants with impaired steroid nucleus modification show giant cell hepatitis, canalicular bile plugs, hepatocyte bile stasis, and portal tract inflammation, with variable severity of fibrosis. Generally, urinary screening for IEBAS uses fast atom bombardment ionization mass spectrometry (FAB-MS) in the USA and Europe and gas chromatography-mass spectroscopy (GC-MS) or liquid chromatography-electrospray ionization tandem mass spectrometry (LC-ESI-MS/MS) in Japan [4] (Table 9.1). Genetic analysis is available for definitive diagnosis [5].

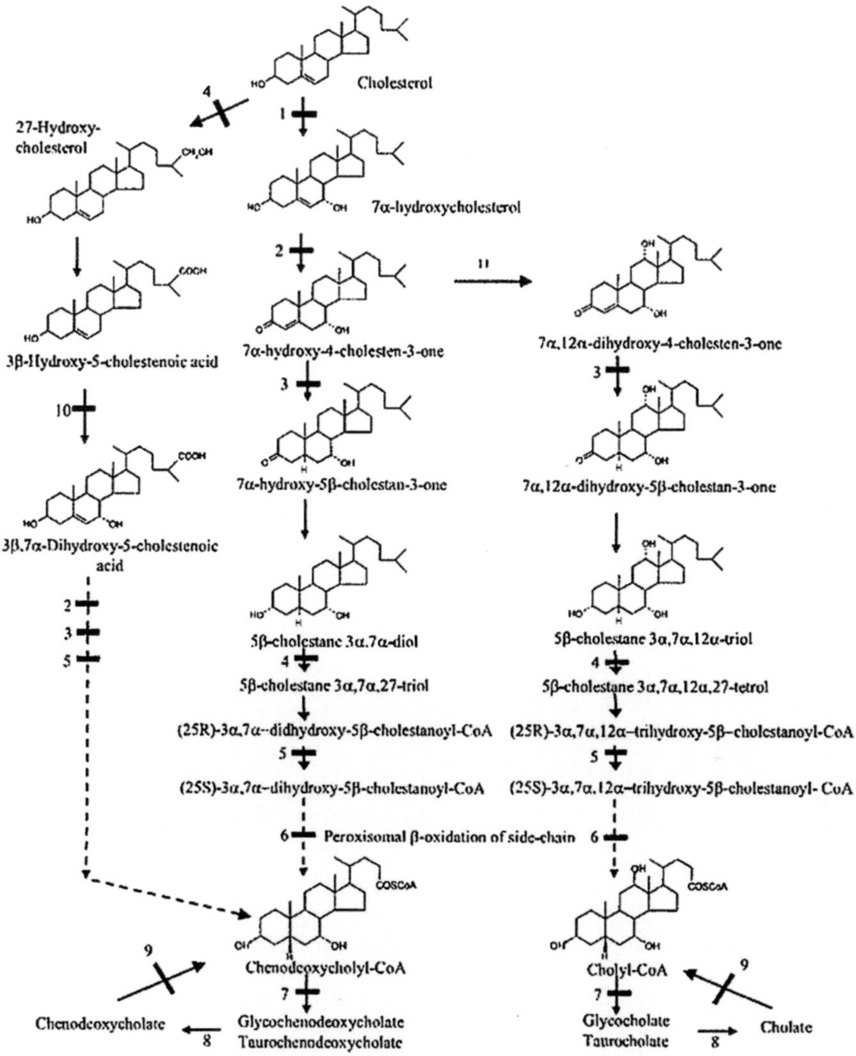

Fig. 9.1 Simplified scheme of the two major pathways for the synthesis of bile acids from cholesterol and for their recycling. The "neutral" pathway starts with conversion of cholesterol to 7α-hydroxycholesterol, while the "acidic" pathway begins with formation of 27-hydroxycholesterol. Numbered bars indicate blockades imposed by enzymatic defects. (*1*) cholesterol 7α-hydroxylase; (*2*) 3β-hydroxy-Δ^5-C_{27}-steroid dehydrogenase/isomerase; (*3*) Δ^4-3-oxosteroid 5β-reductase; (*4*) sterol 27-hydroxylase; (*5*) α-methylacyl CoA racemase; (*6*) proteins involved in peroxisomal biogenesis and β-oxidation; (*7*) bile acid-CoA: amino acid N-acyl transferase; (*8*) bacterial deconjugation in the gut; (*9*) bile acid-CoA ligase; (*10*) oxysterol 7α-hydroxylase; (11) sterol 12α-hydroxylase. Known enzyme defects are depicted by solid bars across the arrows (Adapted from [1])

Table 9.1 Bile acid analysis of the urine using GC/MS in three patients with inborn errors of bile acid synthesis

Patient	*HSD3B7* deficiency (F, 22years)				*SRD5B1* deficiency (M, 6 months)				*CYP7B1* deficiency (F, 6 months)			
	Before		After 3 years		Before		After 4 years		Before		After 1 month	
Treatment	mmol/molCre (%)		mmol/molCre (%)		mmol/molCre (%)		mmol/molCre (%)		mmol/molCre (%)		mmol/molCre (%)	
Total bile acids	115.4		0.8		125.9		6.2		109.5		11.4	
Usual bile acids	2.2	(9.8)	0.2	(30.2)	1.2	(1.0)	0.5	(8.7)	4.9	(9.7)	2.7	(92.9)
UDCA	93.0	–	0.1	–	0.0	–	0.0	–	59.2	–	8.5	–
3-Oxo-Δ^4-bile acids	0.0	(0.0)	0.0	(0.0)	123.9	(98.4)	5.4	(87.0)	2.0	(3.9)	0.0	(1.4)
Monohydroxy-Δ^5-bile acids	0.0	(0.0)	0.1	(11.1)	0.0	(0.0)	0.1	(1.3)	41.7	(82.9)	0.0	(0.0)
Dihydroxy-Δ^5-bile acids	5.0	(22.5)	0.1	(12.7)	0.0	(0.0)	0.0	(0.3)	0.2	(0.3)	0.0	(0.0)
Trihydroxy-Δ^5-bile acids	15.2	(67.7)	0.3	(44.4)	0.0	(0.0)	0.0	(0.0)	0.0	(0.0)	0.0	(0.0)
Others	0.0	(0.0)	0.0	(1.6)	0.8	(0.6)	0.2	(2.7)	1.6	(3.1)	0.2	(5.8)

Two patients, with 3β-hydroxysteroid-Δ^5-C_{27}-steroid dehydrogenase/isomerase (*HSD3B7*) deficiency and Δ^4-3-oxosteroid 5β-reductase (*SRD5B1*) deficiency, underwent oral chenodeoxycholic acid treatment. A patient with oxysterol-7α-hydroxylase (*CYP7B1*) deficiency underwent living donor liver transplantation

9.3 Inborn Errors of Bile Acid Synthesis [3]

9.3.1 Defects Involving Reactions Affecting the Steroid Nucleus

9.3.1.1 3β-Hydroxy-Δ^5-C_{27}-Steroid Dehydrogenase/Isomerase (3βHSD, *HSD3B7*) Deficiency [6]

3βHSD deficiency, the most common bile acid synthetic defect, is caused by mutation in the *HSD3B7* gene on chromosome 16p. The inheritance pattern is autosomal recessive. The major bile acids present in serum and excreted as sulfate esters in the urine are Δ^5-3β,7α-dihydroxy-5-cholenoic and Δ^5-3β,7α,12α-trihydroxy-5-cholenoic acids. About 50 patients with this disorder have been reported. Even adults with this disease have been reported reflecting its relatively mild nature. Some treated patients with this disease have had normal children [7]. Orally administered primary bile acids (CA and/or CDCA) represent an effective treatment that may normalize and growth and development. However, ursodeoxycholic acid (UDCA) is not effective. Bile acid profiles in serum and urine after bile acid therapy show a marked decrease in amounts of unusual bile acids but no decrease in their percentages.

9.3.1.2 Δ^4-3-Oxosteroid 5β-Reductase (5β-Reductase, *SRD5B1*, *AKR1D1*) Deficiency [8, 9]

5β-Reductase deficiency is an autosomal recessive disorder. The affected enzyme, Δ^4-3-oxosteroid-5β-reductase, is encoded by the gene *AKR1D1* (or *SRD5B1*) and converts 7α-hydroxy-4-cholesten-3-one and 7α,12α-dihydroxy-4-cholesten-3-one into 3-oxo-5β analogues. Excretion of large amounts of 3-oxo-Δ^4-bile acids also may be detected in urine from children with severe liver disease arising from causes other than primary defects in bile acid biosynthesis. An alternative clinical presentation, neonatal liver failure resembling neonatal hemochromatosis, also has been described in patients with 5β-reductase deficiency, although no patient with this presentation has been shown to have mutations in the *AKR1D1* gene. Histopathology in patients with 5β-reductase deficiency is typical for neonatal hepatitis, with findings of giant cell hepatitis, pseudoacinar transformation, hepatocellular and canalicular cholestasis, and extramedullary hematopoiesis. Investigation of the urinary steroid profile of patients with this disease showed that tetrahydrocortisone, whose synthesis is catalyzed by 5β-reductase activity in the liver, is decreased; however, no symptoms of adrenal dysfunctional arise, because of compensation by 5β-reductase [10].

9.3.1.3 Oxysterol 7α-Hydroxylase (*CYP7B1*) Deficiency [11]

Deficiency involving the enzyme oxysterol 7α-hydroxylase, which is enclosed by the *CYP7B1* gene, interrupts the alternative acidic pathway for synthesis of the bile acid steroid nucleus. Liver function tests show elevated alanine aminotransferase, but serum TBA and GGT are within the normal range. Large amounts of 3β-monohydroxy-Δ^5 bile acids are detected in serum and urine. Several patients have been reported to be homozygous for nonsense mutations in the *CYP7B1* gene encoding oxysterol 7α-hydroxylase. Further information concerning possible consequences of oxysterol 7α-hydroxylase deficiency has been uncovered by a gene mapping study of hereditary spastic paraplegia [12]. Patients with oxysterol 7α-hydroxylase deficiency have a marked bleeding tendency and are severely ill. Recently, two patients rescued by liver transplantation [13] or CDCA therapy (11 mg/kg/day) [14] have been reported.

9.3.2 Defects Involving Reactions Leading to Side-Chain Modification

9.3.2.1 Sterol 27-Hydroxylase (*CYP27A1*) Deficiency

CYP27A1 deficiency has two possible phenotypes. One is a cholestatic disorder with neonatal [15]. Another is cerebrotendinous xanthomatosis (CTX), which develops in adolescence [16].

A defect in side-chain oxidation via the 25-hydroxylation pathway has been in a reported 9-week-old infant who presented with familial giant cell hepatitis and severe intrahepatic cholestasis. Diagnosis was based upon findings of reduced primary bile acid concentrations and elevated concentrations of specific bile alcohol glucuronides in serum. This boy had consistently normal aminotransferase concentrations. Bile alcohol production was suppressed by primary bile acids, CDCA and CA. Subsequently the patient was diagnosed with CYP27A1 deficiency by demonstrational a mutation in *CYP27A1* [17], after which similar cholestatic disease has been reported in neonates [18].

CTX is a rare inherited lipid storage disease characterized by progressive neurologic dysfunction, dementia, ataxia, and cataracts. This disorder results from abnormal side-chain modification of bile acids, which is caused by mitochondrial sterol 27-hydroxylase deficiency. In patients with CTX, primary bile acid synthesis is reduced, while bile alcohol glucuronide excretion in bile, urine, and stools is increased. Serum and plasma cholesterol concentrations are low or normal, while plasma cholestanol concentrations are markedly elevated. In early childhood, CTX may present with chronic diarrhea and cataracts or with developmental delay/regression. Later in childhood, CTX may present with tendon xanthomata, low IQ, or psychiatric illness. Diagnosis of CTX is established by the finding of a greatly increased plasma cholestanol/cholesterol ratio or a characteristic metabolite in urine, followed by DNA sequencing of *CYP27A1*. Oral CDCA therapy is effective.

9.3.2.2 α-Methylacyl-CoA Racemase (AMACR) Deficiency [19]

AMACR deficiency is an autosomal recessive disorder in which cholesterol side-chain oxidation is inhibited. AMACR is necessary for racemization of trihydroxycholestenoic acid and pristanic acid into their stereoisomers. Conversion of these stereoisomers is necessary for the subsequent step of peroxisomal β-oxidation of the C27 bile acid side chain. AMACR deficiency affects both bile acid and fatty acid synthesis pathways. Histopathologic findings in infants with this disease include giant cell transformation, moderate intralobular cholestasis, scattered necrotic hepatocytes, and foci with multinucleated hepatocytes. Affected infants' liver enzyme activities were normalized by treatment with CA therapy (15 mg/kg/day) and fat-soluble vitamin supplements [19].

9.3.3 Bile Acid Conjugation Defects

Conjugation of CA and CDCA to taurine or glycine, the final step in primary bile acid synthesis, is catalyzed by bile acid-CoA: amino acid N-acyltransferase (BAAT) in the liver, after which the conjugate is excreted via the intestine, where bacterial deconjugation occurs. Reconjugation in the course of the enterohepatic circulation requires two enzymes, bile acid-CoA ligase (*SLC27A5*) and BAAT, in the liver (Fig. 9.1).

9.3.3.1 Bile Acid-CoA: Amino Acid N-Acyltransferase (BAAT) Deficiency [20]

Patients affected by defects in bile acid conjugation present with marked malabsorption and deficiencies of fat-soluble vitamins. These symptoms occur as a consequence of decreased biliary secretion of conjugated bile acids. Severe cholestasis and liver failure also have been described in patients with bile acid conjugation defects. Oral administration of conjugated primary bile acid, such as glycocholic acid (15 mg/kg/day), is a potential treatment for these patients [21].

9.3.3.2 Bile Acid-CoA Ligase (*SLC27A5*) Deficiency [22]

A patient with this disorder developed conjugated hyperbilirubinemia which persisted until the age of 12 months but was unaccompanied by cholestasis. A liver biopsy specimen showed portal-to-portal bridging fibrosis. Analysis of urinary

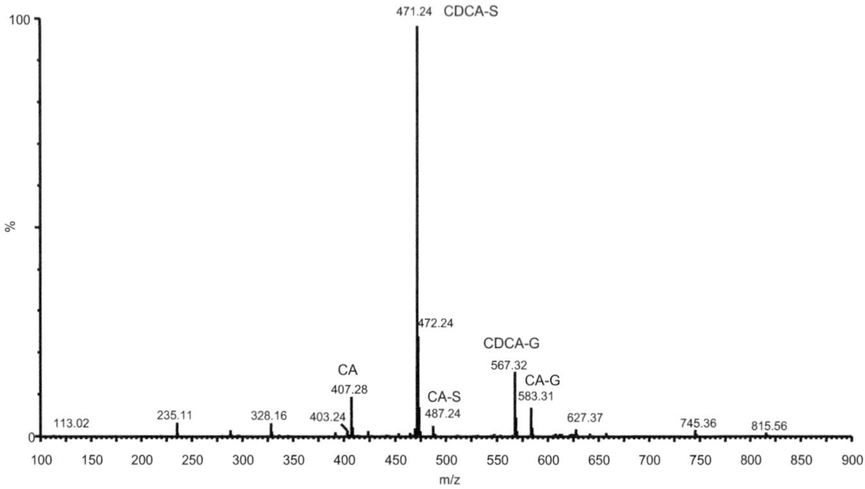

Fig. 9.2 Bile acid electrospray ionization mass spectra in urine of a patient with bile acid amidation defect. Abscissa, mass-charge ratio (m/z); ordinate, intensity of ion current as percentage of intensity of most abundant peak in spectrum (%). Principal peak sites and the species represented are unamidated cholic acid (CA), 407; unamidated chenodeoxycholic acid sulfate (CDCA-S), 471; unamidated cholic acid sulfate CA-S), 487; unamidated chenodeoxycholic acid glucuronide (CDCA-G), 567; unamidated cholic acid glucuronide (CA-G), 583

cholanoids by negative ion electrospray ionization mass spectrometry showed the major cholanoids to be similar to those seen in BAAT deficiency, with the major peak representing unconjugated CA. Most serum bile acids were unconjugated. Sequencing of the BAAT gene showed no mutation, but sequencing of the *SLC27A5* gene, which encodes bile acid-CoA ligase, detected homozygous mutations in a histidine residue. The treatment given was oral UDCA and fat-soluble vitamins. Interestingly, this patient had a homozygous mutation in the bile salt export pump (BSEP, *ABCB11*).

Recently, we encountered a patient with an amidation defect. The specimen dried urine drops on filter paper was sent from Thailand to our institution. Results of bile acid analysis in this material showed a likely amidation defect; almost all bile acids were conjugated to sulfate or glucuronide (Fig. 9.2). Unfortunately, no genetic analysis was performed in this patient.

References

1. Clayton PT. Disorders of bile acid synthesis. J Inherit Metab Dis. 2011;34:593–604.
2. Sundaram S, Bove KE, Lovell MA, Sokol RJ. Mechanisms of disease: inborn errors of bile acid synthesis. Nat Clin Pract Gastroenterol Hepatol. 2008;5:456–68.

3. Setchell KDR, O'Connell NC. Disorders of bile acid synthesis and metabolism: a metabolic basis for liver disease. In: Suchy FJ, Sokol RJ, Balistereri WF, editors. Liver disease in children. New York: Cambridge University Press; 2007. p. 736–66.
4. Muto A, Takei H, Unno A, Murai T, Kurosawa T, Ogawa S, et al. Detection of Δ^4-3-oxo-steroid 5β-reductase deficiency by LC-ESI-MS/MS measurement of urinary bile acids. J Chromatogr B. 2012;900:24–31.
5. Seki Y, Mizuochi T, Kimura A, Takahashi T, Ohtake A, Hayashi S-I, et al. Two neonatal cholestasis patients with mutations in the SRD5B1 (*AKR1D1*) gene: diagnosis and bile acid profiles during chenodeoxycholic acid treatment. J Inherit Metab Dis. 2013;36:565–73.
6. Clayton PT, Leonard JV, Lawson AM, Setchell KDR, Andersson S, Egestad B, et al. Familial giant cell hepatitis associated with synthesis of 3β,7α-dihydroxy- and 3β, 7α,12α–trihydroxy-5-cholenoic acids. J Clin Invest. 1987;79:1031–8.
7. Cheng JB, Jacquemin E, Gerhardt M, Nazer H, Cresteil D, Heubi JE, et al. Molecular genetics of 3β-hydroxy-Δ^5-C_{27}-steroid oxidoreductase deficiency in 16 patients with loss of bile acid synthesis and liver disease. J Clin Endocrinol Metab. 2003;88:1833–41.
8. Setchell KDR, Suchy FJ, Welsh MB, Zimmer-Nechemias L, Heubi JE, Balistreri WF. Δ^4-3-oxosteroid 5β-reductase deficiency described in identical twins with neonatal hepatitis. A new inborn error in bile acid synthesis. J Clin Invest. 1988;82:2148–57.
9. Ueki I, Kimura A, Chen H-L, Yorifuji T, Mori J, Itoh S, et al. SRD5B1 gene analysis needed for the accurate diagnosis of primary 3-oxo-Δ^4-steroid 5β-reductase deficiency. J Gastroenterol Hepatol. 2009;24:776–85.
10. Yanagi T, Mizuochi T, Homma K, Ueki I, Seki Y, Hasegawa T, et al. Distinguishing primary from secondary Δ^4-3-oxosteroid 5β-reductase (*SRD5B1, AKR1D1*) deficiency by urinary steroid analysis. Clin Endocrinol. 2015;82:346–51.
11. Setchell KDR, Schwarz M, O'Connell NC, Lund EG, Davis DL, Lathe R, et al. Identification of a new inborn error in bile acid synthesis: mutation of the oxysterol 7α-hydroxylase gene causes severe neonatal liver disease. J Clin Invest 1998; 102:1690–703.
12. Tsaousidou MK, Ouahchi K, Warner TT, Yang Y, Simpson MA, Laing NG, et al. Sequence alterations within CYP7B1 implicate defective cholesterol homeostasis in motor-neuron degeneration. Am J Hum Genet. 2008;82:510–5.
13. Mizuochi T, Kimura A, Suzuki M, Ueki I, Takei H, Nittono H, et al. Successful heterozygous living donor liver transplantation for an oxysterol 7α-hydroxylase deficiency in a Japanese patient. Liver Transpl. 2011;17:1059–65.
14. Dai D, Mills PB, Footitt E, Gissen P, McClean P, Stahlschmidt J, et al. Liver disease in infancy caused by oxysterol 7α-hydroxylase deficiency: successful treatment with chenodeoxycholic acid. J Inherit Metab Dis. 2014;37:851–61.
15. Clayton PT, Casteels M, Mieli-Vergani G, Lawson AM. Familial giant cell hepatitis with low bile acid concentrations and increased urinary excretion of specific bile alcohols: a new inborn error of bile acid synthesis? Pediatr Res. 1995;37:424–31.
16. Cali JJ, Hsieh CL, Francke U, Russell DW. Mutations in the bile acid biosynthetic enzyme sterol 27-hydroxylase underlie cerebrotendinous xanthomatosis. J Biol Chem. 1991;266:7779–83.
17. Clayton PT, Verrips A, Sistermans E, Mann A, Mieli-Vergani G, Wevers R. Mutations in the sterol 27-hydroxylase gene (CYP27A) cause hepatitis of infancy as well as cerebrotendinous xanthomatosis. J Inherit Metab Dis. 2002;25:501–13.
18. von Bahr S, Björkhem I, van't Hooft F, Alvelius G, Nemeth A, Sjövall J, et al. Mutation in the sterol 27-hydroxylase gene associated with fatal cholestasis in infancy. J Pediatr Gastroenterol Nutr. 2005;40:481–6.
19. Setchell KDR, Heubi JE, Bove KE, O'Connell NC, Brewsaugh T, Steinberg SJ, et al. Liver disease caused by failure to racemize trihydroxycholestanoic acid: gene mutation and effect of bile acid therapy. Gastroenterology. 2003;124:217–32.

20. Carlton VEH, Harris BZ, Puffenberger EG, Batta AK, Knisely AS, Robinson DL, et al. Complex inheritance of familial hypocholanemia with associated mutations in TJP2 and BAAT. Nat Genet. 2003;34:91–6.
21. Heubi JE, Setchell KDR, Jha P, Buckley D, Zhang W, Rosenthal P, et al. Treatment of bile acid amidation defect with glycocholic acid. Hepatology. 2015;61:268–74.
22. Chong CPK, Mills PB, McClean P, Gissen P, Bruce C, Stahlschmidt J, et al. Bile acid-CoA ligase deficiency-a new inborn error of bile acid metabolism. J Inherit Metab Dis. 2012;35:521–30.

Chapter 10
Bile Acids and NAFLD/NASH

Tsuneo Kitamura and Sumio Watanabe

Abstract Bile acids (BAs) have been shown to play physiologic roles in choleresis and digestion. Recent studies, however, reveal that BAs are important signaling molecules as ligand for farnesoid X receptor (FXR) and TGR5 (GPBAR1), a G-protein-coupled receptor, and are involved in the inflammatory responses as well as metabolic regulation of lipid and glucose. BAs also inhibit gut microbial growth through their detergent property, while gut bacteria regulate bile acid biotransformation in the intestine, leading to alterations of lipid, glucose, and energy metabolism. This article reviews recent advances in the understanding of BAs signaling and its regulation of metabolic homeostasis in nonalcoholic fatty liver disease (NAFLD) and nonalcoholic steatohepatitis (NASH).

Keywords Bile acids • Nonalcoholic fatty liver disease (NAFLD) • Nonalcoholic steatohepatitis (NASH) • Farnesoid X receptor (FXR) • TGR5 (GPBAR1)

10.1 NAFLD and NASH

Nonalcoholic fatty liver disease (NAFLD) is a spectrum of chronic liver abnormalities from simple steatosis to nonalcoholic steatohepatitis (NASH), liver cirrhosis, and hepatocellular carcinoma. NASH-related liver cirrhosis, termed burned-out NASH, is an end stage of NAFLD and can be an indication of liver transplantation [1, 2].

T. Kitamura
Department of Gastroenterology, Juntendo University Urayasu Hospital, 2-1-1 Tomioka, Urayasu, Chiba 279-0021, Japan

Department of Gastroenterology, Juntendo University Graduate School of Medicine, 2-1-1 Hongo, Bunkyo-ku, Tokyo 113-8421, Japan

S. Watanabe (✉)
Department of Gastroenterology, Juntendo University Graduate School of Medicine, 2-1-1 Hongo, Bunkyo-ku, Tokyo 113-8421, Japan
e-mail: sumio@juntendo.ac.jp

S. Tazuma, H. Takikawa (eds.), *Bile Acids in Gastroenterology*,
DOI 10.1007/978-4-431-56062-3_10

According to the "evidence-based clinical practice guidelines" [3] by the Japanese Society of Gastroenterology, the definition of nonalcoholic fatty liver disease (NAFLD) is as follows:

> NAFLD is characterized by evidence of hepatic steatosis either by imaging or histology and appropriate exclusion of other liver diseases such as alcoholic liver disease. Epidemiological studies have shown that alcoholic liver disease can occur when the daily alcohol intake exceeds 20 g in women and 30 g in men. Therefore, NAFLD is diagnosed when the alcohol consumption is lower than the aforementioned amounts. NAFLD is associated with obesity, diabetes mellitus, dyslipidemia, and hypertension and is considered the hepatic manifestation of metabolic syndrome. NAFLD is histologically characterized by macrovesicular steatosis and further categorized into NAFL and NASH. NAFL is mostly a benign, nonprogressive clinical entity, while NASH can progress to cirrhosis or even hepatocellular carcinoma (HCC). NASH is histologically characterized by hepatic steatosis associated with evidence of liver cell injury (ballooning degeneration) and inflammation.

NAFLD is closely related to obesity and insulin resistance [4, 5]. The progression of hepatic steatosis to NASH has been suggested to require at least "two hits": hepatic steatosis is the first hit, followed by inflammation as the second hit [6]. Insulin resistance and oxidative stress accelerate the progression from hepatic steatosis to NASH. However, it has been indicated that inflammation may precede steatosis in some cases of NASH, and in certain situations, hepatic steatosis may be considered as "bystander phenomenon" subsequent to inflammatory attacks, including toxic lipids, nutrients, and other signals derived from gut and adipose. Tilg H et al. thus proposed "multiple parallel hits hypothesis" implicating that many hits may act in parallel, finally resulting in liver inflammation [7].

10.2 Bile Acid Receptors and Signaling Molecules

Bile acids (BAs) are physiological detergent molecules, which play a role in the absorption of dietary lipids and vitamins in the gut [8]. BAs have been also suggested to be signaling molecules that regulate lipid, glucose, and energy metabolism. Accumulating evidences have indicated that BAs are important molecules, which may activate signaling pathways to regulate biological processes.

In 1999, it was first reported that BAs are physiological ligands for the farnesoid X receptor (FXR), an orphan nuclear receptor [9–11]. Following this discovery, BAs have been shown to activate other nuclear receptors, pregnane X receptor (PXR) and vitamin D receptor (VDR). BAs also have been reported to activate G-protein-coupled receptor 1 (TGR5/GPBAR1), muscarinic receptor 2 (M2), sphingosine-1-phosphate receptor 2 (S1PR2), and cellular signaling pathways including c-Jun N-terminal kinase (JNK1/JNK2), protein kinase B (AKT), and extracellular signal-regulated protein kinases (ERK1/ERK2) [12, 13].

Among these, much attention has been focused on FXR and TGR5 signaling that are associated with NAFLD and NASH. Activation of FXR or TGR5 lowers hepatic

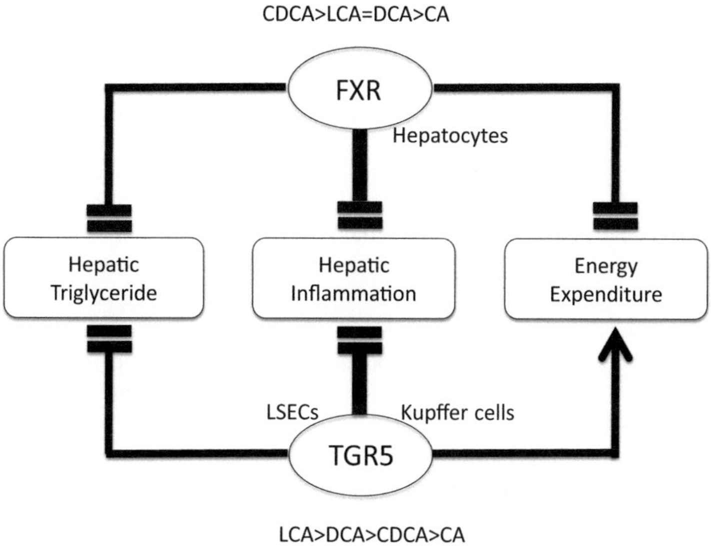

Fig. 10.1 Bile acid receptors (FXR, TGR5) and metabolic regulation in the liver. FXR is expressed in hepatocytes in the liver. TGR5 is expressed in LSECs and Kupffer cells in the liver, but not hepatocytes. The ability of different BAs to activate FXR occurs in the following order *CDCA>LCA=DCA>CA*. TGR5 can be activated by a variety of BAs in the order *LCA>DCA>CDCA>CA*. *FXR* farnesoid X receptor, *TGR5* G-protein-coupled receptor 1, *LSECs* liver sinusoidal endothelial cells

triglyceride levels and inhibits inflammation, suggesting that these two BAs receptors could be candidate for treatment of NAFLD (Fig. 10.1).

10.2.1 Role of FXR in NAFLD and NASH

Both conjugated and unconjugated BAs can activate FXR, and thus BAs may serve as endocrine hormones to regulate metabolism via FXR [14–16]. The ability of different bile acids to activate FXR-α occurs in the following order CDCA>LCA=DCA>CA [17]. FXR is an important regulator of lipid and glucose metabolism as well as inflammatory response. Activated FXR improves lipid and glucose homeostasis and inhibits inflammation.

FXR-null mice developed severe fatty liver, and elevated circulating free fatty acids, which was associated with elevated serum glucose and impaired glucose and insulin tolerance [18].

Inflammation plays an important role in the pathogenesis of NAFLD. $Fxr^{-/-}$ mice display elevated levels of inflammation and develop spontaneous HCC at age of 9–12 months [19]. Diabetes/insulin resistance facilitates the progression

HCC when FXR is deficient [20]. The increased levels of inflammation observed in *Fxr*$^{-/-}$ mice may partly be explained by elevated BAs levels in these mice.

The findings that FXR plays an important role in regulating both lipid homeostasis and inflammation suggest that FXR may modulate the progression of NAFLD. Indeed, *Fxr*$^{-/-}$ mice have increased hepatic TG accumulation. FXR deficiency causes pathologic manifestations of NASH in low-density lipoprotein receptor knockout mice (*Ldlr*$^{-/-}$ mice) after a high-fat feeding; the liver of these mice displayed massive steatosis and inflammatory infiltration [21].

FXR also regulates hepatic fibrosis. FXR is expressed at very low levels on hepatic Kupffer cells, stellate cells, and sinusoidal endothelial cells. FXR activation with 6-ethyl chenodeoxycholic acid (6-ECDCA), an FXR ligand, prevents liver fibrosis in porcine serum-treated rats or rats that underwent bile duct ligation and decreases expression of matrix proteins, including α1-collagen, transforming growth factor β-1 (TGF-β-1), alpha smooth muscle actin (αSMA), and tissue inhibitors of matrix metalloproteinase (MMP) 1 and 2 [22]. Recently, FXR activation has been shown to increase the expression of the microRNA mir29a, which regulates the expression of several extracellular matrix proteins in hepatic stellate cells [23].

It has been reported that in the NAFLD patients, the hepatic expression of FXR is significantly decreased. In this study, the expression of two other nuclear receptors, liver X receptor (LXR) and sterol regulatory element-binding protein 1C (SREBP-1C) that are closely related to fat metabolism and its regulation, was induced [24]. Thus, the reduced FXR expression may play a role in the pathogenesis of human NAFLD.

Interestingly, in two animal models of NASH, serum levels of tauro-β-muricholic and taurocholic acid were increased [25]. Hepatic expression of transporters of bile acids from the circulation to the liver (Slc10a1/Slco1a1) was decreased, whereas those transporters that transfer bile acids to the blood (Abcc1/4) were increased. It has been therefore discussed that if bile acid content is decreased in the liver, vicious circle may aggravate NASH [26], because decreased ligand activation of FXR could lead to triglyceride accumulation and inflammation in the liver.

Another study on 113 NAFLD patients reveals a close association between BA synthesis and plasma BA concentration and the severity of NAFLD [15]. In these patients, both the CYP7A1 and the bile acid transporter Na^+/taurocholate cotransporting polypeptide (NTCP) expression are increased, likely as a result of increased FFA levels [27].

10.2.2 Role of TGR5 (GPBAR1) in NAFLD and NASH

TGR5 is a member of the rhodopsin-like superfamily of G-protein-coupled plasma membrane receptor for BAs, which mediates many of the rapid and non-genomic actions of BAs. TGR5 has been implicated in the control of glucose homeostasis, inflammation, and liver functions. Like FXR, it is originally regarded as an orphan receptor without known ligands [14, 28]. Recently, it has been known that TGR5 can be activated by a variety of bile acids in the order LCA>DCA>CDCA>CA [29].

Activation of TGR5 by bile acids stimulated adenylate cyclase, rapid intracellular cAMP production, and protein kinase A activation. TGR5 plays an important role in BA homeostasis as well as in glucose/lipid homeostasis and energy expenditure. It regulates the expression of genes involved in inflammation, modulates plasma glucose and lipid levels, and increases energy expenditure in skeletal muscle and brown adipose tissue [28, 30–32].

TGR5 is highly expressed along the intestinal tract such as the ileum and colon, which are exposed to high levels of bile acids [29]. It has been shown that bile acid-activated TGR5 stimulated the production of glucagon-like peptide-1 (GLP-1), which promotes insulin secretion and regulates glucose homeostasis, in an enteroendocrine cell line [33]. Despite that the liver is a major bile acid target organ, TGR5 expression in the liver is low. In the liver, TGR5 is expressed in sinusoidal endothelial cells and Kupffer cells, but not in hepatocytes [28, 34].

TGR5 is also expressed in monocytes and macrophages, and in human spleen, suggesting that it plays an anti-inflammatory role in the immune system. Indeed, TGR5 activation has shown protective effects in various inflammation-related diseases in experimental models [29, 35]. Kupffer cells are capable of secreting proinflammatory cytokines, which can contribute to the progression of NAFLD [36]. When Kupffer cells were treated with the synthetic TGR5 agonist INT-777, there was a reduction in the lipopolysaccharide (LPS)-induced production of inflammatory cytokines through the TGR5-cAMP-dependent pathway. INT-777 treatment attenuates the expression of inflammatory mediators by antagonizing NF-κB activity in wild-type mice but not in $Tgr5^{-/-}$ mice [37]. The anti-inflammatory and anti-steatotic properties of TGR5 suggest that TGR5 may protect against the development and progression of NAFLD [38, 39].

10.2.3 Role of Sphingosine-1-Phosphate Receptor 2 in NAFLD and NASH

Sphingosine-1-phosphate (S1P) is a potent bioactive sphingolipid that is involved in a variety of cellular processes, including cell proliferation, differentiation, motility, angiogenesis, inflammation, and malignant transformation [40]. Intracellular S1P is synthesized from sphingosine by sphingosine kinase 1 (SphK1).

Intracellular S1P can directly activate various cellular signaling pathways or be exported out of cells by specific transporters (spinster homologue 2; Spns2) in the cell membrane [41]. Extracellular S1P exerts its function via activating five different G-protein-coupled receptors (S1PR1–5) on the cell membrane to induce various cellular responses [42]. S1PR1 is ubiquitously expressed and plays a key role in angiogenesis, vascular maturation, and immune cell trafficking. Deletion of S1PR1 affects maturation and is embryonically lethal.

Unlike S1PR1, mice deficient in S1PR2 exhibit no phenotypic defects, but develop spontaneous and sporadic seizures [43]. Studies in S1pr2$^{-/-}$ mouse have also shown S1PR2 to be responsible for proper development of the auditory and vestibular systems [44].

S1PR2 is highly expressed in the liver and plays a unique and critical role in the pathophysiology of the liver. The role of S1PR2 in bile acid-mediated hepatic lipid metabolism was identified in recent studies [45]. In primary rodent hepatocytes, conjugated bile acids activate S1PR2, which further activates the downstream ERK1/ERK2 and AKT signaling pathways [45]. Bile acid-mediated activation of ERK1/ERK2 and AKT signaling pathway plays an important role in the regulation of hepatic glucose and lipid metabolism [46, 47]. In primary rat hepatocytes, insulin and bile acids both activated glycogen synthase activity to a similar extent.

Infusion of taurocholate (TCA) into the chronic bile fistula rat rapidly activated the AKT and ERK1/ERK2 signaling pathway and glycogen synthase activity [48]. In addition, TCA induced a rapid downregulation of the gluconeogenic genes, PEP carboxykinase (*Pepck*) and glucose-6-phophatase (*G-6Pase*), and a marked upregulation of small heterodimeric partner (SHP) mRNA in the livers [47]. These results suggest that TCA has insulin-like activity to regulate hepatic glucose metabolism both in vitro and in vivo. A recent study reported that *S1pr2* null mice rapidly develop overt fatty livers on a high-fat diet compared to wild-type mice, suggesting that S1PR2 is an important regulator of hepatic lipid metabolism [49].

10.3 Bile Acids and Gut Microbiota in NAFLD and NASH

BAs and gut microbiota are closely linked through the enterohepatic circulation, which plays a role in communication between the liver and intestine. BAs are produced from cholesterol in the liver, conjugated to amino acid glycine or taurine, and secreted into the small intestine. Conjugated BAs are absorbed in the terminal ileum to return to the liver.

BAs secreted from the liver inhibit gut microbial growth through their detergent property. Gut bacteria also regulate bile acid biotransformation in the intestine, which alters bile acid composition generating secondary bile acids by deconjugation and dehydroxylation (Fig. 10.2). Recent evidence indicates that there is a regulatory relationship between the development of obesity and altered gut microbiota, suggesting that the microbiota can induce NAFLD or its progression toward overt nonalcoholic steatohepatitis [50].

A number of studies showed that germ-free mice were protected against diet-induced obesity compared with the conventionally raised counterparts [51, 52]. Interestingly, germ-free mice receiving cecal microbiota from *ob*/*ob*

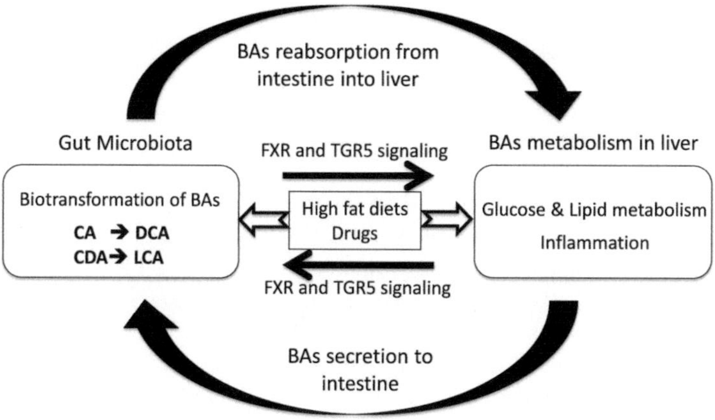

Fig. 10.2 Bile acid and gut microbiota. BAs regulate gut bacteria overgrowth and protect against inflammation. BAs secreted from liver inhibit gut microbial growth through their detergent property. Gut bacteria also regulate bile acid biotransformation in the intestine, which alters bile acid composition generating secondary bile acids by deconjugation and dehydroxylation. High-fat diets and drugs alter bile acid biotransformation and gut microbiota and contribute to pathogenesis of liver-related metabolic diseases

mice had higher energy absorption from food and more weight gain than germ-free mice harboring cecal microbiota from lean mice [52].

Dysbiosis is the major environmental factor, which affects bile acid metabolism, and contributes to diseases not only in the gastrointestinal system but also in chronic diseases including NAFLD, diabetes, and obesity [53]. Treating dysbiosis by modulating bile acid metabolism by gut microbiota may be a therapeutic approach for improving and preventing NAFLD.

10.4 Therapeutic Potential of BAs and Derivatives in NAFLD and NASH

Many reports have described that activation of FXR inhibits inflammation in the liver and intestine, and FXR agonists are potential therapeutic drugs for metabolic and inflammatory diseases. Obeticholic acid (OCA, 6-ethyl-CDCA or INT-747) is a synthetic derivative of chenodeoxycholic acid and a highly potent and selective FXR agonist that has anticholestatic effects [54].

In experimental studies, OCA increases insulin sensitivity, inhibits gluconeogenesis, inhibits lipogenesis, and has anti-inflammatory and antifibrotic properties [55]. OCA ameliorates high-fat diet-induced obesity and insulin resistance in mice, as well as insulin resistance and fatty liver in Zucker rats (*fa*/*fa*) [56]. OCA antagonizes NF-*k*B-stimulated inflammation in the liver [57], modulates innate immunity in animal models of colitis [58], and inhibits and preserves the intestinal barrier in inflammatory bowel disease [59]. The phase II clinical trial of OCA for

NAFLD and T2DM patients showed improved insulin sensitivity, reduced γ-glutamyl-transpeptidase levels (a marker of NASH), and weight loss [60]. Recently, the multicenter, randomized, placebo-controlled trial (FLINT), which was conducted by the NIDDK NASH Clinical Research Network, revealed that OCA improved the histological features of NASH [61].

Since TGR5 signaling inhibits the production of proinflammatory cytokines, drugs targeting to TGR5 also have the potential to treat NAFLD or NASH. A bile acid derivative INT-777 is a selective and potent TGR5 agonist [62, 63]. In animal studies, INT-777 improves glucose tolerance, stimulates GLP-1 secretion from enteroendocrine L cells, and improves insulin sensitivity [31]. TGR5 agonists also reduce and prevent inflammation in the liver [28]. Recently, the FXR and TGR5 dual agonist INT-767 (6α-ethyl-3α,7α,23-trihydroxy-24-nor-5β-cholan-23-sulfate) has been shown to improve NAFLD by modulating hepatic monocyte activity [38].

10.5 Future Perspectives in NAFLD and NASH

Recent research advances in bile acid metabolism and signaling enabled us to understand an important role for bile acids in integration of hepatic lipid, glucose, and energy metabolism. Among them, findings of bile acid receptors have largely contributed to progress in translation of basic research in bile acid metabolism to clinical applications for drug therapies of NAFLD and NASH.

Results of FLINT trial, showing OCA being effective in histological improvement in NASH, are the great first steps of therapeutic strategies, but appear to require further analysis in terms of histological reversibility and long-term follow-up for hepatocellular carcinoma. It is anticipated that new treatment strategies, including nonbile acid-based agonists specific for FXR and TGR5, will be developed for treating NAFLD and NASH.

References

1. Postic C, Girard J. Contribution of de novo fatty acid synthesis to hepatic steatosis and insulin resistance: lessons from genetically engineered mice. J Clin Invest. 2008;118:829–38.
2. Cohen JC, Horton JD, Hobbs HH. Human fatty liver disease: old questions and new insights. Science. 2011;332:1519–23.
3. Watanabe S, Hashimoto E, Ikejima K, Uto H, Ono M, Sumida Y, Seike M, et al. Evidence-based clinical practice guidelines for nonalcoholic fatty liver disease/nonalcoholic steatohepatitis. J Gastroenterol. 2015;50:364–77.
4. Larter CZ, Farrell GC. Insulin resistance, adiponectin, cytokines in NASH: which is the best target to treat? J Hepatol. 2006;44:253–61.
5. Tiniakos DG, Vos MB, Brunt EM. Nonalcoholic fatty liver disease: pathology and pathogenesis. Annu Rev Pathol. 2010;5:145–71.

6. James OF, Day CP. Non-alcoholic steatohepatitis (NASH): a disease of emerging identity and importance. J Hepatol. 1998;29:495–501.
7. Tilg H, Moschen AR. Evolution of inflammation in nonalcoholic fatty liver disease: the multiple parallel hits hypothesis. Hepatology. 2010;52:1836–46.
8. Chiang JY. Bile acid regulation of gene expression: roles of nuclear hormone receptors. Endocr Rev. 2002;23:443–63.
9. Parks DJ, Blanchard SG, Bledsoe RK, Chandra G, Consler TG, Kliewer SA, Stimmel JB, et al. Bile acids: natural ligands for an orphan nuclear receptor. Science. 1999;284:1365–8.
10. Makishima M, Okamoto AY, Repa JJ, Tu H, Learned RM, Luk A, Hull MV, et al. Identification of a nuclear receptor for bile acids. Science. 1999;284:1362–5.
11. Wang H, Chen J, Hollister K, Sowers LC, Forman BM. Endogenous bile acids are ligands for the nuclear receptor FXR/BAR. Mol Cell. 1999;3:543–53.
12. Schaap FG, Trauner M, Jansen PL. Bile acid receptors as targets for drug development. Nat Rev Gastroenterol Hepatol. 2014;11:55–67.
13. de Aguiar Vallim TQ, Tarling EJ, Edwards PA. Pleiotropic roles of bile acids in metabolism. Cell Metab. 2013;17:657–69.
14. Thomas C, Pellicciari R, Pruzanski M, Auwerx J, Schoonjans K. Targeting bile acid signalling for metabolic diseases. Nat Rev Drug Discov. 2008;7:678–93.
15. Zhang Y, Edwards PA. FXR signaling in metabolic disease. FEBS Lett. 2008;582:10–8.
16. Lee FY, Lee H, Hubbert ML, Edwards PA, Zhang Y. FXR, a multipurpose nuclear receptor. Trends Biochem Sci. 2006;31:572–80.
17. Makishima M, Lu TT, Xie W, Whitfield GK, Domoto H, Evans RM, Haussler MR, et al. Vitamin D receptor as an intestinal bile acid sensor. Science. 2002;296:1313–6.
18. Ma K, Saha PK, Chan L, Moore DD. Farnesoid X receptor is essential for normal glucose homeostasis. J Clin Invest. 2006;116:1102–9.
19. Kim I, Morimura K, Shah Y, Yang Q, Ward JM, Gonzalez FJ. Spontaneous hepatocarcinogenesis in farnesoid X receptor-null mice. Carcinogenesis. 2007;28:940–6.
20. Zhang Y, Ge X, Heemstra LA, Chen WD, Xu J, Smith JL, Ma H, et al. Loss of FXR protects against diet-induced obesity and accelerates liver carcinogenesis in ob/ob mice. Mol Endocrinol. 2012;26:272–80.
21. Kong B, Luyendyk JP, Tawfik O, Guo GL. Farnesoid X receptor deficiency induces nonalcoholic steatohepatitis in low-density lipoprotein receptor-knockout mice fed a high-fat diet. J Pharmacol Exp Ther. 2009;328:116–22.
22. Fiorucci S, Antonelli E, Rizzo G, Renga B, Mencarelli A, Riccardi L, Orlandi S, et al. The nuclear receptor SHP mediates inhibition of hepatic stellate cells by FXR and protects against liver fibrosis. Gastroenterology. 2004;127:1497–512.
23. Li J, Zhang Y, Kuruba R, Gao X, Gandhi CR, Xie W, Li S. Roles of microRNA-29a in the antifibrotic effect of farnesoid X receptor in hepatic stellate cells. Mol Pharmacol. 2011;80: 191–200.
24. Yang ZX, Shen W, Sun H. Effects of nuclear receptor FXR on the regulation of liver lipid metabolism in patients with non-alcoholic fatty liver disease. Hepatol Int. 2010;4:741–8.
25. Tanaka N, Matsubara T, Krausz KW, Patterson AD, Gonzalez FJ. Disruption of phospholipid and bile acid homeostasis in mice with nonalcoholic steatohepatitis. Hepatology. 2012;56: 118–29.
26. Gabbi C, Gustafsson JA. Bile acids in nonalcoholic steatohepatitis: inserting nuclear receptors into the circle. Hepatology. 2012;56:2008–9. autthor reply 2009
27. Bechmann LP, Kocabayoglu P, Sowa JP, Sydor S, Best J, Schlattjan M, Beilfuss A, et al. Free fatty acids repress small heterodimer partner (SHP) activation and adiponectin counteracts bile acid-induced liver injury in super obese patients with nonalcoholic steatohepatitis. Hepatology. 2013;57:1394–406.
28. Pols TW, Noriega LG, Nomura M, Auwerx J, Schoonjans K. The bile acid membrane receptor TGR5 as an emerging target in metabolism and inflammation. J Hepatol. 2011;54:1263–72.

29. Kawamata Y, Fujii R, Hosoya M, Harada M, Yoshida H, Miwa M, Fukusumi S, et al. A G protein-coupled receptor responsive to bile acids. J Biol Chem. 2003;278:9435–40.
30. Watanabe M, Houten SM, Mataki C, Christoffolete MA, Kim BW, Sato H, Messaddeq N, et al. Bile acids induce energy expenditure by promoting intracellular thyroid hormone activation. Nature. 2006;439:484–9.
31. Thomas C, Gioiello A, Noriega L, Strehle A, Oury J, Rizzo G, Macchiarulo A, et al. TGR5-mediated bile acid sensing controls glucose homeostasis. Cell Metab. 2009;10:167–77.
32. Pols TW, Nomura M, Harach T, Lo Sasso G, Oosterveer MH, Thomas C, Rizzo G, et al. TGR5 activation inhibits atherosclerosis by reducing macrophage inflammation and lipid loading. Cell Metab. 2011;14:747–57.
33. Katsuma S, Hirasawa A, Tsujimoto G. Bile acids promote glucagon-like peptide-1 secretion through TGR5 in a murine enteroendocrine cell line STC-1. Biochem Biophys Res Commun. 2005;329:386–90.
34. Keitel V, Reinehr R, Gatsios P, Rupprecht C, Gorg B, Selbach O, Haussinger D, et al. The G-protein coupled bile salt receptor TGR5 is expressed in liver sinusoidal endothelial cells. Hepatology. 2007;45:695–704.
35. Keitel V, Donner M, Winandy S, Kubitz R, Haussinger D. Expression and function of the bile acid receptor TGR5 in Kupffer cells. Biochem Biophys Res Commun. 2008;372:78–84.
36. Baffy G. Kupffer cells in non-alcoholic fatty liver disease: the emerging view. J Hepatol. 2009; 51:212–23.
37. Wang YD, Chen WD, Yu D, Forman BM, Huang W. The G-protein-coupled bile acid receptor, Gpbar1 (TGR5), negatively regulates hepatic inflammatory response through antagonizing nuclear factor kappa light-chain enhancer of activated B cells (NF-kappaB) in mice. Hepatology. 2011;54:1421–32.
38. McMahan RH, Wang XX, Cheng LL, Krisko T, Smith M, El Kasmi K, Pruzanski M, et al. Bile acid receptor activation modulates hepatic monocyte activity and improves nonalcoholic fatty liver disease. J Biol Chem. 2013;288:11761–70.
39. Pean N, Doignon I, Garcin I, Besnard A, Julien B, Liu B, Branchereau S, et al. The receptor TGR5 protects the liver from bile acid overload during liver regeneration in mice. Hepatology. 2013;58:1451–60.
40. Maceyka M, Harikumar KB, Milstien S, Spiegel S. Sphingosine-1-phosphate signaling and its role in disease. Trends Cell Biol. 2012;22:50–60.
41. Kawahara A, Nishi T, Hisano Y, Fukui H, Yamaguchi A, Mochizuki N. The sphingolipid transporter spns2 functions in migration of zebrafish myocardial precursors. Science. 2009; 323:524–7.
42. Strub GM, Maceyka M, Hait NC, Milstien S, Spiegel S. Extracellular and intracellular actions of sphingosine-1-phosphate. Adv Exp Med Biol. 2010;688:141–55.
43. MacLennan AJ, Carney PR, Zhu WJ, Chaves AH, Garcia J, Grimes JR, Anderson KJ, et al. An essential role for the H218/AGR16/Edg-5/LP(B2) sphingosine 1-phosphate receptor in neuronal excitability. Eur J Neurosci. 2001;14:203–9.
44. MacLennan AJ, Benner SJ, Andringa A, Chaves AH, Rosing JL, Vesey R, Karpman AM, et al. The S1P2 sphingosine 1-phosphate receptor is essential for auditory and vestibular function. Hear Res. 2006;220:38–48.
45. Dent P, Fang Y, Gupta S, Studer E, Mitchell C, Spiegel S, Hylemon PB. Conjugated bile acids promote ERK1/2 and AKT activation via a pertussis toxin-sensitive mechanism in murine and human hepatocytes. Hepatology. 2005;42:1291–9.
46. Studer E, Zhou X, Zhao R, Wang Y, Takabe K, Nagahashi M, Pandak WM, et al. Conjugated bile acids activate the sphingosine-1-phosphate receptor 2 in primary rodent hepatocytes. Hepatology. 2012;55:267–76.
47. Cao R, Cronk ZX, Zha W, Sun L, Wang X, Fang Y, Studer E, et al. Bile acids regulate hepatic gluconeogenic genes and farnesoid X receptor via G(alpha)i-protein-coupled receptors and the AKT pathway. J Lipid Res. 2010;51:2234–44.

48. Fang Y, Studer E, Mitchell C, Grant S, Pandak WM, Hylemon PB, Dent P. Conjugated bile acids regulate hepatocyte glycogen synthase activity in vitro and in vivo via Galphai signaling. Mol Pharmacol. 2007;71:1122–8.
49. Nagahashi M, Takabe K, Liu R, Peng K, Wang X, Wang Y, Hait NC, et al. Conjugated bile acid-activated S1P receptor 2 is a key regulator of sphingosine kinase 2 and hepatic gene expression. Hepatology. 2015;61:1216–26.
50. Aron-Wisnewsky J, Gaborit B, Dutour A, Clement K. Gut microbiota and non-alcoholic fatty liver disease: new insights. Clin Microbiol Infect. 2013;19:338–48.
51. Backhed F, Ding H, Wang T, Hooper LV, Koh GY, Nagy A, Semenkovich CF, et al. The gut microbiota as an environmental factor that regulates fat storage. Proc Natl Acad Sci U S A. 2004;101:15718–23.
52. Turnbaugh PJ, Ley RE, Mahowald MA, Magrini V, Mardis ER, Gordon JI. An obesity-associated gut microbiome with increased capacity for energy harvest. Nature. 2006;444: 1027–31.
53. Jones ML, Martoni CJ, Ganopolsky JG, Labbe A, Prakash S. The human microbiome and bile acid metabolism: dysbiosis, dysmetabolism, disease and intervention. Expert Opin Biol Ther. 2014;14: 467–82.
54. Pellicciari R, Costantino G, Camaioni E, Sadeghpour BM, Entrena A, Willson TM, Fiorucci S, et al. Bile acid derivatives as ligands of the farnesoid X receptor. Synthesis, evaluation, and structure-activity relationship of a series of body and side chain modified analogues of chenodeoxycholic acid. J Med Chem. 2004;47:4559–69.
55. Adorini L, Pruzanski M, Shapiro D. Farnesoid X receptor targeting to treat nonalcoholic steatohepatitis. Drug Discov Today. 2012;17:988–97.
56. Cipriani S, Mencarelli A, Palladino G, Fiorucci S. FXR activation reverses insulin resistance and lipid abnormalities and protects against liver steatosis in Zucker (fa/fa) obese rats. J Lipid Res. 2010;51:771–84.
57. Wang YD, Chen WD, Wang M, Yu D, Forman BM, Huang W. Farnesoid X receptor antagonizes nuclear factor kappaB in hepatic inflammatory response. Hepatology. 2008;48: 1632–43.
58. Vavassori P, Mencarelli A, Renga B, Distrutti E, Fiorucci S. The bile acid receptor FXR is a modulator of intestinal innate immunity. J Immunol. 2009;183:6251–61.
59. Nijmeijer RM, Gadaleta RM, van Mil SW, van Bodegraven AA, Crusius JB, Dijkstra G, Hommes DW, et al. Farnesoid X receptor (FXR) activation and FXR genetic variation in inflammatory bowel disease. PLoS One. 2011;6:e23745.
60. Mudaliar S, Henry RR, Sanyal AJ, Morrow L, Marschall HU, Kipnes M, Adorini L, et al. Efficacy and safety of the farnesoid X receptor agonist obeticholic acid in patients with type 2 diabetes and nonalcoholic fatty liver disease. Gastroenterology. 2013;145:574–82. e571
61. Neuschwander-Tetri BA, Loomba R, Sanyal AJ, Lavine JE, Van Natta ML, Abdelmalek MF, Chalasani N, et al. Farnesoid X nuclear receptor ligand obeticholic acid for non-cirrhotic, non-alcoholic steatohepatitis (FLINT): a multicentre, randomised, placebo-controlled trial. Lancet. 2015;385:956–65.
62. Pellicciari R, Sato H, Gioiello A, Costantino G, Macchiarulo A, Sadeghpour BM, Giorgi G, et al. Nongenomic actions of bile acids. Synthesis and preliminary characterization of 23- and 6,23-alkyl-substituted bile acid derivatives as selective modulators for the G-protein coupled receptor TGR5. J Med Chem. 2007;50:4265–8.
63. Pellicciari R, Gioiello A, Macchiarulo A, Thomas C, Rosatelli E, Natalini B, Sardella R, et al. Discovery of 6alpha-ethyl-23(S)-methylcholic acid (S-EMCA, INT-777) as a potent and selective agonist for the TGR5 receptor, a novel target for diabesity. J Med Chem. 2009;52: 7958–61.

Chapter 11
Bile Acids and Viral Hepatitis and Hepatocellular Carcinoma

Yasuaki Takeyama and Shotaro Sakisaka

Abstract Serum total bile acid levels are increased in viral hepatitis and correlate with the degree of liver fibrosis and are also high in hepatocellular carcinoma (HCC). In this chapter, we describe how accumulation of bile acids affects hepatitis viruses such as hepatitis B virus (HBV) and hepatitis C virus (HCV) and carcinogenesis of HCC. *Viral hepatitis*: Na^+/taurocholate cotransporting polypeptide (NTCP) is an uptake transporter of bile acids and an HBV entry receptor. Several NTCP inhibitors reduce HBV infection. Bile acids promote HBV replication via nuclear receptor transduction. HBV infection increases bile acid synthesis. In patients with high bile acids, interferon therapy shows higher failure rates in chronic hepatitis C. Bile acids increase HCV replication. *HCC*: Bile acids can induce cell death and inflammation, leading to promotion of carcinogenesis. Bile acid uptake transporters (NTCP and organic anion transporter peptide [OATP]1B3) and bile salt export pump expression are reduced in most cases of HCC. Because OATP1B3 also uptakes gadolinium–ethoxybenzyl–diethylenetriamine pentaacetic acid (Gd–EOB–DTPA), HCC lesions show low signal intensity in the hepatobiliary phase of Gd–EOB–DTPA-enhanced magnetic resonance imaging. *Ursodeoxycholic acid (UDCA)*: UDCA is a hydrophilic bile acid and a safe and effective medical therapy in chronic hepatitis B and C. UDCA improves abnormal liver transaminase levels; however, it cannot eradicate viruses in the liver. UDCA-induced inhibition of DLC1 (deleted in liver cancer 1) protein degradation leads to suppression of HCC cell growth. *DLC1* is a tumor suppressor gene for HCC.

Keywords Bile acids • Hepatitis B virus • Hepatitis C virus • Hepatocellular carcinoma • Hepatobiliary transporter

Y. Takeyama (✉) • S. Sakisaka
Department of Gastroenterology and Medicine, Fukuoka University Faculty of Medicine, 7-45-1 Nanakuma, Jonan-ku, Fukuoka 814-0180, Japan
e-mail: yaz@fukuoka-u.ac.jp

S. Tazuma, H. Takikawa (eds.), *Bile Acids in Gastroenterology*,
DOI 10.1007/978-4-431-56062-3_11

11.1 Introduction

The primary bile acids in humans are cholic acid (CA) and chenodeoxycholic acid (CDCA). Intestinal bacteria dehydroxylate primary bile acids, converting them to secondary bile acids, such as deoxycholic acid (DCA) and lithocholic acid (LCA). The serum concentration of total bile acids reflects the extent to which bile acids reabsorbed from the intestine have escaped extraction on their first passage through the liver. In patients with cholestasis, bile acids such as CDCA and DCA accumulate in hepatocytes and can cause hepatocyte injury, apoptosis, and necrosis. Hence, the level of serum total bile acids is increased in viral hepatitis and correlated with the degree of liver fibrosis [1]. Serum total bile acid levels are also high in hepatocellular carcinoma (HCC) [2]. Serum primary bile acids, CA and CDCA, are increased in advanced cirrhosis [3]. In contrast, serum secondary bile acids, DCA and LCA, are decreased [4]. Serum conjugated bile acids, such as glycocholic acid (GCA), glycochenodeoxycholic acid (GCDCA), taurocholic acid (TCA), taurochenodeoxycholic acid (TCDCA), and glycoursodeoxycholic acid (GUDCA), are increased in liver cirrhosis (LC) type B. Since GCA, GCDCA, TCA, TCDCA, and GUDCA are gradually increased in LC patients with Child–Pugh A, B, and C (Fig. 11.1) [5], GCA, GCDCA, TCA, TCDCA, and GUDCA are useful as potential biomarkers for LC [6].

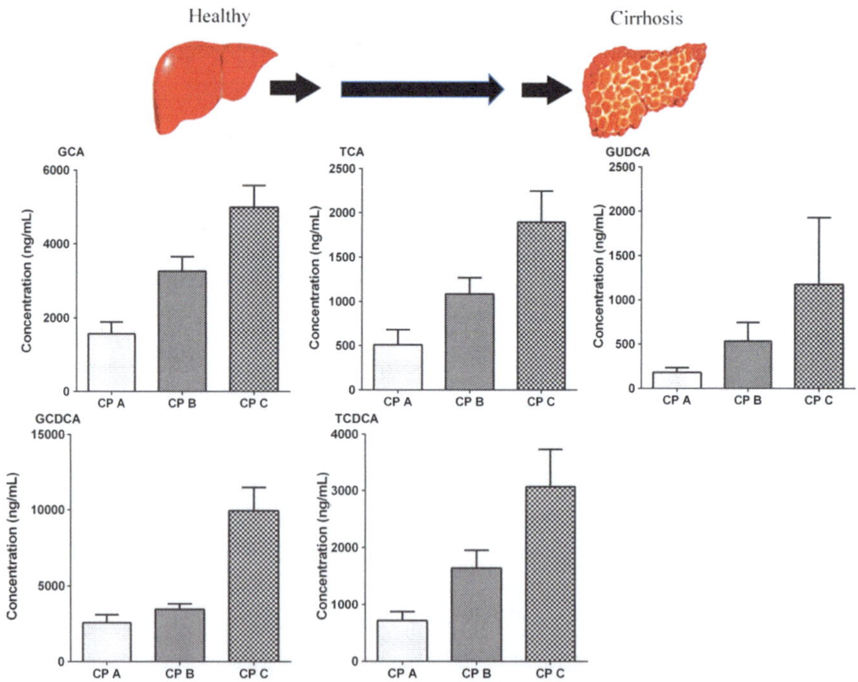

Fig. 11.1 Bar charts of five bile acids that are differentially expressed among patients with Child–Pugh A, B, and C cirrhosis. Serum levels of *GCA*, *GCDCA*, *TCA*, *TCDCA*, and GUDCA are gradually increased among Child–Pugh A, B, and C. *CP A* Child–Pugh A, *CP B*, Child–Pugh B, *CP C*, Child–Pugh C

11.2 Viral Hepatitis B

11.2.1 Etiology

The most common causes of viral hepatitis are persistent hepatotropic viruses such as hepatitis B virus (HBV) and hepatitis C virus (HCV). HBV and HCV infections are a global health problem and the leading causes of chronic hepatitis, which may develop into LC with/without HCC.

The advent of sensitive assays for the detection of HBV and the availability of potent antiviral agents have improved the management of patients with chronic hepatitis B; however, current treatment cannot eradicate the virus. An estimated 350–400 million people are chronically infected with hepatitis B (defined as hepatitis B surface antigen positivity for ≥6 months). More than 780,000 people die every year as a result of complications of hepatitis B, including cirrhosis and HCC (World Health Organization report; http://www.who.int/immunization/diseases/hepatitisB/en/).

Chronic hepatitis B infection can be treated with drugs, including oral antiviral agents or interferon. Treatment can slow the progression of cirrhosis, reduce the incidence of liver cancer, and improve long-term survival. However, in most people, the treatment does not cure hepatitis B infection but only suppresses replication of HBV. In addition, lamivudine, adefovir, entecavir, telbivudine, tenofovir, and tenofovir alafenamide (prodrug of tenofovir) are all nucleoside/nucleotide analogs targeting HBV reverse transcriptase. Hepatic uptake of tenofovir alafenamide is facilitated by organic anion-transporting polypeptide (OATP)1B1 and 1B3, and these transporters also uptake bile acids [7].

11.2.2 HBV Entry Receptor

Na^+/taurocholate cotransporting polypeptide (NTCP) is an HBV entry receptor. NTCP (also known as SLC10A1) is a member of the solute carrier family 10 and localizes to the basolateral membrane of hepatocytes. The key function of NTCP is the Na^+-dependent uptake of bile acids, allowing maintenance of enterohepatic circulation of bile acids. HBV interacts with NTCP through the pre-S1 domain of HBV-encoded large envelope protein [8]. The pre-S1 domain of an HBV-encoded large surface envelope protein plays a role in virus particle entry [9].

siRNA-mediated knockdown of NTCP reduces HBV infection in primary human hepatocytes [10]. NTCP can serve as a therapeutic target. Indeed, myrcludex B, cyclosporin A, and some NTCP inhibitors can inhibit HBV entry by targeting NTCP (Fig. 11.2). Myrcludex B binds to NTCP and inactivates its receptor function for HBV. Cyclosporin A is an immunosuppressant that is classified as a calcineurin inhibitor and inhibits HBV infection by targeting NTCP [11].

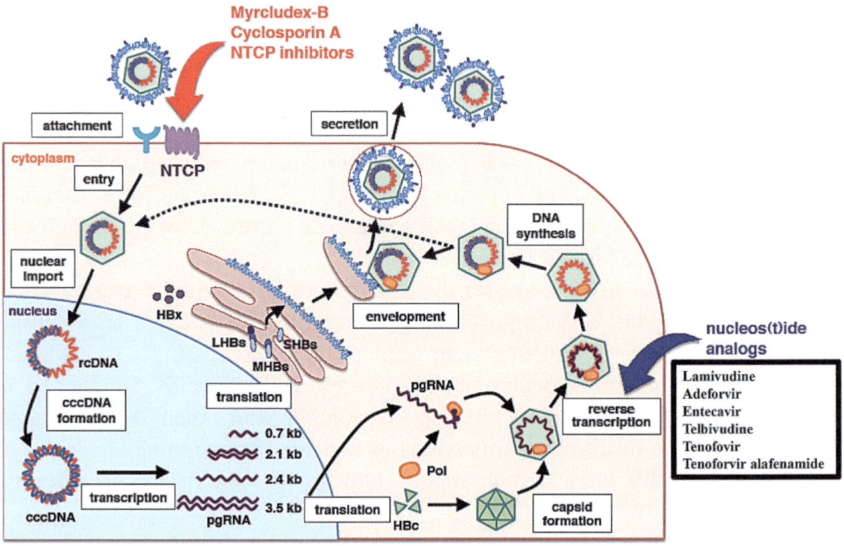

Fig. 11.2 Schematic life cycle of HBV [11]. Myrcludex B, cyclosporin A, and some NTCP inhibitors inhibit the viral entry process by targeting NTCP

11.2.3 Bile Acids Promote HBV Replication

Nuclear receptors regulate HBV promoters and enhancers. Liver-enriched nuclear receptors perform a pivotal role in the regulation of HBV transcription by binding to both HBV enhancer I and enhancer II. The farnesoid X receptor (FXR) is a metabolic nuclear receptor expressed in the liver via regulation of the expression and function of genes involved in bile acid synthesis, uptake, and excretion. FXRα/retinoid X receptor (RXR)α genes have emerged as key factors involved in the maintenance of bile acid and cholesterol homeostasis. FXRα and c-Jun N-terminal kinase (JNK)/c-Jun signal transduction pathway mediate the regulatory effect of bile acids. FXRα/RXRα heterodimeric nuclear receptors can also mediate ligand-dependent HBV transcription and replication when activated by bile acids. CDCA treatment leads to JNK/c-Jun and HBV enhancer I activation that also results in HBV enhancer II induction and enhances the level of HBV biosynthesis [12], through FXRα, which is implicated in the metabolic regulation of HBV transcription [13]. Small heterodimer partner (SHP) is also involved in the bile acid-mediated regulation of HBV gene expression [14]. Bile acids induce SHP, which mediates the inhibitory effects on HBV replication [15, 16].

HBV infection alters the expression of genes in bile acid metabolism, most notably *CYP7A1*, which encodes a key enzyme involved in bile acid synthesis. Hepatic cytochrome P450 (CYP)7A1 expression is increased in chronic HBV patients. FXR nuclear translocation decreases, and expression of its transcriptional

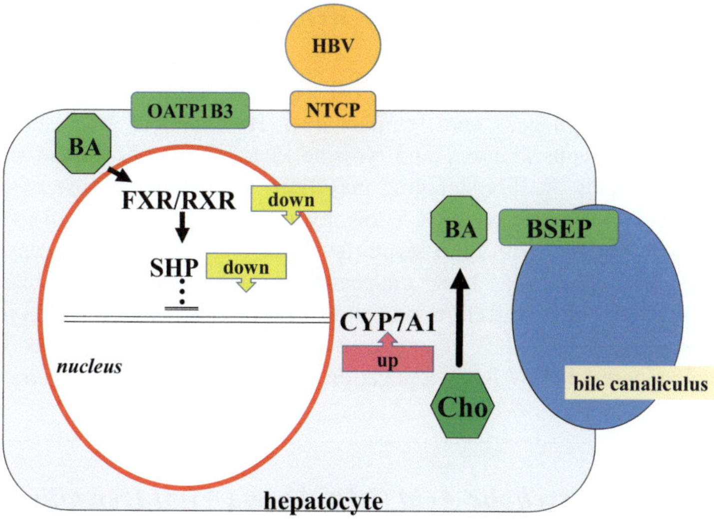

Fig. 11.3 In HBV infection, bile acid synthesis is increased via upregulation of CYP7A1 and downregulation of SHP, which is a transcriptional repressor of CYP7A1. CYP7A1 is a key enzyme involved in bile acid synthesis. NTCP is an HBV entry receptor

target, SHP, is reduced in the liver of HBV-infected patients. SHP is a transcriptional repressor of CYP7A1, and its decrease could explain CYP7A1 induction [17] (Fig. 11.3).

11.3 Viral Hepatitis C

11.3.1 Etiology

Chronic HCV infection is one of the most common chronic liver diseases and accounts for 8,000–13,000 deaths each year [18]. HCV can cause both acute and chronic hepatitis. Fifty to 85 % of patients with HCV infection develop chronic hepatitis C. Five to 30 % of chronically infected individuals develop cirrhosis over a 20–30-year period. Chronic HCV infection often follows a progressive course over many years and can ultimately result in cirrhosis and HCC. Current treatments such as direct-acting antivirals for chronic HCV infection achieve high sustained virological response rates, lower the incidence of side effects, have few drug–drug interactions, and/or shorten the duration of treatment. In the near future, in HCV hepatitis, only acute hepatitis will remain, and chronic hepatitis will disappear and become a rare disease by 2036 [19].

11.3.2 Bile Acids Promote HCV Replication

Bile acids impair interferon (IFN)-α and IFN-β signaling in hepatocytes, natural killer cells, macrophages, and lymphocytes. Hydrophobic bile acids blunt IFN-α-dependent Janus kinase 1 and tyrosine kinase 2 (Tyk2) activation. These effects of bile acids on IFN signaling may limit the therapeutic use of IFNs in hepatitis B and C. The success of HCV therapy with IFN is dependent on serum bile acid levels. In patients with high serum levels of bile acids, IFN therapy shows higher failure rates [20]. Low concentrations of unconjugated bile acids (DCA/CDCA) and high concentrations of conjugated bile acid (GCDCA) increase HCV RNA replication in HCV genotype 1b replicon [21], [22]. Bile acids (CA and CDCA) also increase HCV RNA replication in HCV genotype 2a replicon [23].

11.3.3 Ursodeoxycholic Acid (UDCA) and Viral Hepatitis

Direct-acting antivirals are outstandingly successful in the eradication of HCV, and anti-HBV drugs achieve sustained suppression of HBV. In addition, we have palliative treatment with UDCA for chronic viral hepatitis. In patients with chronic viral hepatitis, including HBV and HCV, UDCA improves serum liver transaminase levels without serious adverse events. However, UDCA does not eradicate viral markers. In addition, there is no compelling evidence showing that these bile acids beneficially affect viral markers, mortality, cirrhosis development, need for liver transplantation, or liver histology in patients with acute or chronic hepatitis B and chronic hepatitis C [24]. UDCA has a direct protective effect on hepatocytes against apoptosis induced by endogenous bile acids and stimulates bile acid secretion, hence reducing retention of toxic bile acids and, therefore, cell injury [25, 26]. The mechanisms of UDCA action include reduction of toxic endogenous bile acids, membrane-stabilizing activity, and immunomodulatory effect. At the mitochondrial level, UDCA inhibits JNK-dependent *Fas* trafficking to the plasma membrane and activates survival signals such as epidermal growth factor receptor and mitogen-activated protein kinase. In addition, UDCA inhibits apoptosis mediated by endoplasmic reticulum stress [27].

11.4 HCC

11.4.1 Etiology

Liver cancer includes two major types: HCC and cholangiocellular carcinoma (CCC). HCC results in between 250,000 and 1 million deaths globally each year. Worldwide, HCC is the sixth most prevalent cancer and the second leading cause of cancer-related death [28]. Many insults that lead to chronic liver damage, such as intoxication, viral infection, cholestasis, or metabolic diseases, increase the risk of HCC. HBV and HCV infections appear to be the most significant causes of HCC worldwide. Chronic HBV infection is the leading cause of HCC in Asia and Africa, and HCV infection is the leading cause of HCC in North America, Europe, and Japan [29]. The annual incidence of HCC in HBV carriers is 0.5–1 % in patients without cirrhosis and 2.5 % per year in patients with cirrhosis. The annual incidence of HCC in HCV-related cirrhotic or pre-cirrhotic liver is reported as 4–8 %.

11.4.2 Bile Acids and Development of HCC

Abnormally high levels of bile acids induce hepatocyte DNA damage, which can increase the mutation rate of tumor suppressor genes and oncogenes. Furthermore, bile acids can induce cell death and inflammation to promote carcinogenesis. Bile acid homeostasis is disrupted in HCC patients with an elevated serum bile acid level as a proposed marker for HCC. However, the underlying mechanisms remain largely unknown. In HCC patients, serum CA, CDCA, and DCA levels are elevated, but serum UDCA level is not elevated [30]. The concentration of CDCA is increased in human HCC tissues [31]. GCDCA contributes to the development of HCC in a mechanism that enhances the antiapoptotic function of myeloid leukemia cell differentiation protein-1 (Mcl-1) [32]. Mcl-1 is a major antiapoptotic member of the Bcl2 family, which has survival and oncogenic properties. In HCC, this is characterized by a marked increase in the CDCA/CA ratio in both serum and urine [33]. This indicates predominant synthesis of CDCA in HCC tissues.

11.4.3 Bile Acid Transporters and HCC

Mutations in the bile salt export pump (BSEP), ABCB11, result in liver tumor formation [34]. BSEP is an efflux transporter that plays an important role in the disposition of bile salts from the liver, and it is predominantly expressed at the apical (canalicular) membranes of hepatocytes [35]. Expression of BSEP is downregulated in HCC cell lines [36]. Furthermore, expression of bile acid uptake transporter NTCP is reduced in most cases of HCC [37].

The elevated bile acid concentrations play a role as an endogenous promoter in hepatocarcinogenesis in rats. *mdr2* gene deletion mice, which have accumulation of bile acids in the liver, display progressive HCC [38]. Multidrug resistance (Mdr)2 (MDR3 in humans) is localized at the canalicular membrane of hepatocytes and is responsible for the ATP-dependent translocation of phosphatidylcholine [35]. Bile acids may directly contribute to the development of HCC in humans.

The absence of FXR and its downstream target SHP results in unsuppressed bile acid synthesis, and the injured liver may fail to complete normal regeneration, leading to repeated cycles of cell necrosis and compensatory proliferation of hepatocytes. This irregular proliferation of hepatocytes is an important factor in promoting hepatocarcinogenesis [39]. FXR, which is necessary for maintaining bile acid homeostasis, prevents bile acid-induced hepatocyte DNA damage and transformation. Therefore, the role of FXR in the promotion of liver regeneration could be an intrinsic mechanism for the prevention of liver carcinogenesis [40].

Bile acids are also ligands for G-protein-coupled bile acid receptor 1 (*GPBAR1*, also known as *TGR5* or membrane-type receptor for bile acids). The receptor is implicated in the suppression of macrophage functions and regulation of energy homeostasis by bile acids. In HCC patients with HBV, serum TGR5 promoter methylation is detected [41]. TGR5 also modulates the activation of signal transducer and activator of transcription (STAT)3. STAT3 is a transcription factor and is traditionally considered to be an oncogene in HCC; however, recent reports demonstrate the antioncogenic functions of STAT3 in HCC development [42, 43]. TGR5 may be a potential tumor suppressor and biomarker in liver cancer.

Fibroblast growth factor (FGF)19 is also implicated in the development of HCC. FGF19 (also called FGF15 in rodents) is an endocrine hormone of the FGF family that regulates bile acid, carbohydrate, and lipid and energy metabolism. EGF19 selectively binds to FGFR4, which can be further enhanced by co-receptor FGFR4–β-Klotho. FGF19–FGFR4 signaling is also implicated in hepatocellular tumorigenesis. In rodents, an engineered FGF19 (M70) fully retains the biological activity of FGF19 and inhibits FGF19-mediated liver tumor formation [44].

OATP1B3 is expressed on the basolateral membranes of hepatocytes and is encoded by the *SLCO1B3* gene. OATP1B3 is a drug transporter mediating the active hepatic uptake of bile acids and gadolinium–ethoxybenzyl–diethylenetriamine pentaacetic acid (Gd–EOB–DTPA). Magnetic resonance images acquired 10–20 min after Gd–EOB–DTPA injection, a period known as the hepatobiliary phase, are useful for HCC detection. HCC shows low signal intensity in the hepatobiliary phase of Gd–EOB–DTPA-enhanced magnetic resonance imaging. OATP1B3 expression is often decreased (or absent) in HCC relative to that of the liver parenchyma [45, 46] (Fig. 11.4).

11.4.4 Senescence-Associated Secretory Phenotype (SASP)

Secondary bile acids, particularly DCA, cause DNA damage through production of reactive oxygen species [47] and are a major risk factor for promoting colon tumorigenesis. In the liver, DCA provokes SASP in senescent hepatic stellate cells [48], which in turn secrete various inflammatory and tumor-promoting factors, thus facilitating HCC development.

Cellular senescence is now recognized as a potent tumor-suppressive mechanism that arrests the growth of cells at risk for malignant transformation. However, recent studies showed that senescent cells develop altered secretory activities that may induce changes in the tissue microenvironment, relaxing its control over cell

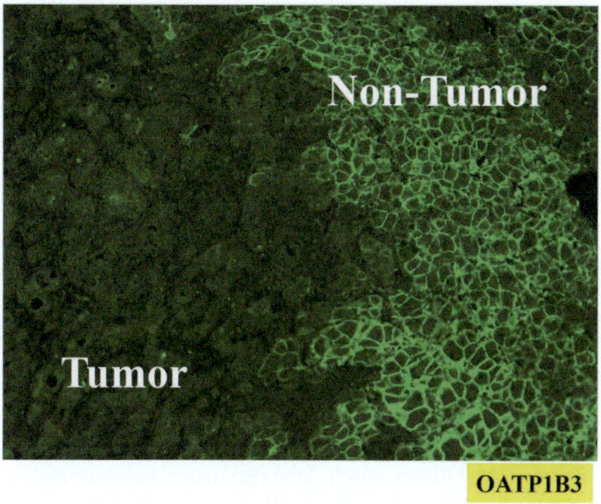

Fig. 11.4 Hepatic OATP1B3 expression in an HCC patient. No OATP1B3 expression was observed in the area of HCC, whereas OATP1B3 expression was observed in the non-tumor area in an immunohistochemical study observed by a laser scanning microscopy (Original magnification: ×200)

behavior and promoting tumorigenesis [49]. SASP represents cellular senescence changes in gene expression that result in secretion of a signature profile of inflammatory cytokines, chemokines, and proteases associated with inflammation and malignancy. SASP is also known as the senescence-messaging secretome [49].

11.4.5 UDCA and HCC

UDCA is a relatively hydrophilic bile acid and is well known to have a hepatocellular protective effect in a variety of liver diseases. In HCV cirrhosis patients, UDCA decreases the risk of HCC [50]. UDCA treatment reduces hepatocarcinogenesis by inducing apoptosis [51]. Moreover, UDCA induces *DLC1*, which is a tumor suppressor gene for HCC, by inhibiting proteasomal DLC1 (deleted in liver cancer 1) degradation in a ubiquitin-independent manner [52]. DLC1 induction participates in UDCA-induced suppression of HCC cellular growth. In HepG2 cells, combined treatment with UDCA and oxaliplatin suppresses carcinogenesis, shifting oxaliplatin-induced necrosis to apoptosis. UDCA also triggers the necrosis-to-apoptosis switch when combined with other platinum-based chemotherapeutic drugs including cisplatin and carboplatin [53].

References

1. Shlomai A, Halfon P, Goldiner I, Zelber-Sagi S, Halpern Z, Oren R, et al. Serum bile acid levels as a predictor for the severity of liver fibrosis in patients with chronic hepatitis C. J Viral Hepat. 2013;20(2):95–102. doi:10.1111/j.1365-2893.2012.01628.x.

2. Chen T, Xie G, Wang X, Fan J, Qiu Y, Zheng X, et al. Serum and urine metabolite profiling reveals potential biomarkers of human hepatocellular carcinoma. Mol Cell Proteomics. 2011;10(7):M110 004945. doi:10.1074/mcp.M110.004945.
3. Kakiyama G, Pandak WM, Gillevet PM, Hylemon PB, Heuman DM, Daita K, et al. Modulation of the fecal bile acid profile by gut microbiota in cirrhosis. J Hepatol. 2013;58(5):949–55. doi:10.1016/j.jhep.2013.01.003.
4. Vlahcevic ZR, Buhac I, Bell Jr CC, Swell L. Abnormal metabolism of secondary bile acids in patients with cirrhosis. Gut. 1970;11(5):420–2.
5. Wang X, Xie G, Zhao A, Zheng X, Huang F, Wang Y, et al. Serum bile acids are associated with pathological progression of hepatitis B-induced cirrhosis. J Proteome Res. 2015; doi:10.1021/acs.jproteome.5b00217.
6. Yin P, Wan D, Zhao C, Chen J, Zhao X, Wang W, et al. A metabonomic study of hepatitis B-induced liver cirrhosis and hepatocellular carcinoma by using RP-LC and HILIC coupled with mass spectrometry. Mol BioSyst. 2009;5(8):868–76. doi:10.1039/b820224a.
7. Murakami E, Wang T, Park Y, Hao J, Lepist EI, Babusis D, et al. Implications of efficient hepatic delivery by tenofovir alafenamide (GS-7340) for hepatitis B virus therapy. Antimicrob Agents Chemother. 2015;59(6):3563–9. doi:10.1128/AAC.00128-15.
8. Nassal M. HBV cccDNA: viral persistence reservoir and key obstacle for a cure of chronic hepatitis B. Gut. 2015;64(12):1972–84. doi:10.1136/gutjnl-2015-309809.
9. Xiao F, McKeating JA, Baumert TF. A bile acid transporter as a candidate receptor for hepatitis B and D virus entry. J Hepatol. 2013;58(6):1246–8. doi:10.1016/j.jhep.2013.01.036.
10. Yan H, Zhong GC, Xu GW, He WH, Jing ZY, Gao ZC et al. Sodium taurocholate cotransporting polypeptide is a functional receptor for human hepatitis B and D virus. Elife. 2012;1. doi:ARTN e000497554/eLife.00049.
11. Watashi K, Urban S, Li W, Wakita T. NTCP and beyond: opening the door to unveil hepatitis B virus entry. Int J Mol Sci. 2014;15(2):2892–905. doi:10.3390/ijms15022892.
12. Reese VC, Oropeza CE, McLachlan A. Independent activation of hepatitis B virus biosynthesis by retinoids, peroxisome proliferators, and bile acids. J Virol. 2013;87(2):991–7. doi:10.1128/JVI.01562-12.
13. Ramiere C, Scholtes C, Diaz O, Icard V, Perrin-Cocon L, Trabaud MA, et al. Transactivation of the hepatitis B virus core promoter by the nuclear receptor FXRalpha. J Virol. 2008;82(21):10832–40. doi:10.1128/JVI.00883-08.
14. Makishima M. Nuclear receptors as targets for drug development: regulation of cholesterol and bile acid metabolism by nuclear receptors. J Pharmacol Sci. 2005;97(2):177–83.
15. Kim HY, Cho HK, Choi YH, Lee KS, Cheong J. Bile acids increase hepatitis B virus gene expression and inhibit interferon-alpha activity. FEBS J. 2010;277(13):2791–802. doi:10.1111/j.1742-4658.2010.07695.x.
16. Reese VC, Moore DD, McLachlan A. Limited effects of bile acids and small heterodimer partner on hepatitis B virus biosynthesis in vivo. J Virol. 2012;86(5):2760–8. doi:10.1128/JVI.06742-11.
17. Oehler N, Volz T, Bhadra OD, Kah J, Allweiss L, Giersch K, et al. Binding of hepatitis B virus to its cellular receptor alters the expression profile of genes of bile acid metabolism. Hepatology. 2014;60(5):1483–93. doi:10.1002/hep.27159.
18. Mohd Hanafiah K, Groeger J, Flaxman AD, Wiersma ST. Global epidemiology of hepatitis C virus infection: new estimates of age-specific antibody to HCV seroprevalence. Hepatology. 2013;57(4):1333–42. doi:10.1002/hep.26141.
19. Kabiri M, Jazwinski AB, Roberts MS, Schaefer AJ, Chhatwal J. The changing burden of hepatitis C virus infection in the United States: model-based predictions. Ann Intern Med. 2014;161(3):170–80. doi:10.7326/M14-0095.
20. Graf D, Haselow K, Munks I, Bode JG, Haussinger D. Inhibition of interferon-alpha-induced signaling by hyperosmolarity and hydrophobic bile acids. Biol Chem. 2010;391(10):1175–87. doi:10.1515/BC.2010.108.
21. Chang KO, George DW. Bile acids promote the expression of hepatitis C virus in replicon-harboring cells. J Virol. 2007;81(18):9633–40. doi:10.1128/JVI.00795-07.

22. Schupp A-K, Graf D. Bile acid-induced modulation of virus replication. Eur J Med Res. 2014;19(Suppl 1):S27. doi:10.1186/2047-783x-19-s1-s27.
23. Chhatwal P, Bankwitz D, Gentzsch J, Frentzen A, Schult P, Lohmann V, et al. Bile acids specifically increase hepatitis C virus RNA-replication. PLoS One. 2012;7(4):e36029. doi:10.1371/journal.pone.0036029.
24. Chen W, Liu J, Gluud C. Bile acids for viral hepatitis. Cochrane Database Syst Rev. 2007;4:CD003181. doi:10.1002/14651858.CD003181.pub2.
25. Carreno V. Review article: management of chronic hepatitis C in patients with contraindications to anti-viral therapy. Aliment Pharmacol Ther. 2014;39(2):148–62. doi:10.1111/apt.12562.
26. Koga Y. Anti-cholestatic and cytoprotective properties of ursodeoxycholic acid Studies in vivo and vitro. Kanzo. 1987;28(12):1597–604. doi:10.2957/kanzo.28.1597.
27. Sola S, Amaral JD, Aranha MM, Steer CJ, Rodrigues CM. Modulation of hepatocyte apoptosis: cross-talk between bile acids and nuclear steroid receptors. Curr Med Chem. 2006;13(25):3039–51.
28. Forner A, Llovet JM, Bruix J. Hepatocellular carcinoma. Lancet. 2012;379(9822):1245–55. doi:10.1016/S0140-6736(11)61347-0.
29. Bruix J, Sherman M. American Association for the Study of Liver D. Management of hepatocellular carcinoma: an update. Hepatology. 2011;53(3):1020–2. doi:10.1002/hep.24199.
30. Zhang W, Zhou L, Yin P, Wang J, Lu X, Wang X, et al. A weighted relative difference accumulation algorithm for dynamic metabolomics data: long-term elevated bile acids are risk factors for hepatocellular carcinoma. Sci Rep. 2015;5:8984. doi:10.1038/srep08984.
31. Nakayama F, Yanagisawa J, Miyazaki H, Itoh M. Bile-acid composition in primary hepatocellular-carcinoma. J Gastroenterol Hepatol. 1987;2(2):149–58. doi:10.1111/j.1440-1746.1987.tb01613.x.
32. Liao M, Zhao J, Wang T, Duan J, Zhang Y, Deng X. Role of bile salt in regulating Mcl-1 phosphorylation and chemoresistance in hepatocellular carcinoma cells. Mol Cancer. 2011;10:44. doi:10.1186/1476-4598-10-44.
33. El-Mir MY, Badia MD, Luengo N, Monte MJ, Marin JJ. Increased levels of typically fetal bile acid species in patients with hepatocellular carcinoma. Clin Sci (Lond). 2001;100(5):499–508.
34. Scheimann AO, Strautnieks SS, Knisely AS, Byrne JA, Thompson RJ, Finegold MJ. Mutations in bile salt export pump (ABCB11) in two children with progressive familial intrahepatic cholestasis and cholangiocarcinoma. J Pediatr. 2007;150(5):556–9. doi:10.1016/j.jpeds.2007.02.030.
35. Takeyama Y, Sakisaka S. Hepatobiliary membrane transporters in primary biliary cirrhosis. Hepatol Res. 2012;42(2):120–30. doi:10.1111/j.1872-034X.2011.00912.x.
36. Chen Y, Song X, Valanejad L, Vasilenko A, More V, Qiu X, et al. Bile salt export pump is dysregulated with altered farnesoid X receptor isoform expression in patients with hepatocellular carcinoma. Hepatology. 2013;57(4):1530–41. doi:10.1002/hep.26187.
37. Zollner G, Wagner M, Fickert P, Silbert D, Fuchsbichler A, Zatloukal K, et al. Hepatobiliary transporter expression in human hepatocellular carcinoma. Liver Int. 2005;25(2):367–79. doi:10.1111/j.1478-3231.2005.01033.x.
38. Katzenellenbogen M, Mizrahi L, Pappo O, Klopstock N, Olam D, Jacob-Hirsch J, et al. Molecular mechanisms of liver carcinogenesis in the mdr2-knockout mice. Mol Cancer Res. 2007;5(11):1159–70. doi:10.1158/1541-7786.MCR-07-0172.
39. Ueno Y, Moriyama M, Uchida T, Arakawa Y. Irregular regeneration of hepatocytes is an important factor in the hepatocarcinogenesis of liver disease. Hepatology. 2001;33(2):357–62. doi:10.1053/jhep.2001.21902.
40. Stanimirov B, Stankov K, Mikov M. Bile acid signaling through farnesoid X and TGR5 receptors in hepatobiliary and intestinal diseases. Hepatobiliary Pancreat Dis Int. 2015;14(1):18–33. doi:10.1016/S1499-3872(14)60307-6.

41. Han LY, Fan YC, Mu NN, Gao S, Li F, Ji XF, et al. Aberrant DNA methylation of G-protein-coupled bile acid receptor Gpbar1 (TGR5) is a potential biomarker for hepatitis B virus associated hepatocellular carcinoma. Int J Med Sci. 2014;11(2):164–71. doi:10.7150/ijms.6745.
42. Schneller D, Machat G, Sousek A, Proell V, van Zijl F, Zulehner G, et al. p19(ARF)/p14(ARF) controls oncogenic functions of signal transducer and activator of transcription 3 in hepatocellular carcinoma. Hepatology. 2011;54(1):164–72. doi:10.1002/hep.24329.
43. Calvisi DF. Dr. Jekyll and Mr. Hyde: a paradoxical oncogenic and tumor suppressive role of signal transducer and activator of transcription 3 in liver cancer. Hepatology. 2011;54(1):9–12. doi:10.1002/hep.24435.
44. Zhou M, Wang X, Phung V, Lindhout DA, Mondal K, Hsu JY, et al. Separating tumorigenicity from bile acid regulatory activity for endocrine hormone FGF19. Cancer Res. 2014;74(12):3306–16. doi:10.1158/0008-5472.CAN-14-0208.
45. Narita M, Hatano E, Arizono S, Miyagawa-Hayashino A, Isoda H, Kitamura K, et al. Expression of OATP1B3 determines uptake of Gd-EOB-DTPA in hepatocellular carcinoma. J Gastroenterol. 2009;44(7):793–8. doi:10.1007/s00535-009-0056-4.
46. Takeyama Y, Tsuchiya N, Kunimoto H, Fukunaga A, Sakurai K, Hirano G, et al. Gadolinium-ethoxybenzyl-diethylenetriamine pentaacetic acid-enhanced magnetic resonance imaging as a useful detection method for advanced primary biliary cirrhosis. Hepatol Res. 2015;45(10):E108–14. doi:10.1111/hepr.12470.
47. Payne CM, Weber C, Crowley-Skillicorn C, Dvorak K, Bernstein H, Bernstein C, et al. Deoxycholate induces mitochondrial oxidative stress and activates NF-kappaB through multiple mechanisms in HCT-116 colon epithelial cells. Carcinogenesis. 2007;28(1):215–22. doi:10.1093/carcin/bgl139.
48. Friedman SL. Hepatic stellate cells: protean, multifunctional, and enigmatic cells of the liver. Physiol Rev. 2008;88(1):125–72. doi:10.1152/physrev.00013.2007.
49. Coppe JP, Desprez PY, Krtolica A, Campisi J. The senescence-associated secretory phenotype: the dark side of tumor suppression. Annu Rev Pathol. 2010;5:99–118. doi:10.1146/annurev-pathol-121808-102144.
50. Tarao K, Fujiyama S, Ohkawa S, Miyakawa K, Tamai S, Hirokawa S, et al. Ursodiol use is possibly associated with lower incidence of hepatocellular carcinoma in hepatitis C virus-associated liver cirrhosis. Cancer Epidemiol Biomark Prev. 2005;14(1):164–9.
51. Oyama K, Shiota G, Ito H, Murawaki Y, Kawasaki H. Reduction of hepatocarcinogenesis by ursodeoxycholic acid in rats. Carcinogenesis. 2002;23(5):885–92.
52. Chung GE, Yoon JH, Lee JH, Kim HY, Myung SJ, Yu SJ, et al. Ursodeoxycholic acid-induced inhibition of DLC1 protein degradation leads to suppression of hepatocellular carcinoma cell growth. Oncol Rep. 2011;25(6):1739–46. doi:10.3892/or.2011.1239.
53. Lim SC, Choi JE, Kang HS, Han SI. Ursodeoxycholic acid switches oxaliplatin-induced necrosis to apoptosis by inhibiting reactive oxygen species production and activating p53-caspase 8 pathway in HepG2 hepatocellular carcinoma. Int J Cancer. 2010;126(7):1582–95. doi:10.1002/ijc.24853.

Chapter 12
Bile Acids and Pancreatic Disease

Morihisa Hirota and Tooru Shimosegawa

Abstract It is generally believed that biliary acute pancreatitis is initiated by contact between bile acid and pancreatic acinar cells due to bile reflux into the pancreatic duct followed by the impaction of a gallstone into the papilla of Vater, although it is still debatable. Several animal models of biliary acute pancreatitis have been established and used to elucidate the molecular mechanisms by which bile acids induce acute pancreatitis. The bile acids enter the acinar cells through transporters on the plasma membrane and induce sustained Ca^{2+} influx into the cytosol from acidic stores in the apical portion and from the endoplasmic reticulum in the basal portion of the cells. The intercellular Ca^{2+} overload leads to acinar cell necrosis subsequent to mitochondrial depolarization. A receptor *Gbpa1*-mediated bile acid signaling has also been demonstrated to play an important role in the bile acid-induced acinar cell injury. Pancreatic fluid secretion from ductal cells is influenced by the bile acids in a concentration-dependent manner, with a stimulatory effect at low concentrations and an inhibitory effect at high concentrations. It is expected to develop a specific medicine to prevent bile acids-induced acute pancreatitis.

Keywords Acute pancreatitis • Biliary acute pancreatitis • Bile acid • Calcium • Necrosis

12.1 Introduction

Gallstones are one of main risk factors for acute pancreatitis [1]. Following alcoholic pancreatitis (33.5%), biliary pancreatitis is the second leading cause (26.9%) of acute pancreatitis in Japan. In females, gallstones are most common cause

M. Hirota
Department of Gastroenterology, Tohoku University Hospital, 1-1 Seiryo-cho, Aoba-ku, Sendai, Miyagi 980-8574, Japan

T. Shimosegawa (✉)
Division of Gastroenterology, Tohoku University Graduate School of Medicine, 1-1 Seiryo-cho, Aoba-ku, Sendai, Miyagi 980-8574, Japan
e-mail: tshimosegawa@int3.med.tohoku.ac.jp

S. Tazuma, H. Takikawa (eds.), *Bile Acids in Gastroenterology*,
DOI 10.1007/978-4-431-56062-3_12

(40.3%) [2]. Although a gallstone that migrates into the common bile duct is regarded as a high risk for acute pancreatitis, the detailed molecular mechanisms by which inappropriate protease activation occurs in acinar cells, exacerbates the inflammatory process, and develops acute pancreatitis have not been precisely elucidated. Three hypotheses are discussed in a review article by Lerch et al. [3]. (A) Obstruction of the pancreatic duct by an impacted gallstone leads to blocked pancreatic outflow triggering pancreatitis. (B) Opie's common channel hypothesis is that a gallstone impacted at the papilla creates communication between the pancreatic and bile duct behind it, through which bile could enter the pancreatic duct and potentially reach the acinar cells. (C) Both bile and pancreatic ducts are obstructed by an impacted gallstone without the potential for bile reflux into the pancreas. The obstruction of pancreatic secretion triggers the disease, but an additional bile duct obstruction would act as an aggravating factor by increasing the circulating or interstitial bile acid concentration [3].

There is increasing evidence that bile acid plays an important role in the pathogenesis of biliary acute pancreatitis. In this chapter, we focus on experimental animal models of biliary acute pancreatitis and recently elucidated molecular mechanisms of the bile acid-induced phenomena in both acinar and ductal cells in the pancreas.

12.2 Experimental Models of Biliary Acute Pancreatitis

12.2.1 Duct Obstruction Model

A duct obstruction model mimics the gallstone obstruction-induced acute pancreatitis in the clinical setting [4]. Either the common biliopancreatic duct or pancreatic duct is ligated to obstruct the outflow of both the bile and pancreatic juice or the pancreatic juice alone in this model. In most animal models, except for opossum, if the pancreatic duct alone is ligated, necrotizing pancreatitis cannot be induced [3]. The animals develop chronic lesions in the pancreas characterized by atrophy and apoptosis of the acinar and ductal tissue [5]. On the other hand, if the common biliopancreatic duct is ligated, the animals develop acute pancreatitis. This model is consistent with Opie's common cannel hypothesis. In this situation, bile reflux enters into the pancreas and the pancreatic intraductal pressure rises. Ligation of the common biliopancreatic duct in rat causes acute pancreatitis with pancreatic necrosis and hemorrhage and a clinical syndrome resembling the multiple organ failure observed in man [5]. On the other hand, conflicting data have been reported about the severity of pancreatitis in this rat model from mild to severe. Moreover, the severity of pancreatitis produced by this model varies depending on whether rabbits, rats, or opossums are used as subjects [4].

12.2.2 Duct Infusion Model

Acute pancreatitis induced by direct cannulation and infusion of bile acid into pancreatic duct is another established experimental animal model for biliary acute pancreatitis. Since 1856 when Bernard developed experimental acute pancreatitis by the infusion of bile and olive oil into a canine pancreas, various bile salts such as sodium chenodeoxycholate (CDC), sodium taurocholate (TC), sodium glycodeoxycholic acid (GDC), sodium taurodeoxycholate (TDC), and taurolithocholic acid 3-sulfate (TLC-S) have been reported to induce acute pancreatitis in different species [6].

Among these bile salts, sodium TC-induced pancreatitis has been most extensively characterized. Between 3% and 6% of sodium TC is effective for inducing acute pancreatitis with edema, hemorrhage, and necrosis in large animals such as rabbit, dogs, and pigs. However, such large animals are less susceptible to the pancreatic injury observed in rats, which is severe enough to induce multiple organ failure involving the lung, kidney, liver, intestine, and brain [4]. Recently genetically manipulated mice have been employed for studies of experimental acute pancreatitis, and TLC-S is favored by researchers over sodium TC for the induction of acute pancreatitis [6].

12.3 Mechanisms of Acinar Cell Injury by Bile Acid

12.3.1 Ca^{2+} Overload Initiates Acinar Cell Injury

Ca^{2+} signals elicited by secretagogues, such as cholecystokinin (CCK) and CCK analogue cerulein, initiate enzyme secretion from the apical membrane of pancreatic acinar cells. It has been reported that hyperstimulation by a secretagogue can induce an abnormal and sustained cytosolic Ca^{2+} concentration ($[Ca^{2+}]_i$) in the apical pole of acinar cell and that pronounced trypsin activation and extensive vacuole formation are localized in the same region [7, 8]. Voronina et al. demonstrated that bile acids such as TLC-S, TC, and TDC induced global Ca^{2+} oscillation in pancreatic acinar cells that was initiated from the apical region and then propagated to the basal region [9]. They suggested that biliary acute pancreatitis could be explained by the potentially toxic $[Ca^{2+}]_i$ overload induced by bile acids.

The molecular mechanisms of bile acid-induced acinar cell injury have been explored. Kim et al. demonstrated bile acid transporters located in the luminal and basolateral membrane of acinar cells, Na^+-dependent transporter Na^+-taurocholate cotransporting polypeptide (Ntcp) and Na^+-independent transporter organic anion-transporting polypeptide (Oatp), respectively. Moreover, they reported that cytosolic bile acid inhibited the sarco/endoplasmic reticulum Ca^{2+} ATPase (SERCA) pump [10]. Fischer et al. reported that phosphatidylinositol 3-kinase (PI3K) and its product phosphatidylinositol (3,4,5)-trisphosphate (PIP_3) facilitated bile acid-induced $[Ca^{2+}]_i$ responses in pancreatic acinar cells through the inhibition of SERCA-dependent Ca^{2+} reloading into the endoplasmic reticulum (ER) and that bile acid-induced trypsinogen activation was mediated by PI3K [11]. Pancreatic acinar cells have a remarkably large amount of Ca^{2+} stores in both the ER, which is located in the basal part of the cells, and the acidic stores, which are exclusively located in the apical part of the cells [12]. Gerasimenko et al. described that bile acids released Ca^{2+} from both the ER and the acidic stores and that TLC-S interacted with both the inositol trisphosphate receptors (IP_3Rs) and ryanodine receptors (RyRs), which are opened through activation of nicotinic acid adenine dinucleotide phosphate (NAADP) [13]. A Ca^{2+} reloading mechanism is also involved in the pathogenesis of acinar cell injury. The principal store-operated calcium entry (SOCE) channel ORAI1, which exists at the plasma membrane, opens and induces Ca^{2+} influx into the ER after the depletion of ER Ca^{2+} through interaction with stromal interaction molecule (STIM) 1 and STIM2. Inhibitors of ORAI1, GSK-7975A, and CM_128, each inhibited all local and systemic features of acute pancreatitis in three mouse models including a TLC-S-induced model. The ORAI channel was identified as potential target for the early treatment of acute pancreatitis [14].

Another mechanism of bile acid signaling in the pancreatic acinar cells through bile acid receptor has been identified. Perides et al. reported that G-protein-coupled, cell surface, bile acid receptor *Gpbal*, which is expressed at the apical pole of acinar cells, might play a critical role in the evolution of bile acid-induced acute pancreatitis, based on the observation of the markedly reduced generation of pathological calcium transients, intracellular activation of digestive zymogens, and cell injury induced by the exposure of TLC-S to the acinar cells of genetically manipulated *Gpbal*-deficient mice [15].

12.3.2 Cell Fate Decision

Mitochondria play a central role in the cell fate decisions leading to either apoptosis or necrosis during the pathogenesis of acute pancreatitis. It has been reported that $[Ca^{2+}]_i$ overload induced by bile acids was sufficient for mitochondrial depolarization and reduced cytosolic and mitochondrial adenosine triphosphate (ATP) in acinar cells [16, 17]. Mitochondrial matrix calcium overload opens mitochondrial permeability transition pore (MPTP), a nonspecific channel formed in the inner mitochondrial membrane that allows passage of particles smaller than 1,500 Da, causing a loss of the mitochondrial membrane potential ($\Delta\Psi m$), which ultimately leads to intercellular ATP depletion and acinar cell necrosis [18–20]. Pharmacological and genetic MPTP inhibition protected $\Delta\Psi m$, ATP production, and autophagy and prevented the acinar cell necrosis from bile acid-induced Ca^{2+} release via IP_3R and RyR. Therefore, the MPTP has been identified as a potential drug target for acute pancreatitis [19]. On the other hand, bile acids induce prolonged intercellular and mitochondrial Ca^{2+}, which leads to a dose-dependent increase in the intercellular and mitochondrial reactive oxygen species (ROS) production. The increased ROS production promotes apoptosis and decreased necrosis [21, 22]. In contrast to Ca^{2+}, ROS had little effect on $\Delta\Psi m$. ROS and Ca^{2+} promote cytochrome c release through mitochondrial outer membrane permeability, resulting in caspase activation and apoptosis [20].

12.3.3 Effect of Bile Acid on Ductal Cell

As well as the pancreatic acinar cells, bile acids affect the ductal cells. Luminal administration of a low dose of CDC (0.1 mM) stimulates ductal HCO_3^- secretion. In contrast, both luminal and basolateral administration of a high dose of CDC (1 mM) strongly inhibited HCO_3^- secretion from ductal cells [23]. The stimulatory effect of a low dose of CDC on HCO_3^- secretion is dependent on Ca^{2+}. In this situation, ductal cells may try to wash out the toxic bile acid and thus defend the acinar cell by increasing fluid and HCO_3^- secretion. On the other hand, a high concentration of CDC leads to epithelial barrier damage, the secretory mechanisms of pancreatic ductal cells are inhibited, and the ducts can no longer act as a defensive wall against the toxic bile [24]. It has been documented that 1 mM of CDC inhibits the pancreatic ductal HCO_3^- secretion. In this situation, mitochondrial damage and intracellular ATP depletion are the most crucial factors in the toxic inhibitory effect of CDC on pancreatic ductal secretion [24, 25].

12.4 Conclusion

The molecular mechanisms of the pathogenesis of biliary acute pancreatitis have been explored. Bile acid-induced $[Ca^{2+}]_i$ overload is a crucial event mediated by IP_3R and RyR on the ER membrane and SOCE channel on the plasma membrane. A bile acid receptor, *Gpbal*, is another important pathway that leads to acinar cell injury. Mitochondria depolarization followed by $[Ca^{2+}]_i$ overload induces intercellular ATP depletion and acinar cell necrosis (Fig.12.1). In ductal cells, a low concentration of bile acids stimulates pancreatic fluid secretion, which may be a protective response to wash out the toxic bile acids before they reach the acinar cells. In contrast, a high concentration of bile acids rather inhibits the pancreatic fluid secretion.

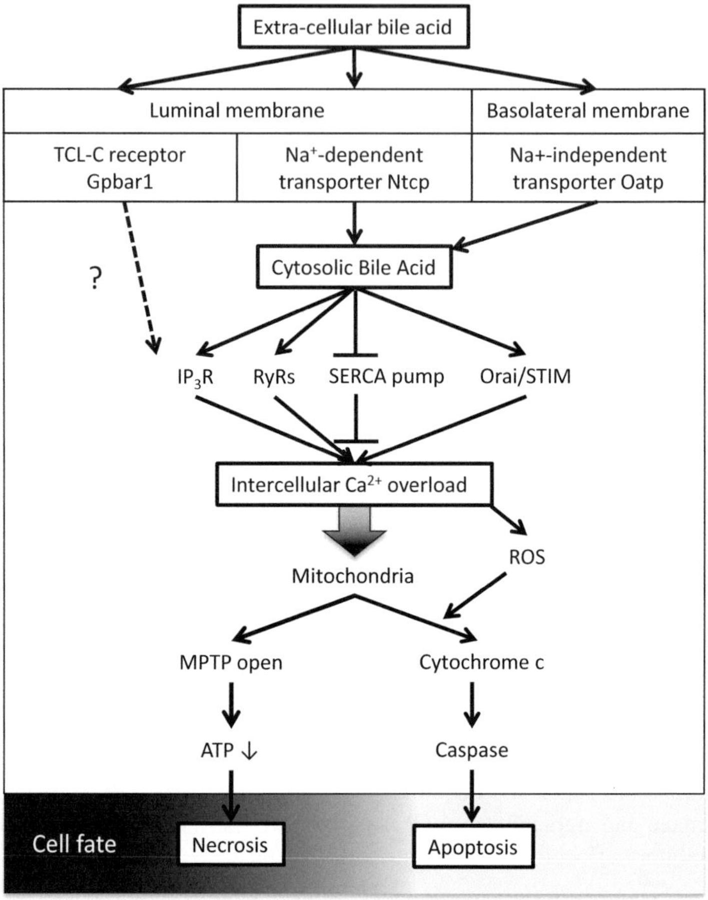

Fig. 12.1 A schema of bile acid signaling in pancreatic acinar cells. Extracellular bile acid enters pancreatic acinar cells through Na^+-dependent transporter Ntcp at the luminal membrane and Na^+-independent transporter Oatp at the basolateral membrane. Cytosolic bile acid induces intracellular Ca^{2+} overload to activate iP3R, RyRs, and Orai channel and to inhibit SERCA pump. Intracellular Ca^{2+} overload induces MPTP opening and subsequent acinar cell necrosis by ATP depletion. On the other hand, ROS and intracellular Ca^{2+} overload can induce acinar cell apoptosis by cytochrome c/caspase pathway, as well. The intercellular signaling of bile acid receptor Gpbar1 in pancreatic acinar cells is still largely unknown. *Gpbar1* G protein-coupled bile acid receptor, *Ntcp* Na^+-taurocholate cotransporting polypeptide, *Oatp* organic anion-transporting polypeptide, *IP_3R* inositol trisphosphate receptor, *RyRs* ryanodine receptors, *SERCA* sarco/endoplasmic reticulum Ca^{2+} ATPase, *STIM* stromal interaction molecule, *ROS* Reactive oxygen species, *MPTP* mitochondrial permeability transition pore, *ATP* adenosine triphosphate

Thus, some of the molecular mechanisms by which bile acids induce acute pancreatitis have been elucidated so far. Importantly, there have been several experimental therapeutic attempts to identify molecular targets for preventing the processes of bile acid-induced acute pancreatitis.

References

1. Lankish PG, Apte M, Banks PA. Acute pancreatitis. Lancet. 2015;386(9988):85–96. doi:10.1016/S0140-6736(14)60649-8.
2. Hamada S, Masamune A, Kikuta K, Hirota M, Tsuji I, Shimosegawa T. Research committee of intractable disease of the pancreas. Nationwide epidemiological survey of acute pancreatitis in Japan. Pancreas. 2014;43(8):1244–8. doi:10.1097/MPA.0000000000000200.
3. Lerch MM, Aghdassi AA. The role of bile acids in gallstone-induced pancreatitis. Gastroenterology. 2010;138(2):429–33. doi:10.1016/j.bpg.2009.02.013.
4. Chan YC, Leung PS. Acute pancreatitis: animal models and recent advances in basic research. Pancreas. 2007;34(1):1–14.
5. Su KH, Cuthbertson C, Christophi C. Review of experimental animal models of acute pancreatitis. HPB. 2006;8(4):264–86. doi:10.1080/13651820500467358.
6. Wan MH, Huang W, Latawiec D, Jiang K, Booth DM, Elliott V, Mukherjee R, Xia Q. HPB. 2012;14(2):73–81. doi:10.1111/j.1477-2574.2011.00408.x.
7. Kruger B, Albrecht E, Lerch MM. The role of intracellular calcium signaling in premature protease activation and the onset of pancreatitis. Am J Pathol. 2000;157(1):43–50.
8. Raraty M, Ward J, Erdemli G, Vaillant C, Neoptolemos JP, Sutton R, Petersen OH. Calcium-dependent enzyme activation and vacuole formation in the apical granular region of pancreatic acinar cells. Proc Natl Acad Sci U S A. 2000;97(24):13126–31.
9. Voronina S, Longbottom R, Sutton R, Petersen OH, Tepikin A. Bile acids induce calcium signals in mouse pancreatic acinar cells: implications for bile-induced pancreatic pathology. J Physiol. 2002;540(Pt 1):49–55.
10. Kim JY, Kim KH, Lee JA, Namkung W, Sun AQ, Ananthanarayanan M, Suchy FJ, Shin DM, Muallem S, Lee MG. Transporter-mediated bile acid uptake causes Ca^{2+}-dependent cell death in rat pancreatic acinar cells. Gastroenterology. 2002;122(7):1941–53.
11. Fischer L, Gukovskaya AS, Penninger JM, Mareninova OA, Friess H, Gukovsky I, Pandol SJ. Phosphatidylinositol 3-kinase facilitates bile acid-induced Ca2+ responses in pancreatic acinar cells. Am J Physiol Gastrointest Liver Physiol. 2007;292(3):G875–86. doi:10.1152/ajpgi.00558.2005.
12. Gerasimenko J, Peng S, Gerasimenko O. Role of acidic stores in secretory epithelia. Cell Calcium. 2014;55(6):346–54. doi:10.1016/j.ceca.2014.04.002.
13. Gerasimenko JV, Flowerdew SE, Voronina SG, Sukhomlin TK, Tepikin AV, Petersen OH, Gerasimenko OV. Bile acids induce Ca2+ release from both the endoplasmic reticulum and acidic intracellular calcium stores through activation of inositol trisphosphate receptors and ryanodine receptors. J Biol Chem. 2006;281(52):40154–63.
14. Wen L, Voronina S, Javed MA, Awais M, Szatmary P, Latawiec D, Chvanov M, Collier D, Huang W, Barrett J, Begg M, Stauderman K, Roos J, Grigoryev S, Ramos S, Rogers E, Whitten J, Velicelebi G, Dunn M, Tepikin AV, Criddle DN, Sutton R. Inhibitors of ORAI1 prevent cytosolic calcium-associated injury of human pancreatic acinar cells and acute pancreatitis in 3 mouse models. Gastroenterology. 2015;149(2):481–92. doi:10.1053/j.gastro.2015.04.015.
15. Perides G, Laukkarinen JM, Vassileva G, Steer ML. Biliary acute pancreatitis in mice is mediated by the G protein-coupled cell surface bile acid receptor *GPBAR1*. Gastroenterology. 2010;138(2):715–25. doi:10.1053/j.gastro.2009.10.052.
16. Voronina SG, Barrow SL, Gerasimenko OV, Petersen OH, Tepikin AV. Effects of secretagogues and bile acids on mitochondrial membrane potential of pancreatic acinar cells. J Biol Chem. 2004; 279(26)279(26):27327–38.
17. Voronina SG, Barrow SL, Simpson AW, Gerasimenko OV, da Silva XG, Rutter GA, Petersen OH, Tepikin AV. Dynamic changes in cytosolic and mitochondrial ATP level in pancreatic acinar cells. Gastroenterology. 2010;138(5):1976–87. doi:10.1053/j.gastro.2010.01.037.

18. Halestrap AP, Richardson AP. The mitochondrial permeability transition: a current perspective on its identity and role in ischemia/reperfusion injury. J Mol Cell Cardiol. 2015;78:129–41. doi:10.1016/j.yjmcc.2014.08.018.
19. Mukherjee R, Mareninova OA, Odinokova IV, Huang W, Murphy J, Chvanov M, Javed MA, Wen L, Booth DM, Cane MC, Awais M, Gavillet B, Pruss RM, Schaller S, Molkentin JD, Tepkin AV, Petersen OH, Pandol SJ, Gukovsky I, Criddle DN, Gukovskaya AC, Sutton R, and NIHR Pancreas Biomedical Research Unit. Mechanism of mitochondrial permeability transition pore induction and damage in the pancreas: inhibition prevent acute pancreatitis by protecting production of ATP. Gut 2015; Jun 12. pil: gutjnl-2014-308553. Doi: 10.1136/gutjnl-2014-308553.
20. Gukovsky I, Pandol SJ, Gukovskaya AS. Organellar dysfunction in the pathogenesis of pancreatitis. Antioxid Redox Signal. 2011;15(10):2699–710. doi:10.1089/ars.2011.4068.
21. Booth DM, Murphy JA, Mukherjee R, Awais M, Neoptolemos JP, Gerasimenko OV, Tepikin AV, Petersen OH, Sutton R, Criddle DN. Reactive oxygen species induced by bile acid induce apoptosis and protect against necrosis in pancreatic acinar cells. Gastroenterology. 2011;140(7):2116–25. doi:10.1053/j.gastro.2011.02.054.
22. Maleth J, Hegyi P, Rakonczay Jr Z, Venglovecz V. Breakdown of bioenergetics evoked by mitochondrial damage in acute pancreatitis: mechanism and consequences. Pancreatology. 2015;15(4 Suppl):S18–22. doi:10.1016/j.pan.2015.06.002.
23. Venglovecz V, Rakonczay Jr Z, Ozsvari B, Takacs T, Lonovics J, Varro A, Gray MA, Argent BE, Hegyi P. Effects of bile acids on pancreatic ductal bicarbonate secretion in guinea pig. Gut. 2008;57(8):1102–12. doi:10.1136/gut.2007.134361.
24. Hegyi P, Pandol S, Venglovecz V, Rakonczay Jr Z. The acinar-ductal tango in the pathogenesis of acute pancreatitis. Gut. 2011;60(4):544–52. doi:10.1136/gut.2010.218461.
25. Maleth J, Venglovecz V, Razga ZS, Tiszlavicz L, Rakonczay Jr Z, Hegyi P. Non-conjugated chenodeoxycholate induced severe mitochondrial damage and inhibits bicarbonate transport in pancreatic ductal cells. Gut. 2011;60(1):136–8. doi:10.1136/gut.2009.192153.

Chapter 13
Bile Acids and Esophageal Cancer

Juntaro Matsuzaki and Hidekazu Suzuki

Abstract The incidence rates of esophageal adenocarcinoma and its precursor lesion, Barrett's esophagus, have increased considerably in Western countries. Duodenogastroesophageal bile reflux is the major cause of this disease. Bile acids induce cytotoxicity in the esophageal epithelium through production of reactive oxygen species and activation of nuclear factor-κB and its downstream signaling pathways. Recent studies have revealed the characteristics of bile acid receptors and transporters in Barrett's esophagus and esophageal adenocarcinoma.

Keywords Barrett's esophagus • Oxidative stress • CDX2 • FXR • TGR5

13.1 Duodenogastroesophageal Bile Reflux Causes Esophageal Adenocarcinoma

Esophageal cancer is the eighth most common cancer worldwide, with 456,000 new cases and 400,000 related deaths in 2012 [1]. The majority of esophageal cancers are classified into two main histological subtypes: esophageal adenocarcinoma (EAC) and esophageal squamous cell carcinoma (ESCC). In recent decades, the incidence of EAC has increased among the white population of high-income countries. This increase is thought to be due to the rising prevalence of obesity. EAC typically arises from the metaplastic columnar epithelium, called Barrett's esophagus (BE), in the lower third of the esophagus. EAC and BE develop as a result of long-standing gastroesophageal reflux disease (GERD). Since bile acids are contained in gastric juices due to duodenogastric reflux, the esophagus of patients with GERD is exposed to a mixture of acid and bile acids. Therefore, the cytotoxic effect of bile acids can play a role in the development of BE and EAC.

J. Matsuzaki
Division of Molecular and Cellular Medicine, National Cancer Center Research Institute, 5-1-1 Tsukiji, Chuo-ku, Tokyo 104-0045, Japan

H. Suzuki (✉)
Medical Education Center, Keio University School of Medicine, 35 Shinanomachi, Shinjuku-ku, Tokyo 160-8582, Japan
e-mail: hsuzuki.a6@keio.jp

S. Tazuma, H. Takikawa (eds.), *Bile Acids in Gastroenterology*,
DOI 10.1007/978-4-431-56062-3_13

In fact, Menges et al. conducted simultaneous 24-h esophageal pH and bile reflux testing and found that acid and bile exposure were more extensive in 23 patients with BE than in 20 patients with esophagitis [2]. Nehra et al. investigated the spectrum of bile acids by using 15-h continuous esophageal aspiration with simultaneous pH monitoring [3]. The predominant bile acids detected were cholic acid (CA), taurocholic acid, and glycocholic acid, but there was a significantly greater proportion of secondary bile acids, deoxycholic and taurodeoxycholic acids (DCA and TDCA, respectively), in patients with BE.

In contrast, the association between ESCC and bile acid reflux is controversial. ESCC arises in squamous epithelial cells and usually occurs in the upper and middle third of the esophagus. Smoking and heavy alcohol consumption are the main factors that increase the risk of ESCC. The incidence of ESCC is declining in developed countries probably due to a decline in tobacco smoking; however, this incidence remains common in Africa and eastern Asia. These characteristics of ESCC imply the difference in underlying etiologies of ESCC and EAC. However, from another perspective, tobacco smoking and heavy alcohol consumption increase the risk of erosive esophagitis and BE, especially in Asians [4]. More interestingly, in several rat duodenal and gastroduodenal contents reflux models, both ESCC and EAC can develop without stimulus from any known carcinogens [5]. Therefore, we can not deny the possibility that bile acids might play a role in the development of ESCC.

In the following sections, we provide an overview of recent studies related to EAC and bile acids.

13.2 Risk of BE in Patients After Resection of the Lower Esophageal Sphincter

Since esophageal reflux of gastric and duodenal contents is facilitated after esophagectomy or gastrectomy, several researchers assessed the relationship between the resection of the esophagus or stomach and development of BE or EAC. Avidan et al. reported that Billroth-1 gastrectomy, Billroth-2 gastrectomy, vagotomy, and pyloroplasty were not associated with BE [6]. However, O'Riordan et al. showed that BE occurs frequently after lower esophagectomy [7]. Among 48 patients with a median follow-up period of 26 months (range = 12–67 months) postesophagectomy, 24 (50%) developed columnar metaplasia, and of these, 13 had specialized intestinal metaplasia. The prevalence of specialized intestinal metaplasia increased over time possibly due to chronic acid and bile exposure. In addition, Tsiouris et al. reported that concomitant fundoplication with resection of the gastroesophageal junction had some protective effect against the development of BE [8]. Thus, the association is still controversial, but careful long-term observation should be recommended for patients after the resection of the lower esophageal sphincter.

13.3 Theories on Cellular Origin of BE

There are two distinct hypotheses on the mechanisms of metaplastic conversion of esophageal squamous epithelium to BE. One possibility is the conversion of differentiated squamous cells or stem cells of the squamous epithelium in the basal cell layer. Alternatively, cells at the gastroesophageal junction or transitional zone may colonize the distal esophagus in response to noxious luminal contents.

There are extensive in vitro evidences that suggest the transdifferentiation of squamous cell lineage to BE. CDX2, a member of the caudal-related homeobox gene family, may play a major role in the development of BE. Since CDX2 regulates intestinal cell differentiation, stomach-specific transgenic overexpression of CDX2 induced intestinal metaplasia in mice stomach [9]. CDX2 is not expressed in squamous epithelial cells in normal human esophagus; however, it is aberrantly expressed in BE [10]. Therefore, several researchers investigated CDX2 expression in esophageal squamous cell cultures during exposure to acid and bile and found a high expression of CDX2 in response to bile acids via the activation of nuclear factor-κB (NF-κB) [11–13]. Kong et al. generated transgenic mice that expressed the CDX2 transgene in esophageal squamous tissues [14]. They found that ectopic CDX2 transgene expression in esophageal squamous cells reduced basal epithelial cell proliferation and barrier function and altered cell morphology in vivo.

On the other hand, recently, two studies on animals models strongly suggested that BE arises from a gastric cardia lineage of BE-like metaplasia. Wang et al. showed that p63-deficient mice rapidly developed intestine-like metaplasia with gene expression profiles similar to BE [15]. Using this model, they reported that Krt7-positive epithelial cells at the squamocolumnar junction are the origin of BE. They concluded that BE does not develop because of genetic alterations but because of competitive interactions between cell lineages driven by opportunity. Quante et al. observed the novel BE-model mice (L2-IL-1β mice) in which human IL-1β was overexpressed in the esophagus [16]. They also showed that the migration of gastric cardia progenitor cells, including leucine-rich repeat-containing G protein-coupled receptor 5-positive cells, may cause BE development. In addition, oral administration of DCA accelerated intestinal metaplasia and dysplasia in this model. However, as mentioned in the previous section, BE and EAC developed even after the resection of esophagogastric junction or total gastrectomy. Thus, if progenitors of BE exist only in the esophagogastric junction or gastric cardia, the development of BE after the surgery cannot be explained.

The other possibilities include multipotent stem cells in the submucosal glands of the esophagus or migrated cells from the bone marrow. However, we need further investigations to conclude the origins of BE.

13.4 Molecular Mechanisms of How Bile Acids Stimulate the Development of EAC

Various in vitro investigations showed that bile acids enhance cell proliferation and confer resistance to apoptosis in BE and EAC cells [17–20]. Tselepis et al. reported that c-myc expression was upregulated in BE and EAC cells during exposure to chenodeoxycholic acid (CDCA) or DCA [21]. The production of reactive oxygen species (ROS) can explain some of these phenotypic changes during the exposure to bile acids. ROS also cause oxidative DNA damages, leading to carcinogenesis [22, 23]. In addition, ROS are known to activate NF-κB and enhance downstream signals, such as epidermal growth factor receptor (EGFR), IL-1β, IL-8, and cyclo-oxygenase (COX)-2 [22, 24–26]. COX-2 was also reported to be regulated by cAMP response-binding protein (CREB) and activation protein-1 (AP-1) through ROS-mediated activation of PI3K/AKT (phosphatidylinositol 3-kinase/protein kinase B) signaling pathway and extracellular signal-related kinases (ERK) 1/2 during exposure to CDCA or DCA [27].

Since ROS production in esophageal epithelial cells was inhibited by diphenyleneiodonium chloride (an NADPH oxidase [NOX] inhibitor) or N(G)-monomethyl-l-arginine (a nitric oxide synthase [NOS] inhibitor), NOX and NOS play roles in ROS production during exposure to bile acids [28]. McAdam et al. reported that DCA induces inducible NOS (iNOS) expression and produces nitric oxide (NO) in esophageal epithelial cells [29]. Hong et al. reported that TDCA increased NOX5-S expression and hydrogen peroxide (H_2O_2) production in EAC cells [17]. They also revealed that TDCA-induced increase in NOX5-S expression might depend on sequential activation of phosphoinositide phospholipase Cγ2 (PI-PLCγ2) and mitogen-activated protein kinases (MAPK)/ERK signaling cascade.

Two types of bile acid receptors have been identified in BE: the cell membrane receptor Takeda G protein-coupled receptor 5 (TGR5) and the nuclear receptor farnesoid X receptor (FXR). Hong et al. observed that TDCA activates TGR5, leading to the upregulation of NOX5-S expression in BE and EAC cells [19]. On the other hand, we observed that oncogenic microRNA-221/222 was upregulated through the activation of FXR during exposure to CA or CDCA in BE and EAC cells. The target of these microRNAs, p27Kip1, was downregulated, and proteasomal degradation of CDX2 was enhanced by the activation of FXR [30]. Thus, both FXR and TGR5 could play roles in the progression from BE to EAC. In addition, the expressions of bile acid transporters, such as the apical sodium-dependent bile acid transporter (ASBT), ileal bile acid-binding protein (IBABP), and multidrug-resistant protein 3 (MRP3), are increased in BE [31], although these functions are not distinguished enough.

13.5 Association of Obesity and the Bile Acid Composition

There is a remarkable association between abdominal obesity and GERD, including BE and EAC. Classically, abdominal obesity was thought to increase intragastric pressure and gastroesophageal pressure gradient. However, Anggiansah et al. observed that esophageal mechanical function was not associated with increased reflux in obese individuals [32]. Alternatively, recent observations have suggested that other mechanisms, including the release of humoral mediators from visceral adipose tissue, may provide a better explanation for the association between obesity and EAC [33].

One of the promising possibilities is the alteration of the bile acid composition related to lifestyle or obesity. Chen et al. investigated the bile acid composition of the bile juice in rats [34] and noted that high dietary animal fat increased the concentration of taurine conjugates in the bile juice. In addition, they carried out esophagojejunostomy for reflux of the duodenal contents and compared sequential morphological changes between rats fed with low soybean-oil diet and those with high cow-fat diet for up to 30 weeks after surgery. The animals with reflux in the high cow-fat group had a significantly higher incidence of BE and Barrett's dysplasia than those in the low soybean-oil group, and the incidence of EAC in the high cow-fat group was also slightly higher than that in the low soybean-oil group. Since bile acid composition is quite different in humans and rodents, more human studies are warranted.

13.6 Protective Effects of Ursodeoxycholic Acid

Peng et al. investigated whether ursodeoxycholic acid (UDCA) protected against DCA-induced injury in patients and in vitro [23]. They took biopsies of BE from 21 patients before and after esophageal perfusion with DCA at baseline and after 8 weeks of oral UDCA treatment. Baseline esophageal perfusion with DCA significantly increased the levels of phospho-H2AX and phospho-p65 in Barrett's metaplasia, whereas oral UDCA increased the levels of glutathione peroxides 1 (GPX1) and catalase in Barrett's metaplasia and prevented DCA perfusion from inducing DNA damage and NF-κB activation. At the cellular level, DCA-induced DNA damage and NF-κB activation were prevented by 24-h pretreatment with UDCA, but not by a combination of UDCA with DCA. UDCA activated nuclear factor erythroid 2-related factor 2 signaling that increased GPX1 and catalase expression, and protective effects of UDCA pretreatment were blocked by siRNA knockdown of these antioxidants. Rizvi et al. investigated the efficacy of the combination of UDCA and aspirin [35]. They showed that UDCA-aspirin combination reduced the risk of adenocarcinoma in animals with reflux, decreased the proliferation of esophageal adenocarcinoma cells, and downregulated a key cell cycle regulator, cyclin-dependent kinase 2 (CDK2). In addition, they noted that GLI1, a hedgehog-regulated transcription factor, was upregulated during esophageal carcinogenesis, and GLI1 could bind to the CDK2 promoter and activate its expression. The UDCA-aspirin combination could downregulate GLI1. Thus, the chemopreventive effect of UDCA is worthy of being verified by an observational study or a clinical trial.

13.7 Conclusions and Future Prospects

Basic as well as clinical studies focusing on bile acids have provided important insights into the development of EAC. ROS production stimulated by bile reflux probably plays a major role in carcinogenesis. Bile acid receptors and transporters also probably are involved. However, there are still many issues at the molecular level that need to be resolved. In addition, recent next-generation sequencing technologies provide additional data on gut microbiota. Since bile acid metabolism is modulated by the gut microbiota, it also possibly plays an important role in the development of EAC. Further studies on bile acids and EAC will provide us novel biomarkers, therapeutic targets, and strategies of lifestyle interventions.

References

1. Arnold M, Soerjomataram I, Ferlay J, Forman D. Global incidence of oesophageal cancer by histological subtype in 2012. Gut. 2015;64(3):381–7. doi:10.1136/gutjnl-2014-308124.
2. Menges M, Muller M, Zeitz M. Increased acid and bile reflux in Barrett's esophagus compared to reflux esophagitis, and effect of proton pump inhibitor therapy. Am J Gastroenterol. 2001;96 (2):331–7. doi:10.1111/j.1572-0241.2001.03515.x.
3. Nehra D, Howell P, Williams CP, Pye JK, Beynon J. Toxic bile acids in gastro-oesophageal reflux disease: influence of gastric acidity. Gut. 1999;44(5):598–602.
4. Matsuzaki J, Suzuki H, Kobayakawa M, Inadomi JM, Takayama M, Makino K, et al. Association of visceral fat area, smoking, and alcohol consumption with reflux esophagitis and Barrett's esophagus in Japan. PLoS One. 2015;10(7):e0133865. doi:10.1371/journal.pone.0133865.
5. Chen KH, Mukaisho K, Ling ZQ, Shimomura A, Sugihara H, Hattori T. Association between duodenal contents reflux and squamous cell carcinoma – establishment of an esophageal cancer cell line derived from the metastatic tumor in a rat reflux model. Anticancer Res. 2007;27(1A):175–81.
6. Avidan B, Sonnenberg A, Schnell TG, Sontag SJ. Gastric surgery is not a risk for Barrett's esophagus or esophageal adenocarcinoma. Gastroenterology. 2001;121(6):1281–5.
7. O'Riordan JM, Tucker ON, Byrne PJ, McDonald GS, Ravi N, Keeling PW, et al. Factors influencing the development of Barrett's epithelium in the esophageal remnant postesophagectomy. Am J Gastroenterol. 2004;99(2):205–11.
8. Tsiouris A, Hammoud Z, Velanovich V. Barrett's esophagus after resection of the gastroesophageal junction: effects of concomitant fundoplication. World J Surg. 2011;35 (8):1867–72. doi:10.1007/s00268-011-1142-3.

9. Silberg DG, Sullivan J, Kang E, Swain GP, Moffett J, Sund NJ, et al. Cdx2 ectopic expression induces gastric intestinal metaplasia in transgenic mice. Gastroenterology. 2002;122 (3):689–96.
10. Eda A, Osawa H, Satoh K, Yanaka I, Kihira K, Ishino Y, et al. Aberrant expression of CDX2 in Barrett's epithelium and inflammatory esophageal mucosa. J Gastroenterol. 2003;38(1):14–22. doi:10.1007/s005350300001.
11. Kazumori H, Ishihara S, Rumi MA, Kadowaki Y, Kinoshita Y. Bile acids directly augment caudal related homeobox gene Cdx2 expression in oesophageal keratinocytes in Barrett's epithelium. Gut. 2006;55(1):16–25. doi:10.1136/gut.2005.066209.
12. Goldman A, Chen HD, Roesly HB, Hill KA, Tome ME, Dvorak B, et al. Characterization of squamous esophageal cells resistant to bile acids at acidic pH: implication for Barrett's esophagus pathogenesis. Am J Physiol Gastrointest Liver Physiol. 2011;300(2):G292–302. doi:10.1152/ajpgi.00461.2010.
13. Huo X, Zhang HY, Zhang XI, Lynch JP, Strauch ED, Wang JY, et al. Acid and bile salt-induced CDX2 expression differs in esophageal squamous cells from patients with and without Barrett's esophagus. Gastroenterology. 2010;139(1):194–203. e1 doi:10.1053/j.gastro.2010. 03.035.
14. Kong J, Crissey MA, Funakoshi S, Kreindler JL, Lynch JP. Ectopic Cdx2 expression in murine esophagus models an intermediate stage in the emergence of Barrett's esophagus. PLoS One. 2011;6(4):e18280. doi:10.1371/journal.pone.0018280.
15. Wang X, Ouyang H, Yamamoto Y, Kumar PA, Wei TS, Dagher R, et al. Residual embryonic cells as precursors of a Barrett's-like metaplasia. Cell. 2011;145(7):1023–35. doi:10.1016/j. cell.2011.05.026.
16. Quante M, Bhagat G, Abrams JA, Marache F, Good P, Lee MD, et al. Bile acid and inflammation activate gastric cardia stem cells in a mouse model of Barrett-like metaplasia. Cancer Cell. 2012;21(1):36–51. doi:10.1016/j.ccr.2011.12.004.
17. Hong J, Behar J, Wands J, Resnick M, Wang LJ, Delellis RA, et al. Bile acid reflux contributes to development of esophageal adenocarcinoma via activation of phosphatidylinositol-specific phospholipase Cgamma2 and NADPH oxidase NOX5-S. Cancer Res. 2010;70(3):1247–55. doi:10.1158/0008-5472.CAN-09-2774.
18. Yen CJ, Izzo JG, Lee DF, Guha S, Wei Y, Wu TT, et al. Bile acid exposure up-regulates tuberous sclerosis complex 1/mammalian target of rapamycin pathway in Barrett's-associated esophageal adenocarcinoma. Cancer Res. 2008;68(8):2632–40. doi:10.1158/0008-5472.CAN-07-5460.
19. Hong J, Behar J, Wands J, Resnick M, Wang LJ, DeLellis RA, et al. Role of a novel bile acid receptor TGR5 in the development of oesophageal adenocarcinoma. Gut. 2010;59(2):170–80. doi:10.1136/gut.2009.188375.
20. Dvorak K, Chavarria M, Payne CM, Ramsey L, Crowley-Weber C, Dvorakova B, et al. Activation of the interleukin-6/STAT3 antiapoptotic pathway in esophageal cells by bile acids and low pH: relevance to Barrett's esophagus. Clin Cancer Res. 2007;13(18 Pt 1):5305–13. doi:10.1158/1078-0432.CCR-07-0483.
21. Tselepis C, Morris CD, Wakelin D, Hardy R, Perry I, Luong QT, et al. Upregulation of the oncogene c-myc in Barrett's adenocarcinoma: induction of c-myc by acidified bile acid in vitro. Gut. 2003;52(2):174–80.
22. Huo X, Juergens S, Zhang X, Rezaei D, Yu C, Strauch ED, et al. Deoxycholic acid causes DNA damage while inducing apoptotic resistance through NF-kappaB activation in benign Barrett's epithelial cells. Am J Physiol Gastrointest Liver Physiol. 2011;301(2):G278–86. doi:10.1152/ajpgi.00092.2011.
23. Peng S, Huo X, Rezaei D, Zhang Q, Zhang X, Yu C, et al. In Barrett's esophagus patients and Barrett's cell lines, ursodeoxycholic acid increases antioxidant expression and prevents DNA damage by bile acids. Am J Physiol Gastrointest Liver Physiol. 2014;307(2):G129–39. doi:10. 1152/ajpgi.00085.2014.

24. Jenkins GJ, D'Souza FR, Suzen SH, Eltahir ZS, James SA, Parry JM, et al. Deoxycholic acid at neutral and acid pH, is genotoxic to oesophageal cells through the induction of ROS: the potential role of anti-oxidants in Barrett's oesophagus. Carcinogenesis. 2007;28(1):136–42. doi:10.1093/carcin/bgl147.
25. McAdam E, Haboubi HN, Griffiths AP, Baxter JN, Spencer-Harty S, Davies C, et al. Reflux composition influences the level of NF-kappaB activation and upstream kinase preference in oesophageal adenocarcinoma cells. Int J Cancer. 2015;136(3):527–35. doi:10.1002/ijc.29029.
26. Cronin J, McAdam E, Danikas A, Tselepis C, Griffiths P, Baxter J, et al. Epidermal growth factor receptor (EGFR) is overexpressed in high-grade dysplasia and adenocarcinoma of the esophagus and may represent a biomarker of histological progression in Barrett's esophagus (BE). Am J Gastroenterol. 2011;106(1):46–56. doi:10.1038/ajg.2010.433.
27. Song S, Guha S, Liu K, Buttar NS, Bresalier RS. COX-2 induction by unconjugated bile acids involves reactive oxygen species-mediated signalling pathways in Barrett's oesophagus and oesophageal adenocarcinoma. Gut. 2007;56(11):1512–21. doi:10.1136/gut.2007.121244.
28. Feagins LA, Zhang HY, Zhang X, Hormi-Carver K, Thomas T, Terada LS, et al. Mechanisms of oxidant production in esophageal squamous cell and Barrett's cell lines. Am J Physiol Gastrointest Liver Physiol. 2008;294(2):G411–7. doi:10.1152/ajpgi.00373.2007.
29. McAdam E, Haboubi HN, Forrester G, Eltahir Z, Spencer-Harty S, Davies C, et al. Inducible nitric oxide synthase (iNOS) and nitric oxide (NO) are important mediators of reflux-induced cell signalling in esophageal cells. Carcinogenesis. 2012;33(11):2035–43. doi:10.1093/carcin/bgs241.
30. Matsuzaki J, Suzuki H, Tsugawa H, Watanabe M, Hossain S, Arai E, et al. Bile acids increase levels of microRNAs 221 and 222, leading to degradation of CDX2 during esophageal carcinogenesis. Gastroenterology. 2013;145(6):1300–11. doi:10.1053/j.gastro.2013.08.008.
31. Dvorak K, Watts GS, Ramsey L, Holubec H, Payne CM, Bernstein C, et al. Expression of bile acid transporting proteins in Barrett's esophagus and esophageal adenocarcinoma. Am J Gastroenterol. 2009;104(2):302–9. doi:10.1038/ajg.2008.85.
32. Anggiansah R, Sweis R, Anggiansah A, Wong T, Cooper D, Fox M. The effects of obesity on oesophageal function, acid exposure and the symptoms of gastro-oesophageal reflux disease. Aliment Pharmacol Ther. 2013;37(5):555–63. doi:10.1111/apt.12208.
33. Almers LM, Graham JE, Havel PJ, Corley DA. Adiponectin may modify the risk of Barrett's esophagus in patients with gastroesophageal reflux disease. Clin Gastroenterol Hepatol. 2015; doi:10.1016/j.cgh.2015.01.009.
34. Chen KH, Mukaisho K, Sugihara H, Araki Y, Yamamoto G, Hattori T. High animal-fat intake changes the bile-acid composition of bile juice and enhances the development of Barrett's esophagus and esophageal adenocarcinoma in a rat duodenal-contents reflux model. Cancer Sci. 2007;98(11):1683–8. doi:10.1111/j.1349-7006.2007.00605.x.
35. Rizvi S, Demars CJ, Comba A, Gainullin VG, Rizvi Z, Almada LL, et al. Combinatorial chemoprevention reveals a novel smoothened-independent role of GLI1 in esophageal carcinogenesis. Cancer Res. 2010;70(17):6787–96. doi:10.1158/0008-5472.CAN-10-0197.

Chapter 14
Bile Acid and Colorectal Cancer

Michiaki Unno

Abstract Colorectal cancer is one of the most common causes of cancer death worldwide. The mechanism of colorectal carcinogenesis is still unknown, so that the prevention of colorectal cancer is strongly desired. The bile acids, cholesterol derivatives, were thought to be implicated in the pathogenesis of many diseases. In particular, secondary bile acids are thought to be associated with the colorectal carcinogenesis regarding the colorectal mucosal proliferation, apoptosis, and oxidative DNA damage. On the other hand, certain bile acids, ursodeoxycholate, might protect against colorectal carcinogenesis. This review will examine the opposing effects on colorectal tumor promotion and tumor inhibition.

Keywords Bile acid • Colorectal cancer • UDCA • Chemoprevention

14.1 Introduction

Colorectal cancer (CRC) is one of the most common causes of cancer death worldwide, with more than 100,000 persons per year developing CRC in Japan [1]. Recent increases in patients with CRC might be associated with the Western diet and obesity. There is a strong evidence that a high-fat diet is positively correlated with the incidence of CRC [2–4].

Bile acids are cholesterol derivatives that play an important role of fat metabolism. Bile acids are amphipathic molecules that contain a sterol nucleus with hydroxyl groups and a side chain with a terminal carboxylic acid. The principal bile acids in humans are cholic acid (CA) and chenodeoxycholic acid (CDCA), which are primary bile acids, and deoxycholic acid (DCA) and lithocholic acid (LCA), which are secondary bile acids, and their glycine and taurine conjugates.

It was thought that the main function of bile acid was to emulsify lipid aggregates and to solubilize them in a hydrophilic environment. However, recently, bile acids were found to serve as signaling molecules, capable of activating the

M. Unno (✉)
Department of Surgery, Tohoku University Graduate School of Medicine, 1-1, Seiryou-machi, Aoba-ku, Sendai, 980-8574 Sendai, Japan
e-mail: m_unno@surg1.med.tohoku.ac.jp

S. Tazuma, H. Takikawa (eds.), *Bile Acids in Gastroenterology*,
DOI 10.1007/978-4-431-56062-3_14

signaling pathway. Therefore, bile acids have been implicated in the pathogenesis of many diseases, especially colorectal cancer.

Bile acids were shown to activate a number of different receptors, including farnesoid X receptor (FXR), pregnane X receptor (PXR), vitamin D receptor (VDR), G protein-coupled receptor (TGR5), and EGFR [5–9]. In addition, bile acids have been shown to activate signaling molecules such as c-Jun N-terminal kinase (JNK), protein kinase B (AKT), and extracellular signal-regulated kinase 1 and 2 (ERK1/2), epidermal growth factor (EGFR), mitogen-activated protein kinase (MAPK), and others [10, 11].

In this review, we first describe the biochemical and physiological roles of bile acids in colorectal carcinogenesis. Next, we summarize the potential protective activity of bile acids, mainly UDCA, against colorectal carcinogenesis.

14.2 Bile Acids and Colorectal Carcinogenesis

DCA was first proposed to be a carcinogen of CRC in 1940 by Cook et al. [12]. They reported the induction of tumors after DCA injection into mice. Since then, many researchers have examined the effect of DCA, CDCA, and LCA on tumor progression or carcinogenesis. In 1999, in a study using mice with a germ line mutation in Apc (Min/+) as a model of familial adenomatous polyposis (FAP), the administration of CDCA increased duodenal tumors [13]. Moreover, some bile acids had a promoting effect on colorectal carcinogenesis after intrarectal instillation of methyl-N ’-nitro-N-nitrosoguanidine (MNNG) [14–16] or N-methyl-N-mitrosourea (MNU) [17]. Based on these experiments in non-mutated rat model systems, it has been generally assumed that bile acids act as promoters, but not as carcinogens, in humans [18].

In general, a Western diet high in fat, low in vegetables, is strongly linked with both a higher incidence of CRC and higher level of fecal bile acid, such as DCA. Ou et al. reported that 3–4 times as much DCA is present in persons who consume a high-fat diet compared to those who maintain a low-fat diet [19]. In addition, patients with colonic adenomas and carcinomas usually present elevated concentrations of serum or fecal bile acids [20, 21]. Epidemiologic studies also reveal an increased risk of colorectal cancer linked to high serum or fecal bile acid concentrations [22].

Moreover, an assessment of human colon biopsies showed that high DCA serum levels positively correlated with increased proliferation rates of colon epithelium [23]. In addition, a study of bromodeoxyuridine labeling of colonic epithelium showed that DCA has a complex influence on mucosal proliferation [24].

On the other hand, bile acids induce apoptosis in colon cells through different mechanisms. The extrinsic apoptotic pathways, for example, Fas and Fas-L, seem to have low relevance regarding bile acid cytotoxicity in the colon because the colon cells may downregulate Fas surface expression or develop a signaling pathway that inhibits the Fas receptor signaling [25]. In contrast, bile acids mainly trigger apoptosis through direct or indirect mitochondrial perturbations, where oxidative stress plays a key role. Bile acid-induced apoptosis through the mitochondrial pathway has been described in many colon cancer cells [25–27]. Regarding HCT-116 cells, bile acid treatment, mainly DCA, promotes the release of cytochrome c from the mitochondria [28].

DCA and other hydrophobic bile acids increase oxidative/nitrosative stress through the generation of reactive oxygen/nitrogen species (ROS/RNS). Some of the generated ROS results from a direct detergent effect of bile acids on membrane enzymes, phospholipase A_2 (PLA_2). PLA2 generates arachidonic acid, and arachidonic acid is acted on by cyclooxygenase and lipooxygenase to release ROS. Finally, the ROS cause oxidative DNA damage.

ROS are also produced by mitochondria. Mitochondria are known to be damaged by bile acids, although the mechanism is not established.

As indicated before, bile acid causes oxidative/nitrosative stress and the release ROS and RNS. Oxidative DNA damage can cause mutations. Bile acids also increase NOS2 expression leading to the increased production of RNS and increased DNA damage.

It was thought that a high level of bile acids would promote DNA damage, mainly by oxidative stress, including mutations that may lead to an aberrant expression of oncogenes or tumor suppressor genes. Another possibility is that the continuous exposure to high levels of bile acids would allow selective growth of cell populations resistant to their apoptotic effect, which is one of the major risk factors for the colorectal carcinogensis [29].

It was been suggested that there is an increased risk of CRC after cholecystectomy due to increased level of secondary bile acid, especially right-sided colon tumors. However, a meta-analysis revealed that the there is no relationship between cholecystectomy and CRC [30]. It might be considered that the risk of right-side colon cancer following the cholecystectomy would be relatively small.

14.3 Chemoprevention of Colorectal Cancer

On the other hand, certain bile acids might protect against colorectal carcinogenesis. Ursodeoxycholate (UDCA) is a bile acid that is present in human bile juice at low concentrations, representing only 3% of total bile acids. UDCA is a 7,-hydroxy epimer of the primary bile acid CDCA and can be isolated from the Chinese medicine Yutan, which is derived from the dried bile of adult Chinese black bears [31]. UDCA was initially used for gallstone dissolution and is also employed as the first-line therapy for primary biliary cirrhosis, as well as for other chronic cholestatic liver diseases [32]. UDCA partially blocks the ileal absorption of endogenous bile acids, thereby promoting high concentrations of both UDCA and endogenous bile acids in the colon [33]. A study using the azoxymethane (AOM) model of experimental colon cancer showed that dietary supplementation with UDCA significantly reduced the number of tumor-bearing rats and abolished the

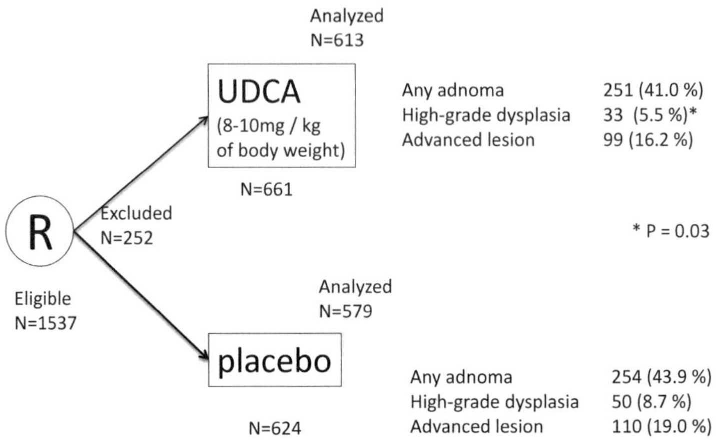

Fig. 14.1 The schema of the randomized control study [36]. Eligible criteria included the removal of one or more colorectal adenomas with a diameter of 3 mm or more during a colonoscopy examination within 6 months before study registration. Of 6570 potential participants, 1537 were eligible for randomized. Of these 1537 participants, 252 were excluded for various reasons. Of these, a total of 1192 underwent at least one colorectal evaluation 6 months of more after randomization and were evaluable for outcome. Finally, 579 in the placebo group and 613 in the UDCA group were analyzed. The primary outcome of this phase III study was the recurrence of colorectal adenomas in 3 years. The results indicated that a nonstatically significant ($P = 0.15$) 12% reduction in the adenoma recurrence rate is associated with UDCA intervention (rate ratio = 0.88, 95% confidence interval (CI) = 0.37–1.05). However, a statistically significant ($P = 0.03$) UDCA related reduction in recurrence of adenoma with high-grade dysplasia (adjusted OR = 0.61, 95% CI = 0.39–0.96).

development of carcinoma [34]. UDCA was also able to inhibit colitis-related mouse colon carcinogenesis [35]. Based on these observations, the idea of using UDCA as a chemopreventative agent for colorectal carcinogenesis was raised.

In humans, the potentially chemoprevention action of UDCA has been investigated in six retrospective studies and four prospective studies [36–45]. In a randomized double-blind placebo-controlled trial (Fig. 14.1), the potentially preventive effect of UDCA on colorectal adenoma recurrence was assessed in 1285 individuals who had undergone adenoma removal [36] and started randomly allocated UDCA or placebo intervention. UDCA was given at doses of 8–10 mg/kg/day vs. placebo for 3 years. Finally, 1192 underwent at least one colorectal evaluation 6 months or more after randomization and were evaluated for the outcomes: 579 in the placebo group and 613 in the UDCA group. The results of the study indicated that UDCA treatment was associated with a nonstatistically significant reduction in total colorectal adenoma recurrence but with a statistically significant 39% reduction in the recurrence of adenoma with high-grade dysplasia. Based on the results, long-term administration of UDCA for more than 5 years should be evaluated in a subpopulation of patients at risk of having a recurrence of highly dysplastic adenomas. A secondary analysis of the trial showed that the patients' gender might also modify the UDCA effect, preventing advanced colorectal adenoma in men while increasing the odds in women with high-fat intakes [46]. These finding suggests that UDCA acts in a complex manner that is not currently well understood.

The UDCA effects were investigated in patients with inflammatory bowel disease (IBD) with primary biliary cirrhosis (PBC). The first study was a retrospective analysis of risk factors for dysplasia in 59 patients with UC-associated PBC. On multivariate analysis, UDCA was negatively associated with the risk of colonic dysplasia.

In the patients with familial adenomatous polyposis (FAP), duodenal adenomas are observed in approximately 90%. Some studies suggest that bile acids may play a role in the development of duodenal adenomas. Therefore, 71 patients with FAP and restorative proctocolectomy were randomized to receive UDCA or a placebo for 2 years. The results indicated that nine (25%) patients in the UDCA group and seven (20%) in the placebo group had a decrease in Spiegelman's score ($p = 0.614$), suggesting that UDCA had no significant effect on the severity of duodenal adenomas in FAP patients [45].

14.4 Future Perspective

In this review, we summarized the two biological effects of the bile acids. The bile acids can induce cellular stresses, oxidative DNA damage, and mitochondrial damage in the epithelial cells in the GI tract. Persistent exposure of the bile acids can result in the development of apoptosis resistant and the modulation of many genes/proteins associated with colorectal carcinogenesis. On the other hand, chemoprevention effect of UDCA has been shown in several clinical studies; however, the efficacy of the UDCA is still under debate. Further basic research into bile acids may provide the new therapy for the CRC.

References

1. Matsuda A, Matsuda T, Shibata A, et al. Cancer incidence and incidence rates in Japan in 2008: a study of 25 population-based cancer registries for the Monitoring of Cancer Incidence in Japan (MCIJ) project. Jpn J Clin Oncol. 2014;44(4):388–96. doi:10.1093/jjco/hyu003.
2. Carroll KK. Dietary fats and cancer. Am J Clin Nutr. 1991;53(4 Suppl):1064S–7S.
3. Butler LM, Wang R, Koh W-P, Stern MC, Yuan J-M, Yu MC. Marine n-3 and saturated fatty acids in relation to risk of colorectal cancer in Singapore Chinese: a prospective study. Int J Cancer. 2009;124(3):678–86. doi:10.1002/ijc.23950.
4. Bernstein C, Holubec H, Bhattacharyya AK, et al. Carcinogenicity of deoxycholate, a secondary bile acid. Arch Toxicol. 2011;85(8):863–71. doi:10.1007/s00204-011-0648-7.
5. Makishima M, Okamoto AY, Repa JJ, et al. Identification of a nuclear receptor for bile acids. Science. 1999;284(5418):1362–5.
6. Wang H, Chen J, Hollister K, Sowers LC, Forman BM. Endogenous bile acids are ligands for the nuclear receptor FXR/BAR. Mol Cell. 1999;3(5):543–53.

7. Staudinger JL, Goodwin B, Jones SA, et al. The nuclear receptor PXR is a lithocholic acid sensor that protects against liver toxicity. Proc Natl Acad Sci U S A. 2001;98(6):3369–74. doi:10.1073/pnas.051551698.
8. Xie W, Radominska-Pandya A, Shi Y, et al. An essential role for nuclear receptors SXR/PXR in detoxification of cholestatic bile acids. Proc Natl Acad Sci U S A. 2001;98(6):3375–80. doi:10.1073/pnas.051014398.
9. Makishima M, Lu TT, Xie W, et al. Vitamin D receptor as an intestinal bile acid sensor. Science. 2002;296(5571):1313–6. doi:10.1126/science.1070477.
10. Hylemon PB, Zhou H, Pandak WM, Ren S, Gil G, Dent P. Bile acids as regulatory molecules. J Lipid Res. 2009;50(8):1509–20. doi:10.1194/jlr.R900007-JLR200.
11. Centuori SM, Gomes CJ, Trujillo J, et al. Deoxycholic acid mediates non-canonical EGFR-MAPK activation through the induction of calcium signaling in colon cancer cells. Biochim Biophys Acta. 2016; doi:10.1016/j.bbalip.2016.04.006.
12. Cook JW, Kennaway EL, Kennaway NM. Serve v100-v159. Nature. 1940;145(3677):627–7. doi:10.1038/145627a0.
13. Mahmoud NN, Dannenberg AJ, Bilinski RT, et al. Administration of an unconjugated bile acid increases duodenal tumors in a murine model of familial adenomatous polyposis. Carcinogenesis. 1999;20(2):299–303.
14. Narisawa T, Magadia NE, Weisburger JH, Wynder EL. Promoting effect of bile acids on colon carcinogenesis after intrarectal instillation of N-methyl-N′-nitro-N-nitrosoguanidine in rats. J Natl Cancer Inst. 1974;53(4):1093–7.
15. Reddy BS, Narasawa T, Weisburger JH, Wynder EL. Promoting effect of sodium deoxycholate on colon adenocarcinomas in germfree rats. J Natl Cancer Inst. 1976;56 (2):441–2.
16. Reddy BS, Watanabe K, Weisburger JH, Wynder EL. Promoting effect of bile acids in colon carcinogenesis in germ-free and conventional F344 rats. Cancer Res. 1977;37(9):3238–42.
17. McSherry CK, Cohen BI, Bokkenheuser VD, et al. Effects of calcium and bile acid feeding on colon tumors in the rat. Cancer Res. 1989;49(21):6039–43.
18. Bernstein H, Bernstein C, Payne CM, Dvorakova K, Garewal H. Bile acids as carcinogens in human gastrointestinal cancers. Mutat Res. 2005;589(1):47–65. doi:10.1016/j.mrrev.2004.08.001.
19. Ou J, DeLany JP, Zhang M, Sharma S, O'Keefe SJD. Association between low colonic short-chain fatty acids and high bile acids in high colon cancer risk populations. Nutr Cancer. 2012;64(1):34–40. doi:10.1080/01635581.2012.630164.
20. Reddy BS, Wynder EL. Metabolic epidemiology of colon cancer. Fecal bile acids and neutral sterols in colon cancer patients and patients with adenomatous polyps. Cancer. 1977;39 (6):2533–9.
21. Bayerdörffer E, Mannes GA, Ochsenkühn T, Dirschedl P, Wiebecke B, Paumgartner G. Unconjugated secondary bile acids in the serum of patients with colorectal adenomas. Gut. 1995;36(2):268–73.
22. Tong JL, Ran ZH, Shen J, Fan GQ, Xiao SD. Association between fecal bile acids and colorectal cancer: a meta-analysis of observational studies. Yonsei Med J. 2008;49 (5):792–803. doi:10.3349/ymj.2008.49.5.792.
23. Ochsenkühn T, Bayerdörffer E, Meining A, et al. Colonic mucosal proliferation is related to serum deoxycholic acid levels. Cancer. 1999;85(8):1664–9.
24. Bartram HP, Scheppach W, Schmid H, et al. Proliferation of human colonic mucosa as an intermediate biomarker of carcinogenesis: effects of butyrate, deoxycholate, calcium, ammonia, and pH. Cancer Res. 1993;53(14):3283–8.
25. Wachs F-P, Krieg RC, Rodrigues CMP, et al. Bile salt-induced apoptosis in human colon cancer cell lines involves the mitochondrial transmembrane potential but not the CD95 (Fas/Apo-1) receptor. Int J Colorectal Dis. 2005;20(2):103–13. doi:10.1007/s00384-004-0616-2.

26. Barrasa JI, Santiago-Gómez A, Olmo N, Lizarbe MA, Turnay J. Resistance to butyrate impairs bile acid-induced apoptosis in human colon adenocarcinoma cells via up-regulation of Bcl-2 and inactivation of Bax. Biochim Biophys Acta. 2012;1823(12):2201–9. doi:10.1016/j.bbamcr.2012.08.008.
27. Payne CM, Weber C, Crowley-Skillicorn C, et al. Deoxycholate induces mitochondrial oxidative stress and activates NF-kappaB through multiple mechanisms in HCT-116 colon epithelial cells. Carcinogenesis. 2007;28(1):215–22. doi:10.1093/carcin/bgl139.
28. Yui S, Saeki T, Kanamoto R, Iwami K. Characteristics of apoptosis in HCT116 colon cancer cells induced by deoxycholic acid. J Biochem. 2005;138(2):151–7. doi:10.1093/jb/mvi106.
29. Payne CM, Bernstein C, Dvorak K, Bernstein H. Hydrophobic bile acids, genomic instability, Darwinian selection, and colon carcinogenesis. Clin Exp Gastroenterol. 2008;1:19–47.
30. Giovannucci E, Colditz GA, Stampfer MJ. A meta-analysis of cholecystectomy and risk of colorectal cancer. YGAST. 1993;105(1):130–41.
31. Ikegami T, Matsuzaki Y. Ursodeoxycholic acid: mechanism of action and novel clinical applications. Hepatol Res. 2007; 0(0):071127144837001–??? doi: 10.1111/j.1872-034X.2007.00297.x.
32. Poupon R. Ursodeoxycholic acid and bile-acid mimetics as therapeutic agents for cholestatic liver diseases: an overview of their mechanisms of action. Clin Res Hepatol Gastroenterol. 2012;36(Suppl 1):S3–S12. doi:10.1016/S2210-7401(12)70015-3.
33. Marteau P, Chazouilléres O, Myara A, Jian R, Rambaud JC, Poupon R. Effect of chronic administration of ursodeoxycholic acid on the ileal absorption of endogenous bile acids in man. Hepatology. 1990;12(5):1206–8.
34. Earnest DL, Holubec H, Wali RK, et al. Chemoprevention of azoxymethane-induced colonic carcinogenesis by supplemental dietary ursodeoxycholic acid. Cancer Res. 1994;54(19):5071–4.
35. Kohno H, Suzuki R, Yasui Y, Miyamoto S, Wakabayashi K, Tanaka T. Ursodeoxycholic acid versus sulfasalazine in colitis-related colon carcinogenesis in mice. Clin Cancer Res. 2007;13(8):2519–25. doi:10.1158/1078-0432.CCR-06-2727.
36. Alberts DS, Martínez ME, Hess LM, et al. Phase III trial of ursodeoxycholic acid to prevent colorectal adenoma recurrence. J Natl Cancer Inst. 2005;97(11):846–53. doi:10.1093/jnci/dji144.
37. Serfaty L, De Leusse A, Rosmorduc O, et al. Ursodeoxycholic acid therapy and the risk of colorectal adenoma in patients with primary biliary cirrhosis: an observational study. Hepatology. 2003;38(1):203–9. doi:10.1053/jhep.2003.50311.
38. Ochsenkühn T, Marsteller I, Hay U, et al. Does ursodeoxycholic acid change the proliferation of the colorectal mucosa?. A randomized, placebo-controlled study. Digestion. 2003;68(4):209–16.
39. Sjöqvist U, Tribukait B, Ost A, Einarsson C, Oxelmark L, Löfberg R. Ursodeoxycholic acid treatment in IBD-patients with colorectal dysplasia and/or DNA-aneuploidy: a prospective, double-blind, randomized controlled pilot study. Anticancer Res. 2004;24(5B):3121–7.
40. Tung BY, Emond MJ, Haggitt RC, et al. Ursodiol use is associated with lower prevalence of colonic neoplasia in patients with ulcerative colitis and primary sclerosing cholangitis. Ann Intern Med. 2001;134(2):89–95.
41. Wolf JM, Rybicki LA, Lashner BA. The impact of ursodeoxycholic acid on cancer, dysplasia and mortality in ulcerative colitis patients with primary sclerosing cholangitis. Aliment Pharmacol Ther. 2005;22(9):783–8. doi:10.1111/j.1365-2036.2005.02650.x.
42. Pardi DS, Loftus EV, Kremers WK, Keach J, Lindor KD. Ursodeoxycholic acid as a chemopreventive agent in patients with ulcerative colitis and primary sclerosing cholangitis. YGAST. 2003;124(4):889–93. doi:10.1053/gast.2003.50156.
43. Eaton JE, Silveira MG, Pardi DS, et al. High-dose ursodeoxycholic acid is associated with the development of colorectal neoplasia in patients with ulcerative colitis and primary sclerosing cholangitis. Am J Gastroenterol. 2011;106(9):1638–45. doi:10.1038/ajg.2011.156.

44. Lindström L, Boberg KM, Wikman O, et al. High dose ursodeoxycholic acid in primary sclerosing cholangitis does not prevent colorectal neoplasia. Aliment Pharmacol Ther. 2012;35 (4):451–7. doi:10.1111/j.1365-2036.2011.04966.x.
45. Parc Y, Desaint B, Fléjou J-F, et al. The effect of ursodesoxycholic acid on duodenal adenomas in familial adenomatous polyposis: a prospective randomized placebo-control trial. Colorectal Dis. 2012;14(7):854–60. doi:10.1111/j.1463-1318.2011.02816.x.
46. Thompson PA, Wertheim BC, Roe DJ, et al. Gender modifies the effect of ursodeoxycholic acid in a randomized controlled trial in colorectal adenoma patients. Cancer Prev Res (Phila). 2009;2(12):1023–30. doi:10.1158/1940-6207.CAPR-09-0234.
47. Alberts SR, Al-Khatib H, Mahoney MR, et al. Gemcitabine, 5-fluorouracil, and leucovorin in advanced biliary tract and gallbladder carcinoma. Cancer. 2004;103(1):111–8. doi:10.1002/cncr.20753.

Chapter 15
Bile Acids and Metabolic Syndrome

Hiroki Taoka and Mitsuhiro Watanabe

Abstract Bile acids (BAs) are not only facilitators of dietary lipid absorption but also important signaling molecules that participate in various metabolic pathways. Some major signaling pathways involving the nuclear BAs receptor farnesoid X receptor (FXR) and the G protein-coupled BAs receptor TGR5/M-BAR have been identified to be the targets of BAs. BAs affect diverse metabolic pathways including glucose metabolism, lipid metabolism, and energy expenditure via these major pathways. Therefore, BA signaling mechanisms are attractive therapeutic targets of the metabolic syndrome. Actually, bile acid-binding resin (BABR) originally used to treat hypercholesterolemia also stimulates incretin secretion and improves glucose metabolism. In addition to BABR, the clinical applications of FXR and TGR5/M-BAR agonists are ongoing for the treatment of metabolic syndrome. The effects of bariatric surgery on glycemic control are also associated with BA metabolism.

In this chapter, we summarize current knowledge of the metabolic regulation mechanisms of BAs and propose BA signaling pathways as a therapeutic target of the metabolic syndrome.

Keywords Farnesoid X receptor • TGR5/M-BAR • Glucose metabolism • Lipid metabolism • Energy metabolism

---

H. Taoka
Graduate School of Media and Governance, Keio University, 5322 Endo, Fujisawa, Kanagawa 252-0882, Japan

M. Watanabe (✉)
Graduate School of Media and Governance, Department of Environment and Information Studies, Keio University, 5322, Fujisawa, Kanagawa 252-0882, Japan

Department of Internal Medicine, Keio University School of Medicine, 35 Shinanomachi, Shinjuku, Tokyo 160-8582, Japan
e-mail: wmitsu@sfc.keio.ac.jp

S. Tazuma, H. Takikawa (eds.), *Bile Acids in Gastroenterology*,
DOI 10.1007/978-4-431-56062-3_15

15.1 Introduction

Bile acids (BAs) are the main constituents of bile and amphipathic molecules, containing both hydrophilic and hydrophobic regions. BAs are synthesized from cholesterol in the liver, stored in the gallbladder, and flow into the small intestine after meal ingestion. Intestinal BAs facilitate digestion and absorption of lipids and fat-soluble vitamins [1].

Recent reports have suggested that BAs are responsible not only for the absorption of lipids but also for signal transduction. Some major signaling mechanisms have been identified including the MAPK pathways, the nuclear hormone receptor farnesoid X receptor (FXR)-mediated pathway, and the G protein-coupled receptor TGR5/M-BAR (also named GPR131)-mediated pathway [2–5]. The main role of the FXR signaling pathway is regulating both BA biosynthesis and enterohepatic circulation to maintain BA homeostasis [6]. In addition, FXR signaling has been known for regulating lipogenesis gene expression and improving hepatic steatosis [7]. Moreover, recent studies have shown that BAs and FXR signaling are associated with the beneficial glycemic effects of bariatric surgery [8–10]. TGR5/M-BAR signaling pathway stimulates energy expenditure in the brown adipose tissue (BAT) and the skeletal muscle [11]. Furthermore, TGR5/M-BAR is involved in inducing incretin secretion, such as glucagon-like peptide-1 (GLP-1) [12]. GLP-1 is secreted by dietary stimulation from enteric L cell and promotes insulin secretion by binding to the GLP-1 receptor in the pancreatic β cell. Further, GLP-1 maintains pancreatic function, and GLP-1 receptor agonists have been developed for the treatment of diabetes [13]. Taken together, BAs not only participate in digestion and absorption of lipids but also in various metabolic pathways. BA signaling participates in various diseases such as cancer, immune disorders, and metabolic syndrome [14–16]. In this chapter, we summarize current knowledges of the metabolic regulation mechanisms via BAs signaling and propose BA signaling pathways can be a therapeutic target of the metabolic syndrome.

15.2 FXR Signaling and Metabolic Syndrome

15.2.1 Glucose Metabolic Regulation of FXR

Glucose induces the expression of *FXR* and *CYP7A1*, and insulin reduces their expression in vitro [17]. Further studies have shown that BAs seem to regulate gluconeogenesis, but the mechanisms remain poorly understood. Some studies have indicated that the expression of phosphoenolpyruvate carboxykinase (*PEPCK*), the rate-limiting enzyme of gluconeogenesis, is suppressed by BAs in human liver cancer cells (HepG2 cells) and murine liver [18–20]. Additionally, other enzymes that participate in gluconeogenesis, such as glucose 6-phosphatase (G6Pase) and fructose 1,6-bisphosphatase 1 (FBP1), are also repressed by BAs [18]. These effects

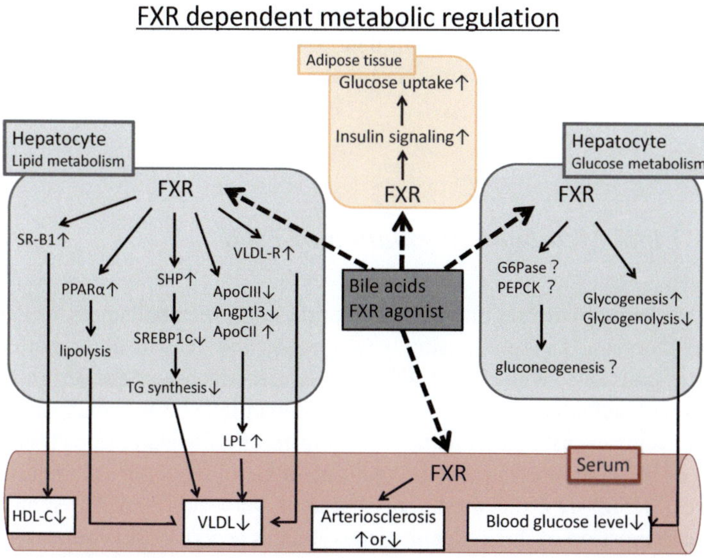

Fig. 15.1 FXR-dependent metabolic regulation. FXR signaling regulates lipid and glucose metabolism. FXR signaling reduces lipogenesis (SREBP1c) and induces fatty acid β oxidation (PPARα) and plasma TG clearance (LPL and VLDL-R), resulting in decreased plasma VLDL levels. Plasma HDL-C uptake is also increased by FXR and SRB1 activity. FXR signaling upregulates glycogenesis and glucose uptake, downregulates glycogenolysis, and reduces blood glucose levels. Hepatic FXR signaling is also associated with gluconeogenesis, but the controlling mechanism is still unclear. *Angptl3* angiopoietin-like protein 3, *ApoCII/CIII* apolipoprotein CII/CIII, *FXR* farnesoid X receptor, *G6Pase* glucose-6-phosphatase, *HDL-C* high-density lipoprotein cholesterol, *LPL* lipoprotein lipase, *PEPCK* phosphoenolpyruvate carboxykinase, *PPARα* peroxisome proliferator-activated receptor α, *SR-B1* scavenger receptor B1, *SREBP1c* sterol regulatory element-binding protein 1c, *TG* triglyceride, *VLDL-R* very low-density lipoprotein receptor

are diminished in both *FXR* and *SHP* knockout mice, supporting the postulate that BAs repress gluconeogenesis in an FXR-SHP-dependent manner [20]. However, others have reported that FXR-dependent signaling induces *PEPCK* expression and increases gluconeogenesis in primary hepatocytes and rat hepatoma cell lines [21]. Furthermore, latest research has revealed that activating intestinal FXR inhibits GLP-1 secretion in L cells [22]. In terms of glycogen synthesis, BAs increase hepatic glycogen synthesis and storage, resulting in decreased blood glucose levels in an FXR-dependent manner (Fig.15.1) [23]. A previous study demonstrated that long-term FXR activation (3 months) with a synthetic FXR agonist, GW4064, worsened glucose intolerance and insulin resistance in high-fat-fed C57BL/6J mice [20, 24]. The mechanism behind the bad effect of GW4064 is lowering the BA pool size following FXR activation. In contrast, some reports have suggested that short-term (10 days) FXR activation by the synthetic FXR agonist GW4064 reduced glycolytic gene expression and improved insulin resistance in *ob/ob* or *db/db* mice [23, 25]. From these data, the difference of the

GW4064 administration period may lead to the opposite result. Actually, long-term administration of BAs, the endogenous natural ligands of FXR, did not decrease the BA pool size and subsequently improved glucose intolerance and insulin resistance [24].

15.2.2 Lipid Metabolic Regulation of FXR

BAs are associated with regulating triglyceride (TG) metabolism as well as cholesterol metabolism. The relationship between BAs and TG was first reported in the treatment of gallstones with CDCA. CDCA treatment decreased the serum TG level in patients with gallstones [26]. In fact, BAs or a synthetic FXR agonist affected TG metabolism via several mechanisms including the FXR-mediated pathway. SHP, the target of FXR, suppressed the upregulation of sterol regulatory element-binding protein-1c (*SREBP-1c*), the master regulator of fatty acid and TG synthesis, to reduce the expression of the lipogenic genes such as acetyl-CoA synthetase, acetyl-CoA carboxylase, stearoyl CoA desaturase 1, and fatty acid synthase [7, 27]. In addition, the TG-lowering effects were attenuated in *SHP* knockout mice, indicating that SREBP-1c-mediated lipogenesis is inhibited in an FXR-SHP-dependent manner [7]. Additionally, FXR activation by BAs increases the expression of apolipoprotein *(Apo)* CII to activate lipoprotein lipase, which stimulates TG hydrolysis in very low-density lipoprotein (VLDL) and chylomicrons and facilitates TG clearance from the serum [28]. The expressions of *ApoCIII* and angiopoietin-like protein 3 (*Angptl3*), inhibiting lipoprotein lipase activity, were repressed by FXR stimulation with BAs [29–31]. In addition, FXR induces the gene expression of the VLDL receptor, which is responsible for plasma TG clearance [32].

BAs also suppress the expression of microsomal triglyceride transfer protein (*MTP*) and *ApoB* by FXR-independent mechanisms to inhibit the formation of VLDL and chylomicrons [33]. Not only VLDL but also high-density lipoprotein (HDL) clearance is suggested to be under the modulation of BAs. The expression of scavenger receptor B1 (*SRB1*), a molecule in charge of hepatic uptake of HDL, is reduced, and HDL-C is elevated in *FXR* knockout mice [34]. In addition, the administration of an FXR ligand increases hepatic *SRB1* expression and decreases HDL-C levels [35].

BAs control other major regulators of lipid metabolism such as PPARα and pyruvate dehydrogenase kinase-4 (PDK4). The nuclear receptor PPARα, which is activated by free fatty acids (FFA), decreases serum TG levels and exerts an important role for controlling enzymes participating in fatty acid oxidation [36]. A study suggested that BAs regulate PPARα directly via FXR in humans, although not in mice [37]. *PDK4* is also upregulated by BAs in an FXR-dependent manner, resulting in the inactivation of pyruvate dehydrogenase, a decrease in glycolysis, and an increase in fatty acid β oxidation (Fig.15.1) [38].

15.2.3 Anti-atherosclerotic Effect of FXR

Some researches show that FXR signaling is associated with onset of atherosclerosis. ApolipoproteinE (*apoE*)-*FXR* double-knockout mice fed with atheroma-induced diet developed severe atherosclerosis [39]. On the other hand, foam cell formation and atherosclerosis development are inhibited in both low-density lipoprotein receptor (*LDLR*)-*FXR* double-knockout mice and *apoE-FXR* double-knockout mice [40, 41]. FXR activation by the synthetic FXR agonist of INT-747 reduced formation of aortic plaque [42]. And more, treatment of synthetic FXR agonist of WAY-362450 also inhibited diet-induced hypertriglyceridemia and aortic lesion formation [43].

15.2.4 Intestinal FXR and Metabolic Regulation

Intestinal FXR has been recently identified as a possible target for improving metabolic syndrome. Intestinal FXR activation induces the expression of fibroblast growth factor (*FGF*)15/19, and several studies have demonstrated that FGF15/19 affects glucose and energy homeostasis. *FGF19* transgenic mice showed increased hepatic β oxidation, reduced adipose tissue weight, and improved glucose tolerance and insulin sensitivity [44]. In mice, hepatic *acetyl-CoA carboxylase 2* (*ACC2*) mRNA was decreased, and the mass of the BAT was increased. ACC2 exists at the mitochondrial membrane and converts acetyl-CoA to malonyl-CoA. ACC2 activation results in an elevation of malonyl-CoA levels, which inhibit carnitine palmitoyl transferase-1 (CPT-1) activation [45]. CPT-1 transfers FFA from the cytoplasm to the mitochondria and induces fatty acid β oxidation. In addition, hyperglycemia is improved upon administration of FGF19 protein in obese mice [46]. Furthermore, activation of intestinal FXR by administration of fexaramine, an FXR agonist, improved obesity and insulin resistance by inducing FGF15, changing the serum BA composition and stimulating systemic TGR5/M-BAR [47]. These results suggest the possibility that metabolic disease is improved through the intestinal FXR-FGF15/19 signaling pathway.

The primary BAs excreted into the intestine become deconjugated BAs and are converted into various secondary BAs by microbial enzymes [48]. In germfree (GF) mice, reduction of gut microbiota facilitating BA deconjugation leads to increased tauro-beta-muricholic acid (T-β-MCA) and decreased beta-muricholic acid. In comparison to conventionally raised mice, FXR-dependent BA synthesis is reduced in GF mice by increasing T-β-MCA of FXR antagonist. Therefore, the microbiota is associated with regulating BA homeostasis via the inhibition of intestinal FXR signaling by changing the BA composition [49]. In contrast to previous reports, recent studies have noted that alteration of the BA composition by microbiota and inhibition of intestinal FXR activity improved lipid and glucose metabolism. Increased T-β-MCA reduced intestinal FXR activation and decreased

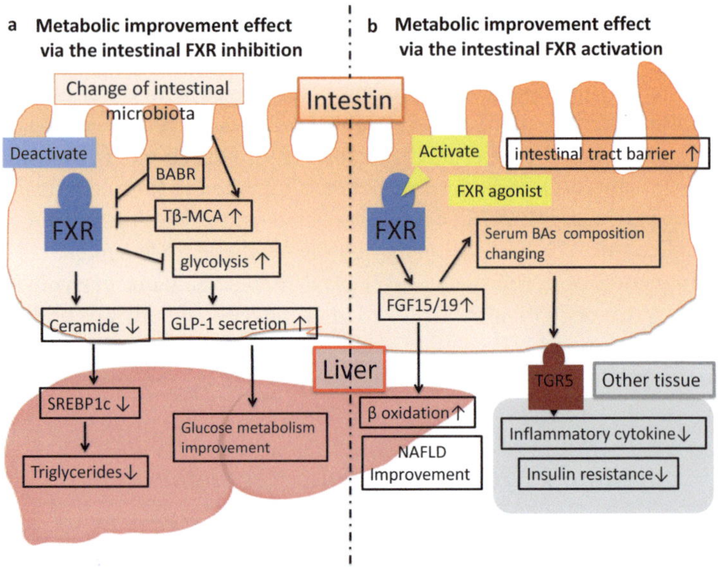

Fig. 15.2 Conflicting mechanisms of metabolic regulation via intestinal FXR activity. (**a**) Inhibiting FXR activation decreases hepatic TG levels and improves glucose metabolism. (**b**) Intestinal FXR activation of FXR agonist leads to FGF15/19 production and improves NAFLD. Synthesized FGF15/19 changes BA metabolism and serum BA composition, which causes TGR5/M-BAR activation, reduced inflammatory cytokine release, and improved insulin resistance. *BABR* bile acid-binding resin, *FGF15/19* fibroblast growth factor 15/19, *FXR* farnesoid X receptor, *NAFLD* nonalcoholic fatty liver disease, *SREBP1c* sterol regulatory element-binding protein 1c, *Tβ-MCA* tauro-β-muricholic acid

serum ceramide levels through repression of ceramide synthesis, which reduced expression of hepatic *SREBP-1c* and resulted in an improvement of obesity and nonalcoholic fatty liver disease (NAFLD) [50–52]. Additionally, intestinal FXR deactivation may also improve glucose metabolism as well as lipid metabolism. FXR activation in L cells decreased glycolysis, proglucagon expression, and cAMP levels [22]. Thus, GLP-1 production and secretion were inhibited [22]. Conflicting opinions suggest that microbiota regulation of BA homeostasis and intestinal FXR activation are involved in controlling hepatic lipid accumulation and glucose metabolism (Fig.15.2). Further studies are needed to clarify the roles of intestinal FXR signaling for improving metabolic diseases.

15.3 TGR5/M-BAR Signaling and Metabolic Syndrome

15.3.1 Glucose Metabolic Regulation of TGR5/M-BAR

BA administration improved metabolism including glucose tolerance and insulin resistance. The beneficial effects of BAs, such as decreasing gluconeogenesis and increasing glycogen synthesis, seem to occur not only via FXR signaling but also via other signaling molecules such as TGR5/M-BAR. TGR5/M-BAR signaling induces GLP-1 secretion in murine enteroendocrine STC-1 cells [53]. Moreover, a semisynthetic TGR5/M-BAR agonist 6-ethyl-23(S)-methylcholic acid (6EMCA or INT-777 [54]) stimulates GLP-1 secretion in both murine and human enteroendocrine cells. In this study, knockdown of *TGR5/M-BAR* by shRNA reduced 6EMCA-induced secretion of GLP-1 in STC-1 cells [12]. A natural TGR5/M-BAR agonist oleanolic acid also improves glucose metabolism [55]. This evidence indicates the importance of TGR5/M-BAR in GLP-1 secretion. An in vivo study with *TGR5/M-BAR* knockout and *TGR5/M-BAR* transgenic mice strongly supports the relationship between TGR5/M-BAR and GLP-1 secretion [56]. Considering the current mechanism, TGR5/M-BAR activation increases cAMP levels and the ATP/ADP ratio, which leads to subsequent plasma membrane depolarization and Ca2+ mobilization, resulting in increased GLP-1 release (Fig.15.3) [12]. Hence, these studies suggested that GLP-1 secretion was stimulated by TGR5/M-BAR signaling in vivo and vitro. BAs and TGR5/M-BAR could become therapeutic targets of diabetes.

15.3.2 Energy Metabolic Regulation in TGR5/M-BAR

BAs have been reported to stimulate adaptive thermogenesis and energy expenditure via TGR5/M-BAR [11]. TGR5/M-BAR activation leads to increased intracellular cAMP levels, activation of PKA, and induction of CREB phosphorylation. This series of signaling activity induces the expression of genes bearing a cAMP-responsive element (CRE) and exists in various tissues (Fig.15.3) [57, 58].

In the BAT, TGR5/M-BAR stimulation increases the intracellular cAMP level and induces cAMP-dependent iodothyronine deiodinase type 2 (*Dio2*) expression, which converts inactive thyroxine (T4) to active 3,5,3′-triiodothyronine (T3) to evoke increased energy expenditure [11, 59]. Dio2 increases the nuclear T3 level without various unwanted side effects caused by increased blood T3 levels. Only 20 % of nuclear T3 is produced and secreted from the human thyroid gland, and the remaining nuclear T3 is supplemented from other tissues. Dio2 supplies approximately 50 % of the T3 in the nucleus including the BAT [60]. The BAT is one of the most important targets of BAs to increase energy expenditure. Although BAT had been regarded as a tissue only in newborn infants, recent studies with FDG-PET revealed the existence of BAT around the neck and shoulders in adult humans,

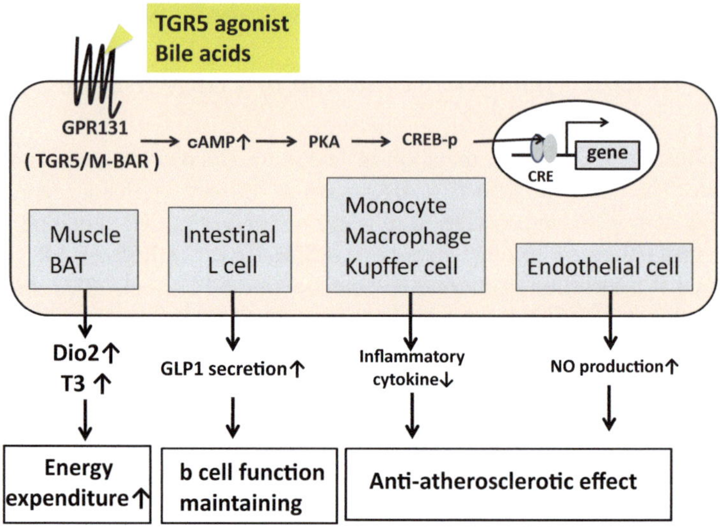

Fig. 15.3 TGR5/M-BAR-dependent metabolic regulation. TGR5/M-BAR activation leads to increased intracellular cAMP levels, the activation of PKA, and induction of CREB phosphorylation. This series of signaling activity induces the expression of genes bearing CRE and exists in various tissues. TGR5/M-BAR signaling induces energy expenditure in the muscle and BAT, increases GLP-1 secretion in the intestinal L cell, and reduces inflammatory cytokine release in immune cells. *CRE* cAMP response element, *CREB-p* cAMP response element-binding protein phosphorylation, *Dio2* deiodinase iodothyronine type II, *eNO* endothelial NO, *T3* triiodothyronine

especially under brief cold exposure [61–63]. Furthermore, several groups have shown the importance of BAT in adult humans. In healthy patients, the amount of BAT is large and its activity is high but is reduced in obese patients [64–66]. In addition, *TGR5/M-BAR* and *Dio2* are co-expressed in human skeletal muscle, suggesting the existence of the thermogenic mechanism in humans [11]. A human genetic study revealed the association between a single nucleotide polymorphism (SNP), rs3731859, of the *TGR5/M-BAR* gene and various metabolic indexes including BMI, waist circumference, intramyocellular lipid, and fasting serum GLP-1 levels [67]. Moreover, a recent study found another type of adipocyte called "beige" cells derived from the white adipose tissue. These adipocytes also respond to cyclic AMP stimulation with high uncoupling protein (*UCP) 1* expression and respiration rates similar to BAT cells [68, 69]. These accumulating findings suggest a therapeutic approach to improve obesity and metabolic syndrome by increasing energy expenditure through TGR5/M-BAR stimulation.

15.3.3 Anti-atherosclerotic Effect of TGR5/M-BAR

BAs are also associated with atherosclerosis [70, 71]. Treatment with TGR5/M-BAR agonist INT-777 represses the activation of inflammatory cytokines such as NF-κB and inhibits foam cell formation and subsequent atherosclerotic plaques (Fig. 15.3). In addition, INT-777 does not inhibit atherosclerosis in *TGR5/M-BAR* knockout mice, supporting that the TGR5/M-BAR activation reduces atherosclerosis [70]. Furthermore, TGR5/M-BAR induces the mRNA expression of endothelial NO synthase (*eNOS*) and activates eNOS by phosphorylation of eNOS at amino acid position 1177 [72]. Recent study have also shown that treatment of TGR5/M-BAR agonist of taurolithocholic acid increases Akt phosphorylation and intracellular Ca^{2+}, which induces NO production and inhibits monocyte adhesion in vascular endothelial cells. This signaling may be associated with anti-atherosclerotic effect of TGR5/M-BAR [73].

15.4 Bile Acids in Clinical Application

15.4.1 Bariatric Surgery

Bariatric surgery may provide another clue to clarify the link between BAs and glucose homeostasis. Bariatric surgery, especially gastric bypass surgery, is an established treatment for obesity and type 2 diabetes mellitus, although the mechanism of its effectiveness is still unclear. Interestingly, the improved glycemic control is observed soon after the operation when the body weight is still unchanged. Therefore, some of the antimetabolic syndrome effects of the surgical intervention are independent of body weight reduction. A recent study suggests that BAs may participate in the immediate effect of bariatric surgery. After gastric bypass, the bile flow is altered, which leads to increased plasma BA levels and incretin secretion [8]. Hormonal factors and the gut microbiota may be involved in the effect of the operation. The gut microbiota is responsible for enteral BA metabolism, and the spectrum of the gut microbiota is affected after gastrointestinal surgery. For example, the predominance of *Firmicutes* was reportedly mitigated, and other species including methanogens and *Prevotellaceae* were also suppressed after bariatric surgery [9]. In addition to these studies, recent research has revealed that FXR is associated with the effect of bariatric surgery [10]. In *FXR* knockout mice, metabolic improvements such as weight loss and improved glucose tolerance were reduced after bariatric surgery. Furthermore, the surgery changed the gut microbial communities differently between wild-type and *FXR* knockout mice. This study suggested that BAs may affect glucose homeostasis via FXR signaling and alterations of the gut microbiota after bariatric surgery.

15.4.2 Bile Acid-Binding Resins

Bile acid-binding resin (BABR) is an effective drug for the treatment of hypercholesterolemia by lowering LDL cholesterol. BABR absorbs BAs in the intestine, thereby preventing their uptake in the ileum, interrupting their enterohepatic circulation, and facilitating their excretion in the feces. The inhibition of enterohepatic circulation leads to a reduction of the BA pool size, repression of FXR-SHP and FGF15/19 signaling, and induction of *CYP7A1* expression and synthesis of BAs from the cholesterol to maintain the BA pool size. A decrease in intrahepatic cholesterol levels activates SREBP-2, which induces the expression of the LDL receptor (*LDLR*) to enhance cholesterol uptake, reducing serum cholesterol levels. In addition to lowering the serum cholesterol effect, there is interaction between BABR and glucose metabolism [74]. In a diet-induced obesity rat model, BABR decreased serum glucose and improved glucose tolerance [75, 76]. In a clinical trial, a first-generation member of BABR cholestyramine improved glycemia by 13 % in patients with type 2 diabetes [77]. In addition, a second-generation BABR colesevelam also improved glucose clearance and increased serum GIP and GLP-1 levels in patients with type 2 diabetes mellitus [78]. These studies clarified that BABR is not absorbed in the body and there are few unwanted side effects. Furthermore, BABR can decrease blood glucose levels only in high-glucose situations and do not affect normal condition. As a result, in January 2008, the Food and Drug Administration (FDA) in the United States approved this drug as a therapeutic drug for diabetes [77, 79–82].

Although how BABR improves diabetes remains unknown, several possible mechanisms have been proposed. BABR-mediated improvement of hepatic insulin sensitivity depends on downregulating the hepatic cholesterol-LXR-IRS2 pathway [83]. In addition, BABRs induce GLP-1 secretion via the activation of TGR5/M-BAR or GPR40, each being activated by BAs binding with BABR or unabsorbed long-chain fatty acids [53, 84, 85]. Further, BABRs affect the composition of the BA pool and peripheral BAs, resulting in an induction of peripheral energy expenditure and improvement of glucose tolerance [74]. The BABR effects of improving diabetes may be explained by the inhibition of intestinal FXR as well as TGR5/M-BAR signaling [22]. BABR inhibits intestinal FXR activation and improves glucose metabolism by increasing proglucagon gene expression and inducing GLP-1 secretion in *ob/ob* mice [22]. These findings suggest that inhibiting FXR in the L cell via BABR could be a new target for diabetes.

15.4.3 Drug Targeting for Bile Acids Receptor

Currently, BABR has been approved by the FDA and has been clinically used as a diabetes treatment drug. The association between bariatric surgery and BAs homeostasis was confirmed. In addition to BABR and bariatric surgery, other clinical applications based on the mechanism of metabolic control via BAs signaling are ongoing. For instance, INT-747 (also named 6-ethyl-CDCA), which is a synthetic FXR agonist, exerts a hepatoprotective effect in patients of primary biliary cirrhosis (PBC) [86–88], and a phase III clinical study has already been completed and confirmed the effect of PBC. In addition to medicine, INT-747 has also entered into a study for NAFLD treatment. A phase II clinical trial for NAFLD has been completed, and an improvement was observed in type 2 diabetes mellitus patients with NAFLD. Clinical trials with TGR5 agonists, such as INT-777, are ongoing, and future studies are expected [12, 54, 89]. Altogether, these clinical applications will elucidate the BA signaling mechanisms that will lead to the improvement of metabolic disorders including obesity and diabetes.

15.5 Conclusion

Today, BAs have become important molecules to control metabolic homeostasis. We mainly discussed the relationship between BA metabolism and signal transmission, such as the FXR and TGR5/M-BAR pathways and the possibility that BAs may improve metabolic diseases. Current evidence shows that BAs regulate lipid, glucose, and energy metabolism via FXR or TGR/M-BAR-mediated pathways. Furthermore, the clinical application of FXR and TGR/M-BAR agonists is ongoing.

Recent studies have focused on intestinal FXR signaling; however, conflicting data have been reported regarding the metabolic regulation of intestinal FXR activity. Further studies are necessary to determine intestinal FXR signaling taking into consideration various factors such as microbiota regulation, BA pool size, and BAs composition.

References

1. Hofmann AF, Borgstroem B. The intraluminal phase of fat digestion in man: the lipid content of the micellar and oil phases of intestinal content obtained during fat digestion and absorption. J Clin Invest. 1964;43:247–57. doi:10.1172/jci104909.
2. Urizar NL, Dowhan DH, Moore DD. The farnesoid X-activated receptor mediates bile acid activation of phospholipid transfer protein gene expression. J Biol Chem. 2000;275 (50):39313–7. doi:10.1074/jbc.M007998200.
3. Maruyama T, Miyamoto Y, Nakamura T, Tamai Y, Okada H, Sugiyama E, et al. Identification of membrane-type receptor for bile acids (M-BAR). Biochem Biophys Res Commun. 2002;298(5):714–9.
4. Makishima M, Okamoto AY, Repa JJ, Tu H, Learned RM, Luk A, et al. Identification of a nuclear receptor for bile acids. Science. 1999;284(5418):1362–5.
5. Parks DJ, Blanchard SG, Bledsoe RK, Chandra G, Consler TG, Kliewer SA, et al. Bile acids: natural ligands for an orphan nuclear receptor. Science. 1999;284(5418):1365–8.

6. Forman BM, Goode E, Chen J, Oro AE, Bradley DJ, Perlmann T, et al. Identification of a nuclear receptor that is activated by farnesol metabolites. Cell. 1995;81(5):687–93. doi:10.1016/0092-8674(95)90530-8.
7. Watanabe M, Houten SM, Wang L, Moschetta A, Mangelsdorf DJ, Heyman RA, et al. Bile acids lower triglyceride levels via a pathway involving FXR, SHP, and SREBP-1c. J Clin Invest. 2004;113(10):1408–18. doi:10.1172/JCI21025.
8. Nakatani H, Kasama K, Oshiro T, Watanabe M, Hirose H, Itoh H. Serum bile acid along with plasma incretins and serum high-molecular weight adiponectin levels are increased after bariatric surgery. Metab: Clin Exp. 2009;58(10):1400–7. doi:10.1016/j.metabol.2009.05.006.
9. Zhang H, DiBaise JK, Zuccolo A, Kudrna D, Braidotti M, Yu Y, et al. Human gut microbiota in obesity and after gastric bypass. Proc Natl Acad Sci U S A. 2009;106(7):2365–70. doi:10.1073/pnas.0812600106.
10. Ryan KK, Tremaroli V, Clemmensen C, Kovatcheva-Datchary P, Myronovych A, Karns R, et al. FXR is a molecular target for the effects of vertical sleeve gastrectomy. Nature. 2014;509(7499):183–8. doi:10.1038/nature13135.
11. Watanabe M, Houten SM, Mataki C, Christoffolete MA, Kim BW, Sato H, et al. Bile acids induce energy expenditure by promoting intracellular thyroid hormone activation. Nature. 2006;439(7075):484–9. doi:10.1038/nature04330.
12. Thomas C, Gioiello A, Noriega L, Strehle A, Oury J, Rizzo G, et al. TGR5-mediated bile acid sensing controls glucose homeostasis. Cell Metab. 2009;10(3):167–77. doi:10.1016/j.cmet.2009.08.001.
13. Holst JJ. The physiology of glucagon-like peptide 1. Physiol Rev. 2007;87(4):1409–39. doi:10.1152/physrev.00034.2006.
14. Ichikawa R, Takayama T, Yoneno K, Kamada N, Kitazume MT, Higuchi H, et al. Bile acids induce monocyte differentiation toward interleukin-12 hypo-producing dendritic cells via a TGR5-dependent pathway. Immunology. 2012;136(2):153–62. doi:10.1111/j.1365-2567.2012.03554.x.
15. Matsuzaki J, Suzuki H, Tsugawa H, Watanabe M, Hossain S, Arai E, et al. Bile acids increase levels of microRNAs 221 and 222, leading to degradation of CDX2 during esophageal carcinogenesis. Gastroenterology. 2013;145(6):1300–11. doi: S0016-5085(13)01154-2 [pii] doi:10.1053/j.gastro.2013.08.008.
16. Yang F, Huang X, Yi T, Yen Y, Moore DD, Huang W. Spontaneous development of liver tumors in the absence of the bile acid receptor farnesoid X receptor. Cancer Res. 2007;67(3):863–7. doi:10.1158/0008-5472.can-06-1078.
17. Duran-Sandoval D, Mautino G, Martin G, Percevault F, Barbier O, Fruchart JC, et al. Glucose regulates the expression of the farnesoid X receptor in liver. Diabetes. 2004;53(4):890–8.
18. Yamagata K, Daitoku H, Shimamoto Y, Matsuzaki H, Hirota K, Ishida J, et al. Bile acids regulate gluconeogenic gene expression via small heterodimer partner-mediated repression of hepatocyte nuclear factor 4 and Foxo1. J Biol Chem. 2004;279(22):23158–65. doi:10.1074/jbc.M314322200.
19. Yamagata K, Yoshimochi K, Daitoku H, Hirota K, Fukamizu A. Bile acid represses the peroxisome proliferator-activated receptor-gamma coactivator-1 promoter activity in a small heterodimer partner-dependent manner. Int J Mol Med. 2007;19(5):751–6.
20. Ma K, Saha PK, Chan L, Moore DD. Farnesoid X receptor is essential for normal glucose homeostasis. J Clin Invest. 2006;116(4):1102–9. doi:10.1172/JCI25604.
21. Stayrook KR, Bramlett KS, Savkur RS, Ficorilli J, Cook T, Christe ME, et al. Regulation of carbohydrate metabolism by the farnesoid X receptor. Endocrinology. 2005;146(3):984–91. doi:10.1210/en.2004-0965.
22. Trabelsi MS, Daoudi M, Prawitt J, Ducastel S, Touche V, Sayin SI, et al. Farnesoid X receptor inhibits glucagon-like peptide-1 production by enteroendocrine L cells. Nat Commun. 2015;6:7629. doi:10.1038/ncomms8629.

23. Zhang Y, Lee FY, Barrera G, Lee H, Vales C, Gonzalez FJ, et al. Activation of the nuclear receptor FXR improves hyperglycemia and hyperlipidemia in diabetic mice. Proc Natl Acad Sci U S A. 2006;103(4):1006–11. doi:10.1073/pnas.0506982103.
24. Watanabe M, Horai Y, Houten SM, Morimoto K, Sugizaki T, Arita E, et al. Lowering bile acid pool size with a synthetic farnesoid X receptor (FXR) agonist induces obesity and diabetes through reduced energy expenditure. J Biol Chem. 2011;286(30):26913–20. doi:10.1074/jbc.M111.248203.
25. Cariou B, van Harmelen K, Duran-Sandoval D, van Dijk TH, Grefhorst A, Abdelkarim M, et al. The farnesoid X receptor modulates adiposity and peripheral insulin sensitivity in mice. J Biol Chem. 2006;281(16):11039–49. doi:10.1074/jbc.M510258200.
26. Fromm H, Eschler A, Tollner D, Canzler H, Schmidt FW. In vivo dissolving of gall-stones: the effect of chenodeoxycholic acid (author's transl). Dtsch Med Wochenschr (1946). 1975;100(32):1619–24. doi:10.1055/s-0028-1106432.
27. Horton JD, Goldstein JL, Brown MS. SREBPs: activators of the complete program of cholesterol and fatty acid synthesis in the liver. J Clin Invest. 2002;109(9):1125–31. doi:10.1172/JCI15593.
28. Kast HR, Nguyen CM, Sinal CJ, Jones SA, Laffitte BA, Reue K, et al. Farnesoid X-activated receptor induces apolipoprotein C-II transcription: a molecular mechanism linking plasma triglyceride levels to bile acids. Mol Endocrinol (Baltimore, Md). 2001;15(10):1720–8. doi:10.1210/mend.15.10.0712.
29. Ginsberg HN, Le NA, Goldberg IJ, Gibson JC, Rubinstein A, Wang-Iverson P, et al. Apolipoprotein B metabolism in subjects with deficiency of apolipoproteins CIII and AI. Evidence that apolipoprotein CIII inhibits catabolism of triglyceride-rich lipoproteins by lipoprotein lipase in vivo. J Clin Invest. 1986;78(5):1287–95. doi:10.1172/jci112713.
30. Claudel T, Inoue Y, Barbier O, Duran-Sandoval D, Kosykh V, Fruchart J, et al. Farnesoid X receptor agonists suppress hepatic apolipoprotein CIII expression. Gastroenterology. 2003;125(2):544–55.
31. Inaba T, Matsuda M, Shimamura M, Takei N, Terasaka N, Ando Y, et al. Angiopoietin-like protein 3 (Angptl3) mediates hypertriglyceridemia induced by the liver X receptor. J Biol Chem. 2003;278(24):21344–51.
32. Sirvent A, Claudel T, Martin G, Brozek J, Kosykh V, Darteil R, et al. The farnesoid X receptor induces very low density lipoprotein receptor gene expression. FEBS Lett. 2004;566(1–3):173–7. doi:10.1016/j.febslet.2004.04.026.
33. Hirokane H, Nakahara M, Tachibana S, Shimizu M, Sato R. Bile acid reduces the secretion of very low density lipoprotein by repressing microsomal triglyceride transfer protein gene expression mediated by hepatocyte nuclear factor-4. J Biol Chem. 2004;279(44):45685–92. doi:10.1074/jbc.M404255200.
34. Sinal CJ, Yoon M, Gonzalez FJ. Antagonism of the actions of peroxisome proliferator-activated receptor-alpha by bile acids. J Biol Chem. 2001;276(50):47154–62. doi:10.1074/jbc.M107000200.
35. Zhang Y, Yin L, Anderson J, Ma H, Gonzalez FJ, Willson TM, et al. Identification of novel pathways that control farnesoid X receptor-mediated hypocholesterolemia. J Biol Chem. 2010;285(5):3035–43. doi:10.1074/jbc.M109.083899.
36. Evans RM, Barish GD, Wang YX. PPARs and the complex journey to obesity. Nat Med. 2004;10(4):355–61. doi:10.1038/nm1025.
37. Pineda Torra I, Claudel T, Duval C, Kosykh V, Fruchart JC, Staels B. Bile acids induce the expression of the human peroxisome proliferator-activated receptor alpha gene via activation of the farnesoid X receptor. Mol Endocrinol (Baltimore, Md). 2003;17(2):259–72. doi:10.1210/me.2002-0120.
38. Savkur RS, Bramlett KS, Michael LF, Burris TP. Regulation of pyruvate dehydrogenase kinase expression by the farnesoid X receptor. Biochem Biophys Res Commun. 2005;329(1):391–6. doi:10.1016/j.bbrc.2005.01.141.

39. Hanniman EA, Lambert G, McCarthy TC, Sinal CJ. Loss of functional farnesoid X receptor increases atherosclerotic lesions in apolipoprotein E-deficient mice. J Lipid Res. 2005;46 (12):2595–604. doi:10.1194/jlr.M500390-JLR200.
40. Zhang Y, Wang X, Vales C, Lee FY, Lee H, Lusis AJ, et al. FXR deficiency causes reduced atherosclerosis in Ldlr-/- mice. Arterioscler Thromb Vasc Biol. 2006;26(10):2316–21. doi:10.1161/01.atv.0000235697.35431.05.
41. Guo GL, Santamarina-Fojo S, Akiyama TE, Amar MJ, Paigen BJ, Brewer Jr B, et al. Effects of FXR in foam-cell formation and atherosclerosis development. Biochim Biophys Acta. 2006;1761(12):1401–9. doi:10.1016/j.bbalip.2006.09.018.
42. Mencarelli A, Renga B, Distrutti E, Fiorucci S. Antiatherosclerotic effect of farnesoid X receptor. Am J Physiol Heart Circ Physiol. 2009;296(2):H272–81. doi:10.1152/ajpheart.01075.2008.
43. Hartman HB, Gardell SJ, Petucci CJ, Wang S, Krueger JA, Evans MJ. Activation of farnesoid X receptor prevents atherosclerotic lesion formation in LDLR-/- and apoE-/- mice. J Lipid Res. 2009;50(6):1090–100. doi:10.1194/jlr.M800619-JLR200.
44. Tomlinson E, Fu L, John L, Hultgren B, Huang X, Renz M, et al. Transgenic mice expressing human fibroblast growth factor-19 display increased metabolic rate and decreased adiposity. Endocrinology. 2002;143(5):1741–7. doi:10.1210/endo.143.5.8850.
45. Abu-Elheiga L, Matzuk MM, Kordari P, Oh W, Shaikenov T, Gu Z, et al. Mutant mice lacking acetyl-CoA carboxylase 1 are embryonically lethal. Proc Natl Acad Sci U S A. 2005;102 (34):12011–6. doi:10.1073/pnas.0505714102.
46. Fu L, John LM, Adams SH, Yu XX, Tomlinson E, Renz M, et al. Fibroblast growth factor 19 increases metabolic rate and reverses dietary and leptin-deficient diabetes. Endocrinology. 2004;145(6):2594–603. doi:10.1210/en.2003-1671.
47. Fang S, Suh JM, Reilly SM, Yu E, Osborn O, Lackey D, et al. Intestinal FXR agonism promotes adipose tissue browning and reduces obesity and insulin resistance. Nat Med. 2015;21(2):159–65. doi:10.1038/nm.3760.
48. Ridlon JM, Kang DJ, Hylemon PB. Bile salt biotransformations by human intestinal bacteria. J Lipid Res. 2006;47(2):241–59. doi:10.1194/jlr.R500013-JLR200.
49. Sayin SI, Wahlstrom A, Felin J, Jantti S, Marschall HU, Bamberg K, et al. Gut microbiota regulates bile acid metabolism by reducing the levels of tauro-beta-muricholic acid, a naturally occurring FXR antagonist. Cell Metab. 2013;17(2):225–35. doi:10.1016/j.cmet.2013.01.003.
50. Li F, Jiang C, Krausz KW, Li Y, Albert I, Hao H, et al. Microbiome remodelling leads to inhibition of intestinal farnesoid X receptor signalling and decreased obesity. Nat Commun. 2013;4:2384. doi:10.1038/ncomms3384.
51. Qi Y, Jiang C, Cheng J, Krausz KW, Li T, Ferrell JM, et al. Bile acid signaling in lipid metabolism: metabolomic and lipidomic analysis of lipid and bile acid markers linked to anti-obesity and anti-diabetes in mice. Biochim Biophys Acta. 2015;1851(1):19–29. doi:10.1016/j.bbalip.2014.04.008.
52. Jiang C, Xie C, Li F, Zhang L, Nichols RG, Krausz KW, et al. Intestinal farnesoid X receptor signaling promotes nonalcoholic fatty liver disease. J Clin Invest. 2015;125(1):386–402. doi:10.1172/jci76738.
53. Katsuma S, Hirasawa A, Tsujimoto G. Bile acids promote glucagon-like peptide-1 secretion through TGR5 in a murine enteroendocrine cell line STC-1. Biochem Biophys Res Commun. 2005;329(1):386–90. doi:10.1016/j.bbrc.2005.01.139.
54. Pellicciari R, Gioiello A, Macchiarulo A, Thomas C, Rosatelli E, Natalini B, et al. Discovery of 6alpha-ethyl-23(S)-methylcholic acid (S-EMCA, INT-777) as a potent and selective agonist for the TGR5 receptor, a novel target for diabesity. J Med Chem. 2009;52(24):7958–61. doi:10.1021/jm901390p.
55. Sato H, Genet C, Strehle A, Thomas C, Lobstein A, Wagner A, et al. Anti-hyperglycemic activity of a TGR5 agonist isolated from Olea europaea. Biochem Biophys Res Commun. 2007;362(4):793–8. doi:10.1016/j.bbrc.2007.06.130.

56. Thomas C, Auwerx J, Schoonjans K. Bile acids and the membrane bile acid receptor TGR5 – connecting nutrition and metabolism. Thyroid. 2008;18(2):167–74. doi:10.1089/thy.2007.0255.
57. Kawamata Y, Fujii R, Hosoya M, Harada M, Yoshida H, Miwa M, et al. A G protein-coupled receptor responsive to bile acids. J Biol Chem. 2003;278(11):9435–40. doi:10.1074/jbc.M209706200.
58. Sato H, Macchiarulo A, Thomas C, Gioiello A, Une M, Hofmann AF, et al. Novel potent and selective bile acid derivatives as TGR5 agonists: biological screening, structure-activity relationships, and molecular modeling studies. J Med Chem. 2008;51(6):1831–41. doi:10.1021/jm7015864.
59. Bianco AC, Salvatore D, Gereben B, Berry MJ, Larsen PR. Biochemistry, cellular and molecular biology, and physiological roles of the iodothyronine selenodeiodinases. Endocr Rev. 2002;23(1):38–89.
60. Bianco AC, Silva JE. Nuclear 3,5,3′-triiodothyronine (T3) in brown adipose tissue: receptor occupancy and sources of T3 as determined by in vivo techniques. Endocrinology. 1987;120(1):55–62. doi:10.1210/endo-120-1-55.
61. Cohade C, Mourtzikos KA, Wahl RL. "USA-Fat": prevalence is related to ambient outdoor temperature-evaluation with 18F-FDG PET/CT. J Nucl Med. 2003;44(8):1267–70.
62. Hany TF, Gharehpapagh E, Kamel EM, Buck A, Himms-Hagen J, von Schulthess GK. Brown adipose tissue: a factor to consider in symmetrical tracer uptake in the neck and upper chest region. Eur J Nucl Med Mol Imaging. 2002;29(10):1393–8. doi:10.1007/s00259-002-0902-6.
63. Saito M. Brown adipose tissue as a regulator of energy expenditure and body fat in humans. Diabetes Metab J. 2013;37(1):22–9. doi:10.4093/dmj.2013.37.1.22.
64. van Marken Lichtenbelt WD, Vanhommerig JW, Smulders NM, Drossaerts JM, Kemerink GJ, Bouvy ND, et al. Cold-activated brown adipose tissue in healthy men. N Engl J Med. 2009;360(15):1500–8. doi:10.1056/NEJMoa0808718.
65. Cypess AM, Lehman S, Williams G, Tal I, Rodman D, Goldfine AB, et al. Identification and importance of brown adipose tissue in adult humans. N Engl J Med. 2009;360(15):1509–17. doi:10.1056/NEJMoa0810780.
66. Virtanen KA, Lidell ME, Orava J, Heglind M, Westergren R, Niemi T, et al. Functional brown adipose tissue in healthy adults. N Engl J Med. 2009;360(15):1518–25. doi:10.1056/NEJMoa0808949.
67. Mussig K, Staiger H, Machicao F, Machann J, Schick F, Schafer SA, et al. Preliminary report: genetic variation within the GPBAR1 gene is not associated with metabolic traits in white subjects at an increased risk for type 2 diabetes mellitus. Metab: Clin Exp. 2009;58(12):1809–11. doi:10.1016/j.metabol.2009.06.012.
68. Seale P, Bjork B, Yang W, Kajimura S, Chin S, Kuang S, et al. PRDM16 controls a brown fat/skeletal muscle switch. Nature. 2008;454(7207):961–7. doi:10.1038/nature07182.
69. Wu J, Bostrom P, Sparks LM, Ye L, Choi JH, Giang AH, et al. Beige adipocytes are a distinct type of thermogenic fat cell in mouse and human. Cell. 2012;150(2):366–76. doi:10.1016/j.cell.2012.05.016.
70. Pols TW, Nomura M, Harach T, Lo Sasso G, Oosterveer MH, Thomas C, et al. TGR5 activation inhibits atherosclerosis by reducing macrophage inflammation and lipid loading. Cell Metab. 2011;14(6):747–57. doi: S1550-4131(11)00425-6 [pii] doi:10.1016/j.cmet.2011.11.006.
71. Wang YD, Chen WD, Yu D, Forman BM, Huang W. The G-protein-coupled bile acid receptor, Gpbar1 (TGR5), negatively regulates hepatic inflammatory response through antagonizing nuclear factor kappa light-chain enhancer of activated B cells (NF-kappaB) in mice. Hepatology (Baltimore, Md). 2011;54(4):1421–32. doi:10.1002/hep.24525.
72. Keitel V, Reinehr R, Gatsios P, Rupprecht C, Gorg B, Selbach O, et al. The G-protein coupled bile salt receptor TGR5 is expressed in liver sinusoidal endothelial cells. Hepatology (Baltimore, Md). 2007;45(3):695–704. doi:10.1002/hep.21458.

73. Kida T, Tsubosaka Y, Hori M, Ozaki H, Murata T. Bile acid receptor TGR5 agonism induces NO production and reduces monocyte adhesion in vascular endothelial cells. Arterioscler Thromb Vasc Biol. 2013;33(7):1663–9. doi:10.1161/atvbaha.113.301565.
74. Watanabe M, Morimoto K, Houten SM, Kaneko-Iwasaki N, Sugizaki T, Horai Y, et al. Bile acid binding resin improves metabolic control through the induction of energy expenditure. PLoS One. 2013;7(8):e38286. doi:10.1371/journal.pone.0038286. PONE-D-11-16446 [pii]
75. Shang Q, Saumoy M, Holst JJ, Salen G, Xu G. Colesevelam improves insulin resistance in a diet-induced obesity (F-DIO) rat model by increasing the release of GLP-1. Am J Physiol Gastrointest Liver Physiol. 2010;298(3):G419–24. doi:10.1152/ajpgi.00362.2009.
76. Chen L, McNulty J, Anderson D, Liu Y, Nystrom C, Bullard S, et al. Cholestyramine reverses hyperglycemia and enhances glucose-stimulated glucagon-like peptide 1 release in Zucker diabetic fatty rats. J Pharmacol Exp Ther. 2010;334(1):164–70. doi:10.1124/jpet.110.166892.
77. Garg A, Grundy SM. Cholestyramine therapy for dyslipidemia in non-insulin-dependent diabetes mellitus. A short-term, double-blind, crossover trial. Ann Intern Med. 1994;121 (6):416–22.
78. Suzuki T, Oba K, Igari Y, Matsumura N, Watanabe K, Futami-Suda S, et al. Colestimide lowers plasma glucose levels and increases plasma glucagon-like PEPTIDE-1 (7-36) levels in patients with type 2 diabetes mellitus complicated by hypercholesterolemia. J Nippon Med Sch. 2007;74(5):338–43.
79. Zieve FJ, Kalin MF, Schwartz SL, Jones MR, Bailey WL. Results of the glucose-lowering effect of WelChol study (GLOWS): a randomized, double-blind, placebo-controlled pilot study evaluating the effect of colesevelam hydrochloride on glycemic control in subjects with type 2 diabetes. Clin Ther. 2007;29(1):74–83. doi:10.1016/j.clinthera.2007.01.003.
80. Bays HE, Goldberg RB, Truitt KE, Jones MR. Colesevelam hydrochloride therapy in patients with type 2 diabetes mellitus treated with metformin: glucose and lipid effects. Arch Intern Med. 2008;168(18):1975–83. doi:10.1001/archinte.168.18.1975.
81. Goldberg RB, Fonseca VA, Truitt KE, Jones MR. Efficacy and safety of colesevelam in patients with type 2 diabetes mellitus and inadequate glycemic control receiving insulin-based therapy. Arch Intern Med. 2008;168(14):1531–40. doi:10.1001/archinte.168.14.1531.
82. Fonseca VA, Rosenstock J, Wang AC, Truitt KE, Jones MR. Colesevelam HCl improves glycemic control and reduces LDL cholesterol in patients with inadequately controlled type 2 diabetes on sulfonylurea-based therapy. Diabetes Care. 2008;31(8):1479–84. doi:10.2337/dc08-0283.
83. Tagawa H, Irie J, Itoh A, Kusumoto Y, Kato M, Kobayashi N, et al. Bile acid binding resin improves hepatic insulin sensitivity by reducing cholesterol but not triglyceride levels in the liver. Diabetes Res Clin Pract. 2015;109(1):85–94. doi:10.1016/j.diabres.2015.04.025.
84. Henry RR, Aroda VR, Mudaliar S, Garvey WT, Chou HS, Jones MR. Effects of colesevelam on glucose absorption and hepatic/peripheral insulin sensitivity in patients with type 2 diabetes mellitus. Diabetes Obes Metab. 2012;14(1):40–6. doi:10.1111/j.1463-1326.2011.01486.x.
85. Porez G, Prawitt J, Gross B, Staels B. Bile acid receptors as targets for the treatment of dyslipidemia and cardiovascular disease. J Lipid Res. 2012;53(9):1723–37. doi:10.1194/jlr.R024794.
86. Pellicciari R, Fiorucci S, Camaioni E, Clerici C, Costantino G, Maloney PR, et al. 6alpha-ethyl-chenodeoxycholic acid (6-ECDCA), a potent and selective FXR agonist endowed with anticholestatic activity. J Med Chem. 2002;45(17):3569–72.
87. Fiorucci S, Antonelli E, Rizzo G, Renga B, Mencarelli A, Riccardi L, et al. The nuclear receptor SHP mediates inhibition of hepatic stellate cells by FXR and protects against liver fibrosis. Gastroenterology. 2004;127(5):1497–512. doi: S0016508504013903 [pii]
88. Fiorucci S, Clerici C, Antonelli E, Orlandi S, Goodwin B, Sadeghpour BM, et al. Protective effects of 6-ethyl chenodeoxycholic acid, a farnesoid X receptor ligand, in estrogen-induced cholestasis. J Pharmacol Exp Ther. 2005;313(2):604–12. doi: jpet.104.079665 [pii] doi:10.1124/jpet.104.079665.

89. Li T, Holmstrom SR, Kir S, Umetani M, Schmidt DR, Kliewer SA, et al. The G protein-coupled bile acid receptor, TGR5, stimulates gallbladder filling. Mol Endocrinol (Baltimore, Md). 2011;25(6):1066–71. doi: me.2010-0460 [pii] doi:10.1210/me.2010-0460.

MIX
Papier aus verantwortungsvollen Quellen
Paper from responsible sources
FSC® C105338

FSC
www.fsc.org

If you have any concerns about our products,
you can contact us on
ProductSafety@springernature.com

In case Publisher is established outside the EU,
the EU authorized representative is:
Springer Nature Customer Service Center GmbH
Europaplatz 3, 69115 Heidelberg, Germany

Printed by Libri Plureos GmbH
in Hamburg, Germany